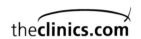

CLINICS IN
CHEST MEDICINE

Sarcoidosis

GUEST EDITORS
Robert P. Baughman, MD
and Marjolein Drent, MD, PhD

September 2008 • Volume 29 • Number 3

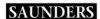

An Imprint of Elsevier, Inc.
PHILADELPHIA   LONDON   TORONTO   MONTREAL   SYDNEY   TOKYO

W.B. SAUNDERS COMPANY
A Division of Elsevier Inc.

1600 John F. Kennedy Boulevard • Suite 1800 • Philadelphia, Pennsylvania 19103

http://www.theclinics.com

CLINICS IN CHEST MEDICINE
September 2008
Editor: Sarah E. Barth

Volume 29, Number 3
ISSN 0272-5231
ISBN-13: 978-1-4160-6279-0
ISBN-10: 1-4160-6279-3

Clinics in Chest Medicine (ISSN 0272-5231) is published quarterly by Elsevier Inc., 360 Park Avenue South, New York, NY 10010-1710. Months of issue are March, June, September, and December. Business and Editorial Offices: 1600 John F. Kennedy Blvd., Suite 1800, Philadelphia, PA 19103-2899. Customer Service Office: 6277 Sea Harbor Drive, Orlando, FL 32887-4800. Periodicals postage paid at New York, NY and additional mailing offices. Subscription prices are $232.00 per year (US individuals), $370.00 per year (US institutions), $113.00 per year (US students), $255.00 per year (Canadian individuals), $444.00 per year (Canadian institutions), $149.00 per year (Canadian students), $297.00 per year (international individuals) $444.00 per year (international institutions), and $149.00 per year (international students). International air speed delivery is included in all *Clinics* subscription prices. All prices are subject to change without notice. **POSTMASTER:** Send address changes to *Clinics in Chest Medicine*, Elsevier Periodicals Customer Service, 6277 Sea Harbor Drive, Orlando, FL 32887-4800. **Customer Service: 1-800-654-2452 (US). From outside the United States, call 1-407-563-6020. Fax: 1-407-363-9661. E-mail: JournalsCustomerService-usa@elsevier.com.**

Reprints. For copies of 100 or more of articles in this publication, please contact the Commercial Reprints Department, Elsevier Inc., 360 Park Avenue South, New York, NY 10010-1710. Tel.: 212-633-3812; Fax: 212-462-1935; E-mail: reprints@elsevier.com.

Clinics in Chest Medicine is covered in *MEDLINE/PubMed (Index Medicus), Current Contents/Clinical Medicine, EMBASE/ Excerpta Medica, Science Citation Index,* and *ISI/BIOMED.*

Printed in the United States of America.

GUEST EDITORS

ROBERT P. BAUGHMAN, MD, Professor of Medicine, Department of Medicine, University of Cincinnati Medical Center, Cincinnati, Ohio

MARJOLEIN DRENT, MD, PhD, Professor of Interstitial Lung Diseases, Department of Respiratory Medicine, Sarcoidosis Management Center, University Hospital Maastricht, Maastricht, The Netherlands

CONTRIBUTORS

JASON J. AKBAR, MD, Department of Radiology, University of Cincinnati Medical Center, Cincinnati, Ohio

UMA S. AYYALA, MD, Assistant Professor of Medicine, Division of Pulmonary and Critical Care Medicine, Mount Sinai Medical Center, New York, New York

E. BARGAGLI, MD, PhD, Respiratory Diseases Section, Department of Clinical Medicine and Immunological Sciences, Siena University, Le Scotte Hospital, Siena, Italy

ROBERT P. BAUGHMAN, MD, Professor of Medicine, Department of Medicine, University of Cincinnati Medical Center, Cincinnati, Ohio

EDWARD S. CHEN, MD, Assistant Professor of Medicine, Division of Pulmonary and Critical Care Medicine, Johns Hopkins University School of Medicine, Baltimore, Maryland

ULRICH COSTABEL, MD, Department of Pneumology/Allergy, Ruhrlandklinik Essen, Essen, Germany

DANIEL A. CULVER, DO, Department of Pulmonary and Critical Care Medicine, Respiratory Institute, Cleveland Clinic, Cleveland, Ohio

JOLANDA DE VRIES, PhD, MSc, Professor of Medical Psychology, Department of Medical Psychology and Neuropsychology, Tilburg University; Department of Medical Psychology, St Elisabeth Hospital, Tilburg; Sarcoidosis Management Center, University Hospital Maastricht, Maastricht, The Netherlands

ENRIQUE DIAZ-GUZMAN, MD, Department of Pulmonary and Critical Care Medicine, Respiratory Institute, Cleveland Clinic, Cleveland, Ohio

MARJOLEIN DRENT, MD, PhD, Professor of Interstitial Lung Diseases, Department of Respiratory Medicine, Sarcoidosis Management Center, University Hospital Maastricht, Maastricht, The Netherlands

RONALD M. DU BOIS, MD, National Jewish Medical Center, Denver, Colorado

CAROL FARVER, MD, Department of Anatomic Pathology, Division of Pathology and Laboratory Medicine, Cleveland Clinic, Cleveland, Ohio

ANNEGRET FISCHER, MSc, Graduate Fellow, Institute of Clinical Molecular Biology, Christian-Albrechts-University, Kiel, Germany

KAROLINE I. GAEDE, PhD, Assistant Professor, Department of Clinical Medicine, Research Center Borstel, Borstel, Germany

ALICIA K. GERKE, MD, Fellow, Division of Pulmonary, Critical Care, and Occupational Medicine, University of Iowa College of Medicine, Iowa City, Iowa

TOMOHIRO HANDA, MD, PhD, Staff, Department of Respiratory Medicine, Graduate School of Medicine, Kyoto University, Kyoto, Japan

SYLVIA HOFMANN, PhD, Postdoctoral Fellow, Institute of Clinical Molecular Biology, Christian-Albrechts-University, Kiel, Germany

GARY HUNNINGHAKE, MD, Professor, Division of Pulmonary, Critical Care, and Occupational Medicine, University of Iowa College of Medicine, Iowa City, Iowa

YUTAKA ITO, MD, PhD, Assistant Professor, Department of Respiratory Medicine, Graduate School of Medicine, Kyoto University, Kyoto, Japan

TAKATERU IZUMI, MD, PhD, Professor Emeritus, Department of Respiratory Medicine, Kyoto University; Central Clinic/Research Center, Kyoto, Japan

DRAGANA JOVANOVIC, MD, PhD, Professor of Pulmonology, Medical School, University of Belgrade; Vth Clinical Department; and Director, Institute of Pulmonary Diseases, University Clinical Center, Belgrade, Serbia

MARC A. JUDSON, MD, Professor of Medicine, Division of Pulmonary and Critical Care Medicine, Medical University of South Carolina, Charleston, South Carolina

KENNETH S. KNOX, MD, Associate Professor of Medicine, Division of Pulmonary and Critical Care Medicine, Indiana University, Richard L. Roudebush VA Medical Center, Indianapolis, Indiana

ELYSE E. LOWER, MD, Professor of Medicine, Interstitial Lung Disease and Sarcoidosis Center, University of Cincinnati Medical Center, Cincinnati, Ohio

A. MAZZI, MD, Respiratory Diseases Section, Department of Clinical Medicine and Immunological Sciences, Siena University, Le Scotte Hospital, Siena, Italy

CRIS A. MEYER, MD, Associate Professor of Radiology, Department of Radiology, University of Cincinnati Medical Center, Cincinnati, Ohio

VIOLETA MIHAILOVIC-VUCINIC, MD, PhD, Professor of Internal Medicine and Pulmonology, Medical School, University of Belgrade; President, Yugoslav Association of Sarcoidosis; Head, Vth Clinical Department, Institute of Pulmonary Diseases, University Clinical Center, Belgrade, Serbia

DAVID R. MOLLER, MD, Associate Professor of Medicine, and Director of the Sarcoidosis Clinic, Division of Pulmonary and Critical Care Medicine, Johns Hopkins University School of Medicine, Baltimore, Maryland

JOACHIM MÜLLER-QUERNHEIM, MD, Professor of Medicine, Department of Pneumology, University Medical Center, Freiburg, Germany

SONOKO NAGAI, MD, PhD, Director and Professor, Central Clinic/Research Center, Kyoto, Japan

AJITH P. NAIR, MD, Fellow, Cardiovascular Institute, Mount Sinai Medical Center, New York, New York

KOUSUKE OHTA, MD, Chief of Health Management, Central Clinic/Research Center, Kyoto, Japan

MARIA L. PADILLA, MD, Professor of Medicine, Division of Pulmonary and Critical Care Medicine, Mount Sinai Medical Center, New York, New York

JOSEPH PARAMBIL, MD, Department of Pulmonary and Critical Care Medicine, Respiratory Institute, Cleveland Clinic, Cleveland, Ohio

ANTJE PRASSE, MD, Postdoctoral Fellow, Department of Pneumology, University Medical Center, Freiburg, Germany

ANTHONY S. ROSE, MD, Division of Pulmonary and Critical Care Medicine, Indiana University, Richard L. Roudebush VA Medical Center, Indianapolis, Indiana

PAOLA ROTTOLI, MD, Professor, Respiratory Diseases Section, Department of Clinical Medicine and Immunological Sciences, Siena University, Le Scotte Hospital, Siena, Italy

MANFRED SCHÜRMANN, MD, Postdoctoral Fellow, Institute of Human Genetics, Medical University of Schleswig-Holstein, University of Lübeck, Lübeck, Germany

STEFAN SCHREIBER, MD, Head and Professor of Medicine, Institute of Clinical Molecular Biology; and Deputy Head, Department of General Internal Medicine, Christian-Albrechts-University, Kiel, Germany

OM P. SHARMA, MD, FRCP, Master FCCP, Professor of Medicine, Division of Pulmonary and Critical Care Medicine, Keck School of Medicine, University of Southern California, LAC+USC Medical Center, Los Angeles, California

RALPH T. SHIPLEY, MD, Professor of Radiology, Department of Radiology, University of Cincinnati Medical Center, Cincinnati, Ohio

MANABU TAMAYA, MD, Division of Respiratory Medicine, First Department of Internal Medicine, Osaka Medical College, Osaka, Japan

MARCUS A. TIELKER, MD, Division of Pulmonary and Critical Care Medicine, Indiana University, Richard L. Roudebush VA Medical Center, Indianapolis, Indiana

ACHALA S. VAGAL, MD, Assistant Professor Radiology, Department of Radiology, University of Cincinnati Medical Center, Cincinnati, Ohio

KENNETH L. WEISS, MD, Associate Professor of Radiology, University of Cincinnati Medical Center, Cincinnati, Ohio

GERNOT ZISSEL, PhD, Assistant Professor, Department of Pneumology, University Medical Center, Freiburg, Germany

CONTENTS

85% to 95% of patients who have sarcoidosis. Approximately 20% to 50% of patients who have sarcoidosis present with respiratory symptoms, including dyspnea, cough, chest pain, and tightness of the chest. The clinical course and manifestations of pulmonary sarcoidosis are protean: spontaneous remission occurs in approximately two thirds of patients; up to 30% of patients have chronic course of the lung disease, resulting in progressive, (sometimes life-threatening) loss of lung function. Morbidity that correlates to sarcoidosis occurs in 1% to 4% of patients.

Although neurosarcoidosis seems to occur in only 5% to 10% of patients who have sarcoidosis, it may lead to significant complications. The diagnosis of neurosarcoidosis usually relies on indirect information from imaging and spinal fluid examination. Although MR imaging remains the most sensitive technique for detecting neurologic disease, other tests, including positron emission tomography scanning and cerebral spinal fluid examination, can provide important information. The role of immunosuppressive agents such as methotrexate, cyclophosphamide, and azathioprine has been expanded, and these agents should be considered for the treatment of some manifestations of neurosarcoidosis. Reports of the antitumor necrosis factor agent infliximab suggest that this drug can be helpful for patients who have neurosarcoidosis.

Sarcoidosis is a systemic disease with a favorable prognosis, high remission rate, and low mortality. Cardiac involvement alters this prognosis. Clinical manifestations most commonly include arrhythmias, conduction abnormalities, and congestive heart failure. Treatment includes immunosuppressant therapy, permanent pacemakers in the setting of conduction abnormalities, and implantable cardioverter-defibrillators in patients at risk for sudden cardiac death. Risk stratification for sudden cardiac death is essential in otherwise asymptomatic patients who have suspected cardiac sarcoidosis.

Sarcoid affecting the skin, eye, or liver can be symptomatic of or cause significant morbidity. When disease is sever, alternative therapies may be needed.

The quality of life and health status are impaired in patients suffering from sarcoidosis, especially in those who have clinical symptoms. Fatigue is an integral part of the clinical picture of sarcoidosis, but is an underestimated problem in clinical practice. Objective test results do not always correlate with the well-being of the patient. Present studies are generally cross-sectional. There is a need for prospective follow-up studies assessing the natural course of patients' disease in relation to symptoms and quality of life.

Not all patients who have sarcoidosis require treatment. For those who require treatment, the outcome of sarcoidosis can be considered conceptually in three broad, and at least partially overlapping, groupings: acute, chronic, and refractory. Although corticosteroids remain the initial drug for most patients who require therapy, several steroid-sparing alternatives have been found effective in treating many aspects of sarcoidosis. Methotrexate is most commonly used cytotoxic agent used for chronic disease, but azathioprine and leflunomide also have been shown to be useful. The tumor necrosis factor antibody infliximab has proved useful in treating refractory sarcoidosis. These various agents led to a treatment strategy for the various aspects of sarcoidosis.

FORTHCOMING ISSUES

RECENT ISSUES

THE CLINICS ARE NOW AVAILABLE ONLINE!

Access your subscription at:
http://www.theclinics.com

ELSEVIER
SAUNDERS

Clin Chest Med 29 (2008) xiii–xiv

CLINICS
IN CHEST
MEDICINE

Preface

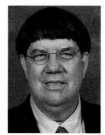
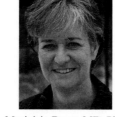

Robert P. Baughman, MD   Marjolein Drent, MD, PhD
Guest Editors

The fascination with sarcoidosis as a disease lies in the failure to identify the cause, its variable presentation, and its unpredictable clinical course. The features of this disease have been known for more than 100 years, which Dr. Sharma discusses in his article. While no specific answer regarding the cause of the disease has been made, we have learned a great deal about sarcoidosis.

One hypothesis is that sarcoidosis is a multi-organ disease representing a specific immune reaction that is triggered by one or more environmental agents (either living or dead). This immune response appears to be modified by genetic predisposition. While this is a fairly broad definition, one can delineate various components of this hypothesis.

From its original description, sarcoidosis has been assumed to be an infection. The granulomatous response found in samples appeared similar to a very common disease of the time, tuberculosis. As tuberculosis has become less frequent, sarcoidosis has become more clearly recognized as a separate disease. Drs. Chen and Moller summarize the work to date that examines the various possible infectious and noninfectious causes of sarcoidosis.

The immune response of sarcoidosis includes the formation of granulomas. This immune response frequently is characterized as Th-1 response. Drs. Gerke and Hunninghake analyze the immune response in terms of its similarity to other Th-1 responses (such as tuberculosis) and differences from other diseases. The variability of the outcome of sarcoidosis seems to be a reflection of the immune response, either in the initial reaction or in its subsequent modification.

Genetic predisposition has been proposed to modify almost every disease encountered by mankind. A rhinovirus that infects a group of office workers ranges from a few who have a runny nose for 2 days to the unfortunate ones who are wheezing and coughing for weeks. Sarcoidosis affects different ethnic groups in different ways, suggesting the influence of genetic background. By using a more homogenous background of patients or families who have the disease, researchers are recognizing that certain genetic factors are increase the risk of the disease, influence organ involvement, or modify the duration of disease. These issues are summarized by Dr. Müller-Quernheim and his colleagues.

One of the challenges of sarcoidosis remains its diagnosis and evaluation. Dr. Judson provides a comprehensive approach to the possible cause of sarcoidosis. He focuses on the multi-organ nature of the disease, emphasizing how this helps to diagnose the disease and make the physician aware of possible extra-thoracic complications of the disease. Dr. Akbar and colleagues provide examples of the information the radiologist can provide about the disease. While the focus is on lung manifestation, imaging of other organs is also highlighted. Dr. Rottoli's group summarizes markers of inflammation as measured in various tissue samples, including bronchoalveolar lavage.

Specific organ involvement is discussed in several articles. Drs. Vucinic and Jovanovic summarize pulmonary involvement in sarcoidosis. Sarcoidosis less frequently affects the heart or central nervous system; however, when these areas are affected, the consequences can be severe and long lasting. Drs. Lower and Weiss provide information about the diagnosis and management of neurosarcoidosis. Dr. Padilla's group focuses on cardiac sarcoidosis, including information about how to screen for potential cardiac disease. Dr. Knox's group highlights the presentation in the three most common extra thoracic organs: liver, skin, and eye.

For the patient who has sarcoidosis, the disease can have a devastating effect on the overall quality of life. Recent instruments for the general quality of life and specific instruments related to the effect of the disease on health have given important insights into sarcoidosis. Drs. De Vries and Drent provide a state of the art summary of this challenging area.

The treatment of sarcoidosis has to be tailored to the individual patient. As new drugs become more widely used in sarcoidosis, clinicians are left with decisions about when to use the older agents (such as prednisone and hydroxychloroquine) versus the newer drugs (such as infliximab or thalidomide). Drs. Baughman, Costabel, and du Bois provide one approach to the patient, which is based on the clinical outcome of a patient: acute, chronic, or refractory. For pulmonary patients, it has been emphasized recently that one reason for

a patient failing to respond to anti-inflammatory drugs is the secondary complication of pulmonary hypertension. Dr. Culver and his group summarize the current knowledge of sarcoidosis associated pulmonary arterial hypertension.

The cause for the variable clinical outcome in sarcoidosis remains a mystery. Dr. Nagai and her colleagues discuss the differences in outcome. One can only assume that genetic background, handling of the etiologic agent by the host, and possibly treatment all have an influence on the clinical outcome.

Although there are still many questions, the practicing physician has plenty of information to diagnose and manage patients who have sarcoidosis. In this issue, we have tried to provide a ready summary of this information.

We thank Elsevier overall, and we thank Sarah Barth in particular for all of her help and encouragement throughout the process of preparing this issue.

Robert P. Baughman, MD
Professor of Medicine
Department of Medicine
University of Cincinnati Medical Center
1001 Holmes, Eden Avenue
Cincinnati, OH 45267-0565, USA

E-mail address: baughmrp@ucmail.uc.edu

Marjolein Drent, MD, PhD
Professor of Interstitial Lung Diseases
Department of Respiratory Medicine
Sarcoidosis Management Center
University Hospital Maastricht
PO Box 5800, 6202 AZ
Maastricht, The Netherlands

E-mail address: m.drent@lung.azm.nl

ELSEVIER
SAUNDERS

CLINICS
IN CHEST
MEDICINE

Clin Chest Med 29 (2008) 357–363

Sarcoidosis Around the World

Om P. Sharma, MD, FRCP, Master FCCP

Division of Pulmonary and Critical Care Medicine, Keck School of Medicine, University of Southern California,
Room 11-900, LAC+USC Medical Center, 1200 North State Street, Los Angeles, CA 90033, USA

Sarcoidosis is an illness that generates tremendous anxiety among persons who suffer from it and interest among the individuals who provide care to them. The disease occurs throughout the world and has been with us for more than 150 years. Its colorful history has been documented before [1,2].

Definition

It is hard to define a disease whose cause is yet to be discovered. Scadding and Mitchell [3] defined sarcoidosis as a disease characterized by the formation in several affected tissues of epithelioid cell tubercles without caseation, although fibrinoid necrosis may be present at the center of a few, proceeding either to resolution or conversion into hyalin fibrous tissue. This definition emphasizes only the histologic features of the illness. The knowledge of the disease is vast, and we need to include not only the clinical but also the radiologic, immunologic, biochemical, and genetic aspects of the illness. The following descriptive definition was provided in the American Thoracic Society, European Respiratory Society, World Association of Sarcoidosis and Other Granulomatous Disorders statement on sarcoidosis in 1999 [4]:

> Sarcoidosis is a multisystem disorder of unknown cause. It commonly affects young and middle-aged adults and frequently presents with bilateral hilar adenopathy, pulmonary infiltration, and ocular and skin lesions. The liver, spleen, lymph nodes, salivary glands, heart, nervous system, muscles, bones, and other organs also may be involved. The diagnosis is established when clinicoradiographic findings are supported by histologic evidence of noncaseating epithelioid cell granulomas. Granulomas of unknown origin and local sarcoid reactions must be excluded. Frequently observed immunologic features are depression of cutaneous delayed-type hypersensitivity and a heightened Th-1 immune response at sites of disease. Circulating immune complexes along with signs of B-cell hyperactivity also may be found.

The beginning

In 1869, Dmitri Mendeleev published the periodic table of elements; John Tyndall discovered the Tyndall effect (namely, that a beam of light passing through colloidal solution can be observed from the side); Pere Armand David, a French missionary in China, described the giant panda; Paul Langerhans dissected the pancreas and discovered the islets of Langerhans; and surgeon Johann Friedrich August von Esmarch demonstrated the use of a prepared first aid bandage on the battlefield. The year 1869 also welcomed to this world Harvey Cushing and Mahatma Gandhi and bid farewell to Hector Berlioz and Augustine Saint-Beuve. Sarcoidologists, however, remember 1869 for the contribution of Jonathan Hutchinson, a British dermatologist who described a 58-year-old coal wharf worker with purple, symmetric skin plaques on the legs and hands that had developed gradually over the preceding 2 years. The lesions were neither tender nor painful. The patient also suffered from gout and finally died of renal failure. This report was most likely the first case of clinically described sarcoidosis. Hutchinson's other fascinating patient was a 64-year-old woman, Mrs. Mortimer, who presented with raised, dusky red skin lesions on the face and forearms. There was no ulceration but some slight scaling. Six months later, the lesions had increased

---

E-mail address: osharma@usc.edu

0272-5231/08/$ - see front matter © 2008 Elsevier Inc. All rights reserved.
doi:10.1016/j.ccm.2008.03.013

in size and extent. The lobule of the ear became affected, and the bridge of the nose became swollen, red, and indurated. Hutchinson [5,6] wrote that the disease differed from tuberculosis and all other forms of lupus lesions and called it Mortimer's malady.

London to Europe

In Oslo in 1897, Caeser Boeck presented to the Medical Society of Christiania a patient with "multiple benign sarkoid [sic] of the skin" and drew attention to its similarity to Mortimer's malady. Boeck [7] showed also the histologic picture of the skin consisting of sharp, well-defined foci of epithelioid cells with giant cells and became the first person to describe histology of sarcoidosis.

Kreibich [8] (1869–1932) was born on May 20, 1869 in Prague and became a professor of dermatology. He described in one of his patients lattice-like rarefactions of the terminal phalanges and became the first to describe bone cysts in sarcoidosis. In France in 1889, Besnier [9] described a patient with violaceous swellings of the nose, ears, and fingers, for which he coined the term "lupus pernio." In 1892, Tenneson [10] reported another example of lupus pernio and described its essential histology of "predominance of epithelioid cells and a variety of giant cells" in the skin lesions. In the reports published by Besnier and Tenneson, cases were not illustrated, but wax models of the appearance of their patients were used to illustrate skin lesions. Darier and Roussy [11] described the cases of five middle-aged women with subcutaneous nodules most frequently on the trunk but occasionally on the legs. In four of these patients, the nodules were biopsied and were shown to have epithelioid cell granulomas.

In Germany, Kuznitzky and Bittorf [12] drew attention to a 27-year-old man with pulmonary manifestations of sarcoidosis and subcutaneous nodules on the legs and arms. Biopsy of the lesions from both sites showed granulomatous histology. The patient had an enlarged spleen, peripheral lymphadenopathy, and albuminuria. Heerfordt [13] (1871–1953) was a Danish ophthalmologist who linked uveitis, enlargement of parotid glands, and paresis of the cranial nerves, especially the seventh nerve, and termed the syndrome "febris uveoparotidea subchronica." He noted that the condition was chronic and frequently complicated by pleocytosis of the cerebrospinal fluid. Heerfordt believed that the syndrome was caused by mumps, however. Jorgen Schaumann [14] (1879–1953), a dermatologist at Saint Goran's Hospital and the Finsen Institute in Stockholm, first proposed a clinicopathologic synthesis of multisystemic sarcoidosis. He called it "lymphogranulomatosis benigna." Sven Löfgren (1910–1978), another Saint Goran's Hospital physician and one of Schaumann's students, brought the mysterious disease of sarcoidosis out of the shadows into the limelight as a common disorder with a good prognosis. The combination of erythema nodosum and hilar adenopathy is currently known as Löfgren's syndrome [15].

Sarcoidosis comes to America

In the earlier decades of the twentieth century, sarcoidosis was not a significant illness; its evidence remained surrounded in the veil of tuberculosis. The disease was not included in the 1907 edition of "Diseases of the Lungs," written by Dr. Robert Babcock and published by D. Appleton and Company of New York. Neither was it to be seen in any of the editions of William Osler's "Textbook of Medicine" or the tomes by Austin Flint and George Pepper. As reported by Osler [16], a 14-year-old African American child admitted to the Johns Hopkins Medical Center had the likely diagnosis of sarcoidosis. The patient had bilateral parotid and lacrimal enlargement, lung disease, and pleural involvement. At autopsy, no evidence of tuberculosis—at that time a common disease—was found.

In 1936, the first significant publication about sarcoidosis in America, a 75-page review from Johns Hopkins Hospital by Warfield Longcope [17], appeared. This event took place almost six decades after the first recorded case of sarcoidosis by Hutchinson. The first epidemiologic study on sarcoidosis appeared in 1950, based on 350 cases detected in US World War II veterans. The annual incidence rates per 100,000 in men differed. In Army inductees, the rates in African Americans and whites were 17.8 and 0.9, respectively, in 350 cases, whereas in Navy recruits, African Americans and whites had the rates of 81.8 and 7.6, respectively, in 134 cases [18]. The most recent data from enlisted Navy men showed an annual incidence rate of 16 for African Americans and 2.5 for whites. In a study of 75 patients from a community of 99.5% whites, the age-adjusted incidence rate of sarcoidosis was 6.1 per 100,000 person-years (5.9 in men and 6.3 in women), with a peak incidence in men in their 30s and in women in their 40s [19].

In 1963, Sven Löfgren sent out a questionnaire to the physicians who were interested in sarcoidosis. The prevalence of pulmonary sarcoidosis based on mass chest radiographic examination varied from 0.2 to 64 cases per 100,000 examinations. No striking difference was seen between urban and rural areas [20]. James and colleagues [21] presented a retrospective analysis of 3676 patients from Europe (London, Reading, Edinburgh, Paris, Lisbon, Novi Sad, Geneca, and Naples), Japan (Tokyo), and the United States (New York, Los Angeles) (Table 1). This extensive survey gave us a profile of cases of sarcoidosis around the world seen in special clinics—many of

the clinics had been in existence for 20 or more years. A slight female predominance was noted (57%). A total of 68% of the patients were younger than 40 years at the time of diagnosis, and their sarcoidosis had been detected via routine chest radiographic screening. Of the patients, 79% were white, 10% were black (47% and 82% of patients in New York and Los Angeles, respectively), and 8% were Japanese, and 17% of the New York patients were Puerto Ricans. This report covered patients from various backgrounds [21]. The findings were as follows:

Erythema nodosum occurred in 28% of the patients in the United Kingdom (mostly white patients), less than 10% in Los Angeles (mostly African Americans), and not at all in Japanese patients.

Ocular lesions were seen in 22% of the Japanese patients but in less than 15% in patients from other areas.

Bilateral hilar adenopathy (stage I) was present in 50% of the patients in most series but was seen as a presenting feature in only 25% of the African American patients.

One third of the African American patients had stage III chest radiographic findings as compared with 15% or less in patients from other series.

Hypergammaglobulinemia occurred in 86% of the African American patients but in only 25% to 30% of patients in other series.

Hypercalcemia was found in approximately 20% of white patients, 11% of African American patients, and 9% of Japanese patients.

Kveim-Siltzbach test results were positive in 80% of the patients.

Although this retrospective study provided a fairly accurate description of sarcoidosis, it did not provide an accurate incidence or prevalence of sarcoidosis. In 1974, in a world review entitled "Course and Prognosis of Sarcoidosis," which was published in the *American Journal of Medicine*, Louis Siltzbach emphasized that there was an extraordinary parallelism in prognosis of sarcoidosis in different ethnic groups who were living in radically different environments and climates. If a patient presented with hilar adenopathy, resolution was to be expected without any treatment, but if lung infiltrates were present, resolution was less likely even with steroid therapy. Depending on the period of observation, the mortality rate caused by sarcoidosis was less than 5% [22].

Table 1
Sarcoidosis around the world: comparison between the world and Eastern Europe

Features	Worldwide	Eastern Europe
Total number	3676	2666
Percentage (%)	100	100
Women	57	57
Black race	10	0.3
Age < 40 y at presentation	68	70
Onset: routine chest radiograph	40	64
Chest radiograph stage 0	8	4
Stage 1	51	58
Stage 2	29	30.5
Stage 3	12	7.5
Intrathoracic involvement	87	96
Lymph node enlargement	22	8
Erythema nodosum	17	11
Other skin lesions	9	5
Ocular disease	15	4
Spleen enlarged	6	1
Parotid	4	2
Nervous system	4	1
Bone cysts	3	3.5
Positive Kveim test result	78	73
Negative tuberculin test result	64	58
Hypergammaglobulinemia	44	44
Hypercalcemia	11	12
Treated with steroids	47	59.5
Resolution of chest radiographic changes	54	55
Mortality caused by sarcoidosis	2.2	1
Mortality caused by other causes	1.1	1

In 2001, A Case Control Etiologic Study of Sarcoidosis (ACCESS), conducted by Baughman and colleagues, finally established the clinical epidemiologic features in 736 patients—53% white and 44% black—with sarcoidosis from ten clinical centers in the United States. There were more women, and they were more likely to have eye lesions, neurologic involvement, and erythema nodosum. Men who were involved were likely to have hypercalcemia. Black patients were more likely to have chronic skin lesions and eye, liver, bone marrow, and lymph node involvement. Organ involvement depended on the race, age, and sex of the patient. The exploration of environmental and occupational factors did not reveal a single, predominant cause of sarcoidosis. Insecticides, agricultural environments, and bioaerosol exposures were associated with sarcoidosis [23,24].

Sarcoidosis in Japan

In Kyoto, Dr. Izumi in the first congress of the newly founded World Association of Sarcoidosis and other Granulomatous Disorders organized a symposium entitled "Population Difference. I: The Clinical Features and Prognosis of Sarcoidosis" to compare and contrast sarcoidosis as it occurs in Japan with the disease seen in other parts of the world. It was found that ocular sarcoidosis was present in 50% of symptomatic Japanese sarcoidosis patients as compared with less than 10% in many countries. Erythema nodosum was rare in Japanese patients [25].

Iwai and colleagues showed that incidence of cardiac sarcoidosis in Japanese patients was significantly higher than that seen in whites and African Americans. In an autopsy study of 503 patients (109 whites, 74 African Americans, 320 Japanese), Iwai and colleagues found myocardial granulomas in 69.1% of the Japanese patients, 18.0% of the whites, and 14.3% of the African American patients. Pulmonary sarcoidosis was the major cause of death in African American patients, but Japanese patients had the highest incidence of death caused by myocardial sarcoidosis [26].

Selroos [27] compared the epidemiologic and clinical features of patients who had sarcoidosis in Finland and Hokkaido, the northern island of Japan. Hokkaido and Finland resemble each other in many respects: both areas have four seasons with cold winters and cool summers, the number of inhabitants is a little more than 5

million in both areas, and the frequency of tuberculosis was similar at the time the study was conducted. The crude prevalence rate for sarcoidosis in Finland was 28.2 per 100,000, and the incidence was 11.4 per 100,000. The corresponding figures for Hokkaido were 5.1 per 100,000 and 0.8 per 100,000. The series consisted of 571 Finnish and 686 Japanese patients seen at one hospital in each region. Among symptomatic patients, respiratory symptoms, erythema nodosum, joint pains, and malaise dominated among Finnish patients, whereas eye symptoms were most frequent in Japanese patients [27].

South Africa

A survey conducted at Groot Schuur Hospital in Capetown revealed a prevalence rate per 100,000 of 17 in colored, 27 in black, and 6 in white patients. Widespread skin lesions, including lupus pernio, plaques, nodules, psoriasiform lesions, and nail dystrophies, were common. Many of these patients with florid skin lesions were misdiagnosed as having leprosy [28].

Eastern Europe

Djuric and colleagues [29] studied the features of sarcoidosis in persons from Novi Sad and Belgrade (Serbia), Debrecen (Hungary), Istanbul (Turkey), Hamburg (Germany), and Warsaw (Poland) along the same lines as the worldwide survey conducted by Siltzbach and colleagues (Table 2). The profile of sarcoidosis in Eastern Europe was similar to that found in other parts of the world. Professor Violeta Vucinic recently made similar observations. Professor Kolek, from University Hospital in Olomouc, analyzed 1487 patients who had sarcoidosis and estimated a mean incidence of 3.68 per 100,000. The clinical picture of Moravian and Silesian sarcoidosis was found to be similar to the rest of Europe. The disease was predominantly benign, with a small number of cases of extrapulmonary disease. The predominance of sarcoidosis in women— with a gender ratio of 2.35 to 1 (70% women, 30% men)—was noted [30].

India

Because of widespread tuberculosis and leprosy, the exact prevalence and incidence of sarcoidosis in India is not known. Until 1981, only 75 cases of systemic sarcoidosis had been reported in India; since that survey it has been increasingly recognized and undoubtedly will

Table 2
Features of sarcoidosis in selected geographic areas

Country/total no.	United States	United Kingdom	Japan	Sweden	Denmark	Finland	Ireland	Germany	Austria	Italy	India	Greece	Hungary
Features (%)	754	320	61	60	77	147	130	346	97	99	61	62	199
Women	58	64	51	48	45	59	46	58	66	59	41	71	59
White	23	55	0	98	100	100	100	99	100	100	100	100	100
Black	66	39	0	0	0	0	0	1	0	0	0	0	0
Japanese/Oriental	2	6	100	2	0	0	0	0	0	0	0	0	0
Age (y)													
≤ 20	4	0	0	0	8	0	6	04	2	03	11	05	2
20–39	66	96	54	82	58	50	72	59	43	60	30	18	47
40–59	25	04	39	17	27	49	18	34	38	35	52	53	47
60	5	0	7	2	7	4	4	3	17	02	07	24	4
Constitutional symptoms	34	81	18	66	21	66	04	46	24	35	90	21	0
Respiratory	70	84	14	64	31	66	24	35	50	40	88	46	35
Ocular	20	11	50	8	5	8	17	06	04	03	17	07	0
Skin	20	31	11	28	15	31	40	57	50	15	13	36	97
Joint involvement	18	21	0	42	11	29	04	69	10	05	60	18	0
Adenopathy	17	0	11	2	2	08	04	13	08	18	37	16	0
Chest radiograph													
Stage 0	7	0	1	0	0	01	03	01	00	18	0	8	0
Stage I	37	27	64	32	45	48	30	69	65	44	23	56	83
Stage II	33	52	20	52	47	35	45	22	24	19	43	26	12
Stage III	23	21	15	16	8	16	22	08	11	19	34	10	5

Data from Refs. [20,22,25,27].

become a commonplace disorder once tuberculosis is totally subdued. Patterns of presentation, tissue involvement, and results of laboratory and radiologic investigations are surprisingly similar to those noted in other parts of the world (Table 3) [31].

Spain

Levinsky and colleagues [32] reported that the incidence of sarcoidosis of 1.3/100,000 in Spain was lower than that in other European countries. Mana and colleagues [33] analyzed 423 cases of sarcoidosis seen in Barcelona between 1972 and 1988. The most significant feature was the high incidence of erythema nodosum, which occurred in 48% of the patients; almost half of the patients with Löfgren's syndrome were diagnosed during the spring months. The pulmonary and extrapulmonary manifestations of the disease were similar to those reported in other series from Europe [33].

Australia

In a prospective study that involved 72 patients, Allen [34] concluded that ocular and neurologic manifestations of sarcoidosis were more frequent in the studied population because they were actively sought in contrast to many earlier retrospective studies. A little more than one third of the patients required corticosteroids.

Israel

Topilski and colleagues [35] followed 40 patients who were diagnosed at the Tel Aviv Medical Center in Israel for 6 years. They showed that prognosis of the patients was excellent: 37 of 40 patients recovered.

Table 3
Percentage comparison of sarcoidosis in India compared with the worldwide series

Features	India (%)	Worldwide series (%)
Women	41	57
Intrathoracic involvement	98	87
Skin lesions	20	26
Ocular lesions	10	15
Parotid enlargement	7	4
Nervous system involvement	10	4
Positive Kveim test result	89	78
Negative tuberculin test result	71	64
Hypercalcemia	47	11
Hypergammaglobulinemia	44	44

China

Luo Wei and colleagues [36] analyzed 223 patients (59% women) with histologic evidence of sarcoidosis reported from different provinces of China. The lungs were involved in all patients; 33.3% had stage I disease, 62.3% had stage II disease, and 4.6% had stage III sarcoidosis. The authors also reported that 51.9% of the patients had high serum angiotensin-converting enzyme. Tuberculin test results were positive in 13% to 15% of patients, who had no evidence of active tuberculosis. The authors concluded that the prevalence of sarcoidosis compared with the prevalence of tuberculosis was not high in China [36].

Iran

Between 1974 and 1992, Amoli and colleagues [37] studied 240 cases (38.4% men and 61.6% women) of sarcoidosis in Iran. Almost all the cases were referred because of symptoms; only three cases were found on routine examination. Cough (50.4%), dyspnea (30%), skin lesions (22.8%), fever (16%), weight loss (15.2%), joint pain (12%), peripheral lymphadenopathy (22%), and eye symptoms (8.4%) were the common signs and symptoms. Three patients died of associated neoplasms [37].

Summary

More than a century ago, Jonathan Hutchinson, a dermatologist, identified the first case of sarcoidosis at King's College Hospital in London. In the decades before and after the turn of the nineteenth century, several publications independently witnessed the blossoming of this dermatologic curiosity into a multisystemic immunologic disorder, currently called sarcoidosis. The disease occurs worldwide. Its frequency, pulmonary and extrapulmonary manifestations, response to treatment, and prognosis are extraordinarily similar. Despite the resemblance, certain inexplicable distinctive features of the disease are related to geography and race. Blacks have a higher incidence of chronic skin lesions, Scandinavians have a higher frequency of erythema nodosum, ocular and myocardial sarcoidosis manifestations are uniquely common in Japanese patients, Italians tend to have abnormal calcium metabolism, and Indians have the highest occurrence of constitutional manifestations of fever, weight loss, joint pain, and adenopathy. Although genetics and racial background influence the presentation, course, and prognosis of the disease, epidemiology data from many countries suffer from fundamental problems in finding and diagnosing sarcoidosis. The scientific enquiry into the cause of sarcoidosis gained significant momentum in the latter part of the twentieth century and continues relentlessly into the current decade of the twenty-first century. By contrast, the progress in epidemiology remains slow, and the cause of the disease remains elusive.

References

[1] Sharma O. Sarcoidosis: a historical perspective. Clin Dermatol 2007;25:232–41.

[2] James D, Sharma O. From Hutchinson to now: a historical glimpse. Curr Opin Pulm Med 2002;8: 416–23.

[3] Scadding JG, Mitchell D. Sarcoidosis. 2nd edition. London: Chapman and Hall; 1985. p. 36–42.

[4] Hunninghake G, Costabel U, Ando M, et al. ATS/ERS/WASOG statement on sarcoidosis. Sarcoidosis Vasc Diffuse Lung Dis 1999;16:149–73.

[5] Hutchinson J. Anomalous diseases of skin and fingers: case of livid papillary psoriasis? Illustrations of clinical surgery. London: J and A Churchill; 1877. p. 42–3.

[6] Hutchinson J. Mortimer's malady: a form of lupus pernio. Arch Surg (London) 1898;9:307–15.

[7] Boeck C. Multiple benign sarcoid of the skin. Norsk Mag Laegevid 1899;14:1321–45.

[8] Kreibich K. Über lupus pernio. Arch Dermatol Syph 1904;71:3–12.

[9] Besnier E. Lupus pernio de la face. Ann Dermatol Syphiligr (Paris) 1889;10:33–6.

[10] Tenneson H. Lupus pernio. Ann Dermatol Syphiligr (Paris) 1889;10:333–6.

[11] Darier J, Roussy G. Des sarcoides sus cutanees. Arch Med Exp D'Anat Path 1906;18:1–50.

[12] Kuznitzky E, Bittorf A. Boecksches sarkoid mit beteiligung innerer organe. MMW Munch Med Wochenschr 1915;62:1349–53.

[13] Heerfordt CF. Über eine febris uveo-parotidea subchronica. Graefes Arch Ophthalmol 1909;70: 254–8.

[14] Schaumann J. Lymphogranulomatosis benigna in the light of prolonged clinical observations and autopsy findings. Br J Dermatol 1936;48:399–446.

[15] Löfgren S. Primary pulmonary sarcoidosis. Acta Med Scand 1953;145:424–55.

[16] Osler W. On chronic symmetrical enlargement of the salivary and lachrymal glands. Am J Med Sci 1898; 11:1–4.

[17] Longcope W. The generalized form of Boeck's sarcoid. Trans Assoc Am Physicians 1936;51:94–102.

[18] Sarcoidosis among U.S. Navy enlisted men, 1965–1993. MMWR Morb Mortal Wkly Rep 1997;46: 539–43.

[19] Henke C, Henke G, Elveback L, et al. The epidemiology of sarcoidosis in Rochester, Minnesota: a population-based study and survival. Am J Epidemiol 1986;123:840–5.

[20] Bauer H, Löfgren S. International study of pulmonary sarcoidosis in mass radiography. Acta Med Scand 1964;425(Suppl):103–5.

[21] James D, Neville E, Siltzbach L, Turiaf J, et al. A worldwide review of sarcoidosis. Ann N Y Acad Sci 1976;278:321–36.

[22] Siltzbach L, James D, Neville E, et al. Course and prognosis of sarcoidosis around the world. Am J Med 1974;57:847–52.

[23] Baughman R, Teirstein A, Judson M, et al. Clinical characteristics of patients in a case control study of sarcoidosis. Am J Respir Crit Care Med 2001;164: 1885–9.

[24] Newman L, Rose C, Bresnitz R, et al. A case control etiologic study of sarcoidosis: environmental and occupational risk factors. Am J Respir Crit Care Med 2004;170:1324–30.

[25] Izumi T. Population differences in clinical features and prognosis of sarcoidosis throughout the world: international survey report. Sarcoidosis 1992; 9(Suppl 1):105–18.

[26] Iwai K, Sekiguchi M, Hosoda Y, et al. Racial difference in cardiac sarcoidosis observed at autopsy. Sarcoidosis 1994;11(Suppl 1):248–51.

[27] Selroos O. Differences in sarcoidosis around the world: what they tell us. In: Baughman R, editor. Sarcoidosis: lung biology in health and disease, vol. 210. New York: Francis & Taylor; 2006. p. 47–64.

[28] Morrison J. Sarcoidosis in Bantu. Br J Dermatol 1974;90:649–54.

[29] Djuric B, Handi I, Vezendi S, et al. Sarcoidosis in six European cities. In: Jones Williams W, Davies B, editors. Sarcoidosis. Cardiff (Wales): Alpha and Omega Press; 1980. p. 527–31.

[30] Kolek V. Epidemiology of sarcoidosis in Moravia and Silesia. Sarcoidosis 1994;11(Suppl 1):263–4.

[31] Gupta S, Dutta S, Kar S, et al. Sarcoidosis in different regions of India: an analytical study. Sarcoidosis 1992;9(Suppl 1):271–2.

[32] Levinsky L, Cumminskey J, Romer F, et al. Sarcoidosis in Europe: a cooperative study. Ann N Y Acad Sci 1976;278:335–46.

[33] Mana J, Morera J, Fite E, et al. Sarcoidosis in Spain. Sarcoidosis 1994;11(Suppl 1):259–62.

[34] Allen R, Martin A, Zimmerman P. A prospective clinical study of sarcoidosis in Australian patients. Sarcoidosis 1994;11(Suppl 1):253–4.

[35] Topilski M, Fireman E, Greif E. Course and prognosis of sarcoidosis in the Tel Aviv area, Israel. Sarcoidosis 1994;11(Suppl 1):255–8.

[36] Luo Wei C, Wang F, Yu R, et al. Sarcoidosis in China. Sarcoidosis 1992;9(Suppl 1):281–2.

[37] Amoli K, Rezai-Adi R, Masjei M, et al. Sarcoidosis in Iran: a study of 250 cases. Sarcoidosis 1992; 9(Suppl 1):272–4.

ELSEVIER
SAUNDERS

Clin Chest Med 29 (2008) 365–377

CLINICS
IN CHEST
MEDICINE

Etiology of Sarcoidosis

Edward S. Chen, MD*, David R. Moller, MD

*Division of Pulmonary and Critical Care Medicine, Johns Hopkins University School of Medicine,
5501 Hopkins Bayview Circle, Baltimore, MD 21224, USA*

Research over the past decade has advanced our understanding of the pathogenesis of sarcoidosis and provided new insights into potential causes of this disease. It is important to remember that any etiologic agent of sarcoidosis must be capable of causing the pathologic hallmark of systemic noncaseating granulomas and the heterogeneous clinical features of sarcoidosis. In addition, etiologic agents must be compatible with immunologic features, including polarized T-helper 1(Th1) cytokine profiles and oligoclonal T cell expansions consistent with antigen driven processes. Genes from the major histocompatibility (MHC) locus involved with immune responses are known to contribute to disease susceptibility. Because of this background, various environmental exposures, both inorganic and organic, as well as microbial triggers have been the targets of study. The recently completed ACCESS (A Case Control Etiologic Study of Sarcoidosis) study provides data supporting the likelihood that specific environmental exposures associated with microbe-rich environments modestly increase the risk of developing sarcoidosis. Directed research into specific microbial etiologies of sarcoidosis provide evidence that mycobacterial DNA and protein antigens are present in sarcoidosis tissues and are the target of T and B cell responses, suggesting these microbes are an important etiologic factor. Propionibacterial organisms have also been shown to be present in sarcoidosis tissues, though the role of these commensal organisms remains uncertain given their normal presence as endogenous flora. Even with these studies, there remains a lack of consensus on the etiology of sarcoidosis. This challenge is likely to be overcome only with additional research that incorporates clinical, genetic, immunologic, environmental, and microbiologic profiles in groups of patients, supplemented with testing of candidate pathogenic agents in experimental models that recapitulate critical features of this disease.

Requirements for an etiologic agent of sarcoidosis

Etiologic agents must be capable of inducing the basic histologic hallmarks of sarcoidosis and account for the clinical heterogeneity and immunologic features of this disease. The epithelioid granuloma is the pathologic hallmark of this disease, a distinct but not disease-specific pattern of inflammation characterized by compact, discrete granulomas [1]. Epithelioid granulomas, as in other types of granulomas (eg, caseating, foreign body), are presumed to form around a nidus of poorly soluble or insoluble material by the spatial assembly of multiple cell types, including mononuclear phagocytes, fibroblasts and, in sarcoidosis, lymphocytes. This structure represents an ancient and preserved pathologic response that acts as a physical barrier to shield adjacent tissue from possible injury and, in the case of infectious agents, prevent dissemination [2]. In sarcoidosis, the epithelioid granulomatous response is associated with local proinflammatory cytokine production and evidence of enhanced T cell immunity at sites of inflammation.

Candidate etiologic agents must be capable of inducing the various clinical manifestations and provide a mechanism for the different clinical

This article was supported by NIH grants HL71100 for E. Chen, and HL68019 and HL83870 for D. Moller.

* Corresponding author.

E-mail address: chenedwa@jhmi.edu (E.S. Chen).

outcomes in sarcoidosis. Sarcoidosis involves the lungs in over 90% of cases, and granulomatous inflammation is found in other organs in a majority of patients [1,3]. Other environmentally exposed organs, such as the skin and eyes, are affected in 20% to 30% of patients. Granulomatous inflammation is also present in internal organs not directly exposed to the environment, such as the liver in most patients [4]. These clinical manifestations indicate that sarcoidosis is a systemic disorder [1]. Clinically apparent organ involvement is typically restricted to a few organs, and these manifestations are usually defined early in the course of disease. In the ACCESS study, only approximately 20% of cases had new organ involvement after a 2-year follow-up [5]. Over 50% of patients with sarcoidosis will eventually experience a remission of disease activity, usually within the first 2 to 3 years [1].

After disease remission, subsequent relapses are rare. Sarcoidosis patients who do not undergo remission usually have a progressive monophasic course of the underlying granulomatous inflammation unless treated, as opposed to a true "waxing-waning" course typified by many autoimmune diseases. Currently used therapies with anti-inflammatory or immunosuppressive medications are effective in suppressing the granulomatous inflammation, but do not induce remission or cure of the sarcoidosis. Opportunistic infections are exceedingly rare in patients with sarcoidosis treated with corticosteroids, suggesting there is no general host defense defect in patients with sarcoidosis. And despite corticosteroid or immunosuppressive therapy, often for many years, there is no clinical evidence for the emergence of active infections by any of the microbial agents that have been implicated in the etiology of sarcoidosis. These clinical features must be reconciled for any candidate etiologic agent that must operate within the confines of a susceptible host response in causing systemic sarcoidosis.

Proposed etiologic agents of sarcoidosis must also account for basic immunologic features of this disease. Immunohistochemical studies demonstrate T-lymphocytes at sites of granulomatous inflammation, typically with CD4+ T cells around the center of the granuloma and CD8+ T cells surrounding the periphery of the granuloma [1]. In a seminal study, Hunninghake and Crystal [6] reported the increased proportion of CD4+ T cells in the lungs of patients with pulmonary sarcoidosis, consistent with enhanced T cell responses in the lung. This finding was instrumental in changing the widely held belief at the time that sarcoidosis was associated with suppressed T cell immunity, as noted by peripheral lymphopenia and cutaneous anergy. Clinical evidence that CD4+ T cells are central to the pathogenesis of sarcoidosis is provided by the observation that patients with sarcoidosis who develop HIV-related immunodeficiency do not show progressive sarcoidosis, whereas patients with pre-existing HIV later found to have sarcoidosis typically have CD4 counts greater than 200 [7]. Multiple studies provide evidence that the T cell response in sarcoidosis is polarized toward dominant Th1 cytokine production, with increased expression of interferon gamma (INFγ), tumor necrosis factor alpha (TNFα), interleukin (IL)-2, and the Th1-promoting immunoregulatory cytokines IL-12 and IL-18 [8].

Clinical observations suggest that polarized Th1 immunity is a necessary component for the development of sarcoidosis. For example, Th1-promoting biologic response modifiers, such as the interferons or IL-2, are associated with an increased risk of developing new onset or recrudescent sarcoidosis [9,10]. HIV-positive patients who undergo treatment with highly active antiretroviral therapy with immune reconstitution may also develop new onset or recurrent multisystem sarcoidosis, particularly involving the lungs and skin [11]. TNFα and other proinflammatory cytokines and chemokines have critical roles in promoting granulomatous inflammation, but these mediators are nonspecific and have been shown to enhance granulomatous inflammation driven by either Th1 or Th2 cytokine expression [12]. Polarized Th1 profiles at sites of inflammation in sarcoidosis are seen at the time of diagnosis and are documented to extend for many years of known disease. Whether there is a switch from a Th1 to more profibrotic Th2 cytokine dominance in later stages of sarcoidosis notable for progressive fibrosis is not yet known.

A separate immunologic feature of sarcoidosis is the finding that T cells at sites of inflammation in sarcoidosis display a restricted repertoire of T cell receptor (TCR) αβ or γδ genes [13]. The most striking example of this immunologic feature is the increased frequency of AV2S3 (Vα2.3)-positive T cells in human leukocyte antigen (HLA)-DRB1*0301 patients with sarcoidosis [14]. Investigators from the United States, Europe, and Japan also report biased expression of specific TCR genes, though none report such restricted T cell heterogeneity as found in the

Swedish population [15,16]. These findings are consistent with the concept that specific αβ-positive T cells have undergone oligoclonal expansion in response to conventional antigens. These basic immunologic features (Th1 polarization, oligoclonal T cell expansions) are found in patients with sarcoidosis despite widely varying clinical manifestations. Because adaptive Th1 immune responses to putative tissue antigens must involve critical interactions with the innate immune system, defining these interactions are of major interest to further our understanding of the pathogenesis of sarcoidosis. One report has linked toll-like receptor 2 gene (TLR2) polymorphisms with chronic sarcoidosis activity and enhanced induction of IL-2 and TNFα expression by peripheral blood mononuclear cells by TLR2 agonists [17]. Whether the local adaptive and innate immune responses of sarcoidosis are induced by the same etiologic agent at the time of initial exposure, or respond to temporally independent agents as a necessary precursor to the development of sarcoidosis, remains unknown.

Genetic and host factors

There is substantial evidence to support a genetic basis for the susceptibility to developing sarcoidosis and in the determination of clinical phenotype (see the article by Muller-Quernheim elsewhere in this issue). Importantly, both genetic association studies and family studies have identified genes involved in the immune response to be responsible for this altered genetic susceptibility. The most consistent data provide for the association of sarcoidosis risk with class I and II HLA molecules [18]. Two genome-wide analyses also implicate a role for genes within the MHC locus in sarcoidosis [19,20]. Interestingly, genetic linkage studies have identified the butyrophilin-like 2 gene (BTNL2), a gene localized in the MHC region, as a susceptibility factor for the development of sarcoidosis risk, though it is still not conclusive whether the link involves the BTNL2 gene or other genes in linkage disequilibrium within the MHC locus [21,22]. Environmental-genetic interactions are likely to be important but to date remain poorly defined. In one study, Iannuzzi and colleagues [23] attempted to identify associations between environmental exposures and the DQB1*02 (protective) and DQB1*06 (susceptibility) alleles using the ACCESS study data. Exposures to high humidity and water damage were found to enhance the protective effect of the DQB1*0201 allele, but no environmental exposures interacted with the DQB1*0602 susceptibility allele. How these gene variants might interact with environmental agents to alter risk of sarcoidosis remains uncertain.

Environmental agents could interact with genetic factors to enhance host susceptibility to sarcoidosis directly by providing necessary disease-causing antigens or by preconditioning host responses to specific environmental antigens. For example, activation of toll-like receptors by their respective ligands can promote Th1 responses through the induction of IL-12 [17,24,25]. In this way, environmental exposures to bacteria, dusts, or other environmental agents that activate the innate immune system could precondition a susceptible host to respond in a highly polarized, antigen specific Th1 immune response to potential etiologic antigens and agents (Fig. 1). Such a scenario could account for the association of sarcoidosis with certain environmental exposures singled out by epidemiologic studies, yet these exposures fail to provide a direct mechanistic basis for explaining the clinical and immunologic features of systemic sarcoidosis.

Single or multiple etiologic agents?

Before considering specific etiologic agents, one question to consider is whether, in an individual patient, the oligoclonal Th1 immune responses in sarcoidosis are directed against a single or few specific tissue antigens or are a marker of a more generalized dysregulated Th1 immune response driven by multiple, even changing, environmentally derived or endogenous tissue antigens. Several clinical examples support the first possibility: (1) studies of T cell antigen receptor distribution in sarcoidosis suggest that the oligoclonal T cell response is directed to a single or very few number of conventional antigens [13,14]; (2) associations of sarcoidosis susceptibility with specific HLA alleles is better explained by adaptive immune responses to a limited number of antigens than to a more broad-based antigenic response; and (3) chronic beryllium disease (CBD) is an example of how a single antigen (hapten) can induce an oligoclonal, Th1-driven pulmonary granulomatous pneumonitis with histologic and immunologic features that mimic sarcoidosis (see "Environmental sarcoidosis-like pulmonary diseases" section, below).

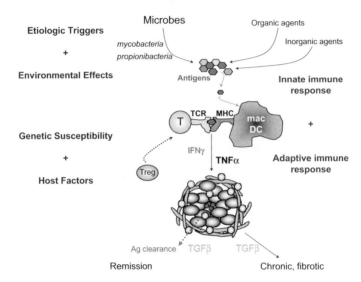

Fig. 1. Hypothetical model of the interactions between environmental, microbial, and immunologic factors that result in granulomatous inflammation in sarcoidosis.

Support for the concept that there is a generalized dysregulated T cell response to multiple antigens in sarcoidosis includes the following:

The recently identified genetic linkage between sarcoidosis and BTNL2, a protein with homology with B-7 costimulatory molecules, would be expected to have a more generalized effect on T cell responses via non-antigen-specific mechanisms [21,22];

The recent demonstration that CD4+ CD25brightFoxP3+ regulatory T lymphocytes, with significant antiproliferative but effete anticytokine effects, are increased at sites of inflammation in sarcoidosis granulomas and in the circulation, are likely to have an effect on T cell responses with little regard to antigen specificity [26];

Regional differences in sunlight exposure and active vitamin D levels that parallel the geographic north-south distribution of sarcoidosis could implicate a nonantigen-specific mechanism by altering immune responses to infectious and environmental agents in general [27].

One phenomenon that continues to offer insights into sarcoidosis etiology is the Kveim (Kveim-Siltzbach) reaction. In this reaction, intradermal injection of sarcoidosis tissue extracts (usually spleen or lymph node) induce a local granulomatous reaction identical to granulomas in affected organs. This observation, initially made by investigators in the 1940s and subsequently confirmed by worldwide studies, indicates that 50% to 80% of sarcoidosis patients have a positive Kveim reaction in early stages of their disease [28]. The Kveim reaction site is infiltrated with CD4+ T cells, with restricted T cell receptor heterogeneity, consistent with antigen driven accumulation [29]. Kveim reactions can be induced from similar preparations made from sarcoidosis bronchoalveolar lavage (BAL) cells or peripheral blood monocytes, suggesting systemic dissemination of the responsible agent by mononuclear phagocytes [30]. The unusual biochemical properties of a Kveim reagent were recently exploited by the authors' group to identify candidate tissue antigens that are present in sarcoidosis tissues and targets of the adaptive immune system in sarcoidosis patients (see "Mycobacteria and sarcoidosis" section below) [31]. Together, studies of the Kveim reaction support the hypothesis that a common antigen or set of compounds induce granulomatous inflammation in most patients with sarcoidosis, and that these antigens are contained in mononuclear phagocytes.

Characterizing potential etiologic agents of sarcoidosis

Environmental agents that can be considered as potential etiologic agents can be classified into inorganic or organic (noninfectious) environmental agents and microbial organisms.

Environmental agents

Different rates of sarcoidosis incidence and prevalence among different geographic regions of the world are consistent with the view that environmental exposures are important determinants of risk of developing sarcoidosis. Epidemiologic studies from the 1950s to 1970s associated sarcoidosis with specific environments, such as rural residence, exposure to pine pollen, pica, or the lumber industry [32]. More recent studies suggest that fireplaces, wood stoves, and home mold exposure are associated with increased risk of sarcoidosis [33]. Occupations, such as military personnel, fire rescue workers, and health care workers have also been associated with higher risk of developing sarcoidosis [34,35]. These studies have lacked validation by larger studies with well-defined, matched control groups.

The multicenter, United States-based ACCESS study was designed to test both a priori hypotheses based on prior studies and to generate new hypotheses regarding the potential for specific environmental and occupational exposures to alter risk of sarcoidosis risk [36]. The study enrolled over 700 biopsy-proven sarcoidosis cases with age, sex, race, and geographically matched control subjects that were identified through random-digit dialing selection. The prestudy goal was to identify risk factors with greater than a twofold risk (odds ratio) when more than 5% of subjects were exposed. The study failed to identify any such exposures that met these criteria. However, the study identified several environmental exposures with more modest positive odds ratios (approximately 1.5) including the following: agricultural employment, mold or mildew, musty odors at work, and pesticide-using industries. There was a strong and robust negative association between tobacco use and sarcoidosis, supporting previous studies that reported a reduced risk of developing sarcoidosis in smokers. Reduced risk was also associated with several exposures linked to allergic (Th2) responses, such as exposure to household cat, animal dust, and feather or down pillow exposures. The primary analysis of the ACCESS study failed to identify an association (positive or negative) between sarcoidosis and several previously hypothesized exposures, such as nonoccupational wood dusts, occupational metals, silica, or in individuals who were employed in dusty trades or had rural residence from birth to 10 years of age. The ACCESS study had insufficient power (prevalence of exposures in control subjects less than 5%) to test associations of sarcoidosis risk among firefighters, military personnel, or occupational wood dust exposures. The ACCESS investigators suggested that an increased risk of developing sarcoidosis may be associated with "dirty" microbe-rich environments, but that a dominant environmental factor could not be identified [36].

Following this initial report, two further publications provide additional analyses of the ACCESS data. One study recoded occupational histories using Standard Industrial Classification and Standard Occupational Classification [37]. Univariate analysis found positive associations of sarcoidosis risk with occupationally related exposures to elementary and secondary schools, building material, garden supplies, mobile homes, hardware, and industrial organic dusts, the latter association also supported by multivariate analysis. Negative associations were found with more isolating occupations in the service industry (childcare, information clerks, personal service attendant, rehabilitation services) and with metal dust or fume exposure, the latter finding also supported by multivariate analysis. A second study performed a cross-sectional analysis to determine whether pulmonary or systemic manifestations of sarcoidosis were associated with a subset of 12 candidate exposures [38]. Univariate analysis identified several factors that were associated with a clinical phenotype dominated by pulmonary sarcoidosis, including occupational organic dust exposure, military service, wood burning at home, and wood or metal dust exposure; this analysis associated higher rates of sarcoidosis to these exposures among individuals within lower income groups. This study also suggested that some exposures have different effects with respect to race. For example, exposure to wood burning was associated with a lower prevalence of systemic sarcoidosis only in African Americans. In aggregate, these studies support a role for specific environmental exposures in altering the risk of developing sarcoidosis.

Environmental sarcoidosis-like pulmonary diseases

Chronic beryllium disease provides a well-studied example of a granulomatous lung disease induced by airborne exposure to an inorganic chemical [39]. The epithelioid granulomatous inflammation in the lung in CBD is histologically identical to that found in pulmonary sarcoidosis. The development of CBD is strongly associated with immunologic sensitization to beryllium salts, most commonly detected by assays of blood T cell proliferation, or more recently, INFγ-producing enzyme-linked immunospot (ELISPOT) assays [39]. This immunologic sensitization is characterized by the localization of beryllium-specific effector memory T cells in the lung and circulating central memory T cells in the blood that produce Th1 cytokines such as INFγ and IL-2 [40–42].

Published surveys have detected a prevalence of beryllium sensitivity in 10% to 15% of occupationally-exposed workers, and the frequency of CBD among newly identified beryllium-sensitive individuals is 10% to 60% [43,44]. Although the actuarial risk of developing CBD among sensitized individuals remains unknown, CBD is most strongly associated with the HLA-DPB1 allele that contains a glutamate at position 69 [45]. Though the granulomatous pneumonitis in CBD mimics sarcoidosis, it remains unlikely that beryllium exposure is a significant cause of systemic sarcoidosis. CBD is not associated with distinct extra-pulmonary syndromes that are part of the spectrum of disease of sarcoidosis, and the ACCESS study found no data to support an increased risk of sarcoidosis with these types of exposures [36]. Notwithstanding this likelihood, CBD is an important and known cause of chronic granulomatous pneumonitis that should be rigorously approached by a detailed occupational history and immunologic testing for beryllium sensitivity in individuals with potential exposures [46]. Metal dusts of zirconium, nickel, and chromium may also induce granulomatous or interstitial lung disease and should be considered in the differential diagnosis of pulmonary sarcoidosis [47]. One recent report supports the association of exposure to man-made mineral fibers and the development of sarcoidosis-like granulomas based on their findings of fiber deposits in 6 of 14 lung tissue samples from patients who reported a history of occupational man-made mineral fiber exposure [48].

Granulomatous inflammation of the lung can be caused by exposure to airborne organic agents. Hypersensitivity pneumonitis (HP) is usually readily distinguished from pulmonary sarcoidosis from differences in radiographic and histologic features, and the presence of extra-pulmonary manifestations may make a diagnosis of sarcoidosis straightforward [49]. The ACCESS study provided little support for overlapping causative agents between sarcoidosis and known HP causing exposures [36]. However, occasionally

overlapping clinical features may make a confident diagnosis difficult and the question of whether similar exposures can cause either HP or sarcoidosis remains conceptually possible. For example, it is difficult to differentiate hypersensitivity pneumonitis from granulomatous infectious pneumonitis in metalworkers exposed to nontuberculous mycobacteria contaminating their metalworking fluid [50]. This overlapping clinical syndrome raises the possibility that mycobacterial organisms may induce different types of granulomatous responses (infectious, HP-like, sarcoidosis-like) in different situations, likely depending on specific host responses and forms of exposures.

Recently, a higher than expected incidence of sarcoidosis was detected among New York City firefighters during the first year after the World Trade Center disaster [51]. In this study, the investigators reported 13 cases in the first year following the incident (incidence 86 per 100,000) compared with 13 cases in the following 4 years (22 per 100,000) and 11 cases in the preceding 15 years (15 per 100,000). Within this new cohort, the investigators noted that many of the New York City firefighters had granulomatous inflammation that was limited to the chest, with impairment of lung function that was mild and difficult to discern from other causes of reactive airway disease. Only a minority of these cases (8 of 26) required corticosteroid therapy. The investigators used the term "sarcoidosis-like granulomatous lung disease" to indicate the uncertainty of whether the excess number of cases represented patients with "systemic sarcoidosis" that conform to current consensus definitions. Regardless of classification, this study adds to other prior reports of higher rates of sarcoidosis in firefighters, to suggest that environmental exposures from this occupation is a risk factor for the development of sarcoidosis.

There is a lack of consensus of whether the granulomatous lung inflammatory processes caused by these inorganic or organic dust exposures should be lumped under the "sarcoidosis" spectrum, or whether their lack of systemic disease and other typical manifestations of sarcoidosis argue for maintaining these diseases under a grouping of "sarcoidosis-like pulmonary disease" [52]. Further clarification of the potential role of these agents in causing sarcoidosis likely awaits an improved understanding of the pathogenetic mechanisms induced by these agents. Unfortunately, experimental models using exposures to beryllium compounds and other inorganic metal exposures have not recapitulated the typical epithelioid granulomatous inflammation in the lung and other organs found in sarcoidosis. Recent reports that intratracheally instilled carbon nanotubes can induce granulomatous pneumonitis in mice support the possibility that noninfectious organic particles may induce some features of pulmonary sarcoidosis, but the lack of other systemic manifestations and the presence microscopically visible aggregates of particles that are not typically seen in sarcoidosis argue against this model as relevant to the pathobiology of systemic sarcoidosis [53].

Microbial agents

An infectious cause for sarcoidosis has been proposed since the first descriptions of this disease, based on the clinical and histologic overlap between sarcoidosis and infectious granulomatous lung diseases [54]. Newer technologies, such as polymerase chain reaction (PCR) methods for nucleic acid detection and immunologic methods, such as ELISPOT, have provided new approaches to the assessment of a role for microbial agents in sarcoidosis. With these technologies, evidence is mounting for a role for specific microbial agents in the development of sarcoidosis.

Mycobacteria and sarcoidosis

The longest held hypothesis regarding the etiology of sarcoidosis is one that links mycobacterial infection with sarcoidosis. Early reports that acid-fast organisms could be detected in some sarcoidosis tissues have not been confirmed, and run contrary to the absence of acid-fast organism staining on routine clinical biopsy specimens. The possibility that remnants of mycobacterial organisms are present in sarcoidosis tissue samples has been suggested by immunohistochemical studies, but these results have also not been widely reproduced [55]. Mycobacterial cell wall components, such as tuberculostearic acid, have been reported in sarcoidosis, but wider confirmation of these data has not been reported [56]. Although epidemiologic studies have failed to identify a clinical association between sarcoidosis and either Bacille Calmette Guerin vaccination or active tuberculosis, other studies report the presence of circulating antibodies to mycobacterial antigens in sarcoidosis, suggesting prior exposure to mycobacterial organisms [57–59].

More recently, PCR methods have been employed to assess the presence of DNA or RNA from mycobacterial or other organisms in sarcoidosis tissues. Results from over two dozen studies have varied, with reports of mycobacterial nucleic acids being detected in 0 to greater than 80% of sarcoidosis tissue samples [60,61]. In one recent study, Drake and colleagues [62] reported detection of mycobacterial rRNA in 60% of sarcoidosis tissue samples from United States patients using nested PCR. A study from Greece detected mycobacteria by PCR in 33 of 46 (71%) sarcoidosis tissue samples [63]. One study from Spain reported finding mycobacterial DNA in 9 of 23 (39%) sarcoidosis tissue samples [64], in contrast to another study from Spain that reported a lack of mycobacterial DNA in all of 78 sarcoidosis tissue samples [65]. In aggregate, a meta-analysis of these studies suggests that greater than 26% of sarcoidosis tissues have evidence of mycobacterial DNA, a more than 9- to 19-fold increased odds over nonsarcoidosis control tissues, strongly indicating that mycobacterial infection is associated with sarcoidosis [61].

Recently, the authors' research group addressed the question of detecting candidate pathogenic antigens in sarcoidosis by using a limited proteomic approach [31]. This approach was based solely on the hypothesis that pathogenic tissue antigens in sarcoidosis would be poorly soluble with biochemical characteristics similar to those of the Kveim reagent and that these antigens could be detected with sarcoidosis sera [66]. Tissue homogenates were prepared from sarcoidosis biopsies and control nondiseased tissue, and sera from sarcoidosis patients was used to detect candidate tissue antigens. The authors found a limited number of tissue antigens in sarcoidosis but not control tissue homogenates. Using mass spectrometry and protein immunoblotting, the authors identified one of these antigenic bands as derived from the *Mycobacterium tuberculosis* catalase-peroxidase protein (mKatG). The presence of mycobacterial *katG* DNA in archived sarcoidosis biopsies was confirmed by in situ hybridization in 38% of sarcoidosis samples using probes for *katG* DNA and mycobacterial 16s rRNA. Using recombinant mKatG protein, there was evidence for circulating IgG directed to mKatG in approximately 50% of sarcoidosis patients, indicating an adaptive immune response to this specific mycobacterial protein in sarcoidosis. Given that this approach was not predicated on any specific hypothesis regarding a microbial etiology of sarcoidosis, the identification of a relevant specific mycobacterial protein antigen in sarcoidosis provides support for a mycobacterial link to sarcoidosis etiology.

Subsequent studies have extended these results, documenting that patients with sarcoidosis mount Th1 responses to mKatG and other mycobacterial proteins with greater frequency than control populations. For example, using ELISPOT to detect IFNγ expression, Drake and colleagues [67] demonstrated peripheral blood mononuclear cell (PBMC) responses to an mKatG peptide in 13 of 26 sarcoidosis, 0 of 6 purified protein derivative (PPD)-negative controls, and 7 of 8 PPD-positive controls. This group also reported IFNγ responses in PBMC of sarcoidosis patients to early secreted antigenic tartget-6, mycobacterial superoxide dismutase A, and mycobacterial antigen 85A, suggesting T cell responses to a range of mycobacterial antigens in sarcoidosis [68,69]. Given that multiple approaches continue to link exposure to mycobacterial organisms to sarcoidosis, it seems likely that these organisms play a role in the pathogenesis of sarcoidosis in a subgroup of sarcoidosis. The specific pathogenetic mechanisms responsible for causing the pathobiology of sarcoidosis distinct from a host response to an active or latent mycobacterial infection remain uncertain.

Propionibacteria and sarcoidosis

Homma and colleagues [70] described the isolation of *Propionibacterium acnes* by culture from 78% of sarcoidosis tissue samples in 1978, suggesting a role for this commensal organism in sarcoidosis. This initial study was followed by a series of studies from Japanese investigators that confirmed the presence of propionibacterial DNA in sarcoidosis tissues from both Japanese and European biopsies [71]. However, *P. acnes* DNA was also reported in 57% of control tissues, including those from healthy individuals, raising questions whether this commensal organism is playing a pathogenic role [72]. Ebe and colleagues [73] demonstrated antibody responses to RP35, a 255 amino acid fragment of *P. acnes* trigger factor protein, in approximately 40% of sarcoidosis BAL samples versus less than 5% of control BAL samples, suggesting that adaptive responses to *P. acnes* proteins may be pathologic in some individuals. Although tetracycline antibiotics, such as minocycline, that kill *P. acnes* may be effective in treating a small fraction of patients with cutaneous sarcoidosis [74], there are no reports demonstrating benefit with treatment using other antibiotics that are microbicidal to propionibacterial

organisms. Minocycline has anti-inflammatory properties that could also explain the positive effects in sarcoidosis [75]. Interestingly, *P. acnes* is capable of induce granulomatous-like reactions in experimental models, and these reactions are blunted by a variety of antibiotics (minocycline, clindamycin, gentamicin) [76,77]. Thus, a role of *P. acnes* or other priopionibacterial organisms in promoting sarcoidosis granulomatous inflammation remains an intriguing possibility, though the underlying mechanisms and specific host factors required to cause the pathobiology of sarcoidosis remain to be determined.

Viruses, rare pathogens, and sarcoidosis

A viral etiology of sarcoidosis has been proposed, based on the presence of serum antibodies to a variety of viruses such as herpes-like viruses (Epstein-Barr virus, herpes simplex virus, human herpes virus-8) in subsets of patients with sarcoidosis [78]. There is little other supporting evidence for this possibility, and these findings could be related to the nonclonal hypergammaglobulinemia frequently observed in sarcoidosis. Because viral infections are not known to cause typical epithelioid sarcoidosis-like granulomas, it is conceivable that viral particles might interact with host proteins (eg, antibody-antigen complex) to create a nidus for granuloma formation, though such a pathogenesis remains theoretic and other mechanisms would be needed to explain chronic sarcoidosis. One potential exception would be if an antiviral immune response resulted in autoimmunity by molecular mimicry. Such a scenario could explain features of autoimmunity sometime seen in sarcoidosis (eg, nongranulomatous uveitis), but how this mechanism would cause chronic granulomatous inflammation is not obvious. There remains the possibility that viral infections could precede or induce an immunologic milieu in the host that increases susceptibility to sarcoidosis if followed by exposure to a second pathogenic environmental exposure.

A variety of other human pathogens, including fungi, spirochetes, Borrelia species and *Tropheryma whipplei* (causative agent of Whipple disease) have been suggested as mimics or potential causes of sarcoidosis [79]. Infections from these agents can cause granulomatous reactions that may be particularly difficult to distinguish from sarcoidosis [80]. Cell-wall deficient organisms derived from *Mycobacteria*, rickettsia, and chlamydia species have also been implicated in sarcoidosis based on limited data. All of these studies lack confirmation by well-controlled laboratory and epidemiologic studies. For example, a recent blinded study using the blood from matched cases and control subjects from the ACCESS study found that the isolation of cell-wall deficient organisms was as frequent in healthy controls as in sarcoidosis patients [81].

Active versus latent infection,
or microbial remnants?

Given increasing evidence that implicate a role for mycobacterial or propionibacterial organisms in sarcoidosis, one persistent question is the status of these microbes in sarcoidosis. Despite the presence of microbial DNA in sarcoidosis tissues that indicate prior infection, there is no clinical evidence that sarcoidosis patients are at higher risk of recurrent active mycobacterial (or propionibacterial infection), even in the face of chronic corticosteroid or immunosuppressive therapy [82]. For example, Fite and colleagues detected mycobacterial DNA in 9 of 23 sarcoidosis tissue samples, and they report that none of these patients developed evidence of active mycobacterial infection over a follow-up period of up to 12 years [64]. Similar results can be confirmed from the authors' study: no sarcoidosis patient with mKatG protein or DNA in their biopsy tissues or with circulating anti-mKatG IgG or T cell responses to mKatG have developed active mycobacterial infection in 5 to 10 years of follow-up, despite a majority undergoing chronic treatment (authors' observations). Thus, "reactivation" of latent mycobacterial infection is not a feature of sarcoidosis. Similarly, no clinical trial has demonstrated the utility of antibiotics alone in the treatment of systemic sarcoidosis. An exception might include anecdotal evidence that the tetracyclines, antimalarials, or dapsone are beneficial in a small subset of cutaneous sarcoidosis. However, these observations could be explained by anti-inflammatory or immunomodulatory effects of these antibiotics, as other antibiotics with similar antimicrobial spectrums do not appear to be effective [75,83]. Although these observations suggest that systemic sarcoidosis is not caused by ongoing active or reactivated infection, there are other observations that indicate the responsible agent for sarcoidosis is transmittable. For example, there are reports of granulomatous inflammation being transmitted via bone marrow transplantation from individuals with sarcoidosis [84,85].

Granulomatous inflammation is also known to develop in lung and heart allografts following transplantation in patients with sarcoidosis [86,87]. Using in situ hybridization, Milman and colleagues [88] reported in one female patient with recurrent allograft sarcoidosis that the origin of the granuloma macrophages were from the male donor. Of interest, Klemen and colleagues [89] demonstrated the presence of nontuberculosis mycobacterial DNA within granulomas in three sarcoidosis patients who experienced sarcoidosis in their transplanted lung. These studies support the conclusion that granuloma-inducing agents and antigens are present in mononuclear phagocytes sarcoidosis, but that active infection is not part of the package.

The pathobiology of sarcoidosis—a hypothetical synthesis

The clinical and immunologic hallmarks of sarcoidosis must be reconciled with potential etiologic agents that foster disease susceptibility and induce systemic granulomatous inflammation. Recent studies confirm the presence of mycobacterial antigens and DNA in a subset of patients, that a majority of patients (at least in the United States and Sweden) have antimycobacterial T and B cell responses to mycobacterial antigens, and do not have evidence of reactivation of mycobacterial infection despite chronic anti-inflammatory or immunosuppressive therapy. One possibility to explain these features is to postulate that sarcoidosis is a pathobiologic outcome of a host response that is effective in killing the invading mycobacterial organisms, but that also results in the deposition of microbial antigens that persist in tissues in a poorly soluble state, perhaps aggregated with specific host proteins (see Fig. 1). This pathobiologic response is characterized by a highly polarized Th1 response—effective in killing, but ineffective in antigen removal. Because established granulomas have been shown to be traps for newly deposited mycobacteria [90], chronic disease may be the result of these early, established sarcoidosis granulomas trapping newly circulating organisms, which could include nontuberculous mycobacterial and propionibacterial organisms or specific antigens derived from them. The deposited antigens may have physiochemical properties (insolubility, resistance to protease degradation) that allow the material to persist for years as a nidus for granuloma formation. Host factors based on genetic-environmental interactions would enhance a potential sarcoidosis outcome by establishing the proper immunologic milieu that precedes exposure to etiologically relevant microbes.

Future studies can be designed to test these hypotheses. Expression profiling studies of sarcoidosis and active mycobacterial infections can be evaluated to examine differences in host and mycobacterial responses. For example, expression-profiling studies have shown significant alterations in mycobacterial gene expression in isolates obtained from cavitary lesions versus more distant areas of lung, indicating that host-pathogen interactions modify the mycobacterial transcriptome [91]. Immunologic profiles in sarcoidosis patients can be further defined to examine specific T and B cell responses to candidate pathogenic antigens to test correlations with specific clinical phenotypes and outcomes. The development of preclinical models can test whether the induction of specific immune responses to these antigens will lead to specific pathologic outcomes. Although these models may not recapitulate the complete pathobiology of sarcoidosis, they may assist in the development of potential immunotherapeutic approaches to this disease.

References

[1] Statement on sarcoidosis. Joint Statement of the American Thoracic Society (ATS), the European Respiratory Society (ERS) and the World Association of Sarcoidosis and Other Granulomatous Disorders (WASOG) adopted by the ATS Board of Directors and by the ERS Executive Committee, February 1999. Am J Respir Crit Care Med 1999; 160(2):736–55.

[2] Saunders BM, Cooper AM. Restraining mycobacteria: role of granulomas in mycobacterial infections. Immunol Cell Biol 2000;78(4):334–41.

[3] Baughman RP, Teirstein AS, Judson MA, et al. Clinical characteristics of patients in a case control study of sarcoidosis. Am J Respir Crit Care Med 2001;164(10 Pt 1):1885–9.

[4] Baird MM, Bogoch A, Fenwick JB. Liver biopsy in sarcoidosis. Can Med Assoc J 1950;62(6):562–5.

[5] Judson MA, Baughman RP, Thompson BW, et al. Two year prognosis of sarcoidosis: the ACCESS experience. Sarcoidosis Vasc Diffuse Lung Dis 2003; 20(3):204–11.

[6] Hunninghake GW, Crystal RG. Pulmonary sarcoidosis: a disorder mediated by excess helper T-lymphocyte activity at sites of disease activity. N Engl J Med 1981;305(8):429–34.

[7] Morris DG, Jasmer RM, Huang L, et al. Sarcoidosis following HIV infection: evidence for CD4+ lymphocyte dependence. Chest 2003;124(3):929–35.

[8] Moller DR, Forman JD, Liu MC, et al. Enhanced expression of IL-12 associated with Th1 cytokine profiles in active pulmonary sarcoidosis. J Immunol 1996;156(12):4952–60.

[9] Nakajima M, Kubota Y, Miyashita N, et al. Recurrence of sarcoidosis following interferon alpha therapy for chronic hepatitis C. Intern Med 1996;35(5): 376–9.

[10] Logan TF, Bensadoun ES. Increased disease activity in a patient with sarcoidosis after high dose interleukin 2 treatment for metastatic renal cancer. Thorax 2005;60(7):610–1.

[11] Foulon G, Wislez M, Naccache JM, et al. Sarcoidosis in HIV-infected patients in the era of highly active antiretroviral therapy. Clin Infect Dis 2004;38(3): 418–25.

[12] Chiu BC, Freeman CM, Stolberg VR, et al. Cytokine-chemokine networks in experimental mycobacterial and schistosomal pulmonary granuloma formation. Am J Respir Cell Mol Biol 2003;29(1): 106–16.

[13] Grunewald J, Eklund A. Role of CD4+ T cells in sarcoidosis. Proc Am Thorac Soc 2007;4(5): 461–4.

[14] Grunewald J, Wahlstrom J, Berlin M, et al. Lung restricted T cell receptor AV2S3+ CD4+ T cell expansions in sarcoidosis patients with a shared HLA-DRbeta chain conformation. Thorax 2002; 57(4):348–52.

[15] Silver RF, Crystal RG, Moller DR. Limited heterogeneity of biased T-cell receptor V beta gene usage in lung but not blood T cells in active pulmonary sarcoidosis. Immunology 1996;88(4):516–23.

[16] Sawabe T, Shiokawa S, Sugisaki K, et al. Accumulation of common clonal T cells in multiple lesions of sarcoidosis. Mol Med 2000;6(9):793–802.

[17] Veltkamp M, Wijnen PA, van Moorsel CH, et al. Linkage between Toll-like receptor (TLR) 2 promotor and intron polymorphisms: functional effects and relevance to sarcoidosis. Clin Exp Immunol 2007;149(3):453–62.

[18] Luisetti M, Beretta A, Casali L. Genetic aspects in sarcoidosis. Eur Respir J 2000;16(4):768–80.

[19] Schurmann M, Reichel P, Muller-Myhsok B, et al. Results from a genome-wide search for predisposing genes in sarcoidosis. Am J Respir Crit Care Med 2001;164(5):840–6.

[20] Iannuzzi MC, Iyengar SK, Gray-McGuire C, et al. Genome-wide search for sarcoidosis susceptibility genes in African Americans. Genes Immun 2005; 6(6):509–18.

[21] Valentonyte R, Hampe J, Huse K, et al. Sarcoidosis is associated with a truncating splice site mutation in BTNL2. Nat Genet 2005;37(4):357–64.

[22] Rybicki BA, Walewski JL, Maliarik MJ, et al. The BTNL2 gene and sarcoidosis susceptibility in

African Americans and Whites. Am J Hum Genet 2005;77(3):491–9.

[23] Iannuzzi MC, Maliarik MJ, Poisson LM, et al. Sarcoidosis susceptibility and resistance HLA-DQB1 alleles in African Americans. Am J Respir Crit Care Med 2003;167(9):1225–31.

[24] Berenson LS, Ota N, Murphy KM. Issues in T-helper 1 development—resolved and unresolved. Immunol Rev 2004;202:157–74.

[25] Dabbagh K, Lewis DB. Toll-like receptors and T-helper-1/T-helper-2 responses. Curr Opin Infect Dis 2003;16(3):199–204.

[26] Miyara M, Amoura Z, Parizot C, et al. The immune paradox of sarcoidosis and regulatory T cells. J Exp Med 2006;203(2):359–70.

[27] Hunninghake GW. Sarcoidosis; Past, Present and Future. ATS 2006 International Conference, Amberson Lecture. San Diego, May 21, 2006.

[28] Siltzbach LE. The Kveim test in sarcoidosis. A study of 750 patients. JAMA 1961;178:476–82.

[29] Klein JT, Horn TD, Forman JD, et al. Selection of oligoclonal V beta-specific T cells in the intradermal response to Kveim-Siltzbach reagent in individuals with sarcoidosis. J Immunol 1995;154(3):1450–60.

[30] Holter JF, Park HK, Sjoerdsma KW, et al. Nonviable autologous bronchoalveolar lavage cell preparations induce intradermal epithelioid cell granulomas in sarcoidosis patients. Am Rev Respir Dis 1992; 145(4 Pt 1):864–71.

[31] Song Z, Marzilli L, Greenlee BM, et al. Mycobacterial catalase-peroxidase is a tissue antigen and target of the adaptive immune response in systemic sarcoidosis. J Exp Med 2005;201(5):755–67.

[32] Dunner E, Williams JH Jr. Epidemiology of sarcoidosis in the United States. Am Rev Respir Dis 1961; 84(5Pt 2):163–8.

[33] Kajdasz DK, Lackland DT, Mohr LC, et al. A current assessment of rurally linked exposures as potential risk factors for sarcoidosis. Ann Epidemiol 2001; 11(2):111–7.

[34] Sarcoidosis among U.S. Navy enlisted men, 1965–1993. MMWR Morb Mortal Wkly Rep 1997; 46(23):539–43.

[35] Prezant DJ, Dhala A, Goldstein A, et al. The incidence, prevalence, and severity of sarcoidosis in New York City firefighters. Chest 1999;116(5):1183–93.

[36] Newman LS, Rose CS, Bresnitz EA, et al. A case control etiologic study of sarcoidosis: environmental and occupational risk factors. Am J Respir Crit Care Med 2004;170(12):1324–30.

[37] Barnard J, Rose C, Newman L, et al. Job and industry classifications associated with sarcoidosis in A Case-Control Etiologic Study of Sarcoidosis (ACCESS). J Occup Environ Med 2005;47(3):226–34.

[38] Kreider ME, Christie JD, Thompson B, et al. Relationship of environmental exposures to the clinical phenotype of sarcoidosis. Chest 2005;128(1):207–15.

[39] Newman LS, Mroz MM, Balkissoon R, et al. Beryllium sensitization progresses to chronic beryllium disease: a longitudinal study of disease risk. Am J Respir Crit Care Med 2005;171(1):54–60.

[40] Fontenot AP, Canavera SJ, Gharavi L, et al. Target organ localization of memory CD4(+) T cells in patients with chronic beryllium disease. J Clin Invest 2002;110(10):1473–82.

[41] Pott GB, Palmer BE, Sullivan AK, et al. Frequency of beryllium-specific, TH1-type cytokine-expressing CD4+ T cells in patients with beryllium-induced disease. J Allergy Clin Immunol 2005;115(5): 1036–42.

[42] Fontenot AP, Palmer BE, Sullivan AK, et al. Frequency of beryllium-specific, central memory CD4+ T cells in blood determines proliferative response. J Clin Invest 2005;115(10):2886–93.

[43] Sackett HM, Maier LA, Silveira LJ, et al. Beryllium medical surveillance at a former nuclear weapons facility during cleanup operations. J Occup Environ Med 2004;46(9):953–61.

[44] Kreiss K, Mroz MM, Newman LS, et al. Machining risk of beryllium disease and sensitization with median exposures below 2 micrograms/m3. Am J Ind Med 1996;30(1):16–25.

[45] Saltini C, Richeldi L. A genetic marker for chronic beryllium disease. Med Lav 1995;86(3):226–8.

[46] Muller-Quernheim J, Gaede KI, Fireman E, et al. Diagnoses of chronic beryllium disease within cohorts of sarcoidosis patients. Eur Respir J 2006; 27(6):1190–5.

[47] Kelleher P, Pacheco K, Newman LS. Inorganic dust pneumonias: the metal-related parenchymal disorders. Environ Health Perspect 2000;108(Suppl 4): 685–96.

[48] Drent M, Bomans PH, Van Suylen RJ, et al. Association of man-made mineral fibre exposure and sarcoidlike granulomas. Respir Med 2000;94(8): 815–20.

[49] Churg A, Muller NL, Flint J, et al. Chronic hypersensitivity pneumonitis. Am J Surg Pathol 2006; 30(2):201–8.

[50] Respiratory illness in workers exposed to metalworking fluid contaminated with nontuberculous mycobacteria–Ohio, 2001. MMWR Morb Mortal Wkly Rep 2002;51(16):349–52.

[51] Izbicki G, Chavko R, Banauch GI, et al. World Trade Center "sarcoid-like" granulomatous pulmonary disease in New York City Fire Department rescue workers. Chest 2007;131(5):1414–23.

[52] Rossman MD, Kreider ME. Is chronic beryllium disease sarcoidosis of known etiology? Sarcoidosis Vasc Diffuse Lung Dis 2003;20(2):104–9.

[53] Shvedova AA, Kisin ER, Mercer R, et al. Unusual inflammatory and fibrogenic pulmonary responses to single-walled carbon nanotubes in mice. Am J Physiol Lung Cell Mol Physiol 2005;289(5): L698–708.

[54] El-Zammar OA, Katzenstein AL. Pathological diagnosis of granulomatous lung disease: a review. Histopathology 2007;50(3):289–310.

[55] Alavi HA, Moscovic EA. Immunolocalization of cell-wall-deficient forms of *Mycobacterium tuberculosis* complex in sarcoidosis and in sinus histiocytosis of lymph nodes draining carcinoma. Histol Histopathol 1996;11(3):683–94.

[56] Hanngren A, Odham G, Eklund A, et al. Tuberculostearic acid in lymph nodes from patients with sarcoidosis. Sarcoidosis 1987;4(2):101–4.

[57] Sutherland I, Mitchell DN, Hart PD. Incidence of Intrathoracic Sarcoidosis among Young Adults Participating in a Trial of Tuberculosis Vaccines. Br Med J 1965;2(5460):497–503.

[58] Grange JM, Gibson J, Nassau E, et al. Enzyme-linked immunosorbent assay (ELISA): a study of antibodies to Mycobacterium tuberculosis in the IgG, IgA and IgM classes in tuberculosis, sarcoidosis and Crohn's disease. Tubercle 1980;61(3):145–52.

[59] Milman N, Andersen AB. Detection of antibodies in serum against *M. tuberculosis* using western blot technique. Comparison between sarcoidosis patients and healthy subjects. Sarcoidosis 1993;10(1):29–31.

[60] Hance AJ. The role of mycobacteria in the pathogenesis of sarcoidosis. Semin Respir Infect 1998; 13(3):197–205.

[61] Gupta D, Agarwal R, Aggarwal AN, et al. Molecular evidence for the role of mycobacteria in sarcoidosis: a meta-analysis. Eur Respir J 2007;30(3): 508–16.

[62] Drake WP, Pei Z, Pride DT, et al. Molecular analysis of sarcoidosis tissues for mycobacterium species DNA. Emerg Infect Dis 2002;8(11):1334–41.

[63] Gazouli M, Ikonomopoulos J, Trigidou R, et al. Assessment of mycobacterial, propionibacterial, and human herpes virus 8 DNA in tissues of Greek patients with sarcoidosis. J Clin Microbiol 2002; 40(8):3060–3.

[64] Fite E, Fernandez-Figueras MT, Prats R, et al. High prevalence of *Mycobacterium tuberculosis* DNA in biopsies from sarcoidosis patients from Catalonia, Spain. Respiration 2006;73(1):20–6.

[65] Marcoval J, Benitez MA, Alcaide F, et al. Absence of ribosomal RNA of *Mycobacterium tuberculosis* complex in sarcoidosis. Arch Dermatol 2005; 141(1):57–9.

[66] Chase MW, Siltzbach LE. Concentration of the active principle resopnsible for the Kveim reaction. In: Turiaf J, Chabot J, editors. La sarcoïdose. Paris: Masson et Cie; 1967.

[67] Drake WP, Dhason MS, Nadaf M, et al. Cellular recognition of *Mycobacterium tuberculosis* ESAT-6 and KatG peptides in systemic sarcoidosis. Infect Immun 2007;75(1):527–30.

[68] Carlisle J, Evans W, Hajizadeh R, et al. Multiple Mycobacterium antigens induce interferon-gamma production from sarcoidosis peripheral blood mononuclear cells. Clin Exp Immunol 2007;150(3):460–8.

[69] Hajizadeh R, Sato H, Carlisle J, et al. *Mycobacterium tuberculosis* Antigen 85A induces Th-1 immune responses in systemic sarcoidosis. J Clin Immunol 2007;27(4):445–54.

[70] Homma JY, Abe C, Chosa H, et al. Bacteriological investigation on biopsy specimens from patients with sarcoidosis. Jpn J Exp Med 1978;48(3):251–5.

[71] Eishi Y, Suga M, Ishige I, et al. Quantitative analysis of mycobacterial and propionibacterial DNA in lymph nodes of Japanese and European patients with sarcoidosis. J Clin Microbiol 2002;40(1): 198–204.

[72] Ishige I, Eishi Y, Takemura T, et al. *Propionibacterium acnes* is the most common bacterium commensal in peripheral lung tissue and mediastinal lymph nodes from subjects without sarcoidosis. Sarcoidosis Vasc Diffuse Lung Dis 2005;22(1):33–42.

[73] Ebe Y, Ikushima S, Yamaguchi T, et al. Proliferative response of peripheral blood mononuclear cells and levels of antibody to recombinant protein from *Propionibacterium acnes* DNA expression library in Japanese patients with sarcoidosis. Sarcoidosis Vasc Diffuse Lung Dis 2000;17(3):256–65.

[74] Bachelez H, Senet P, Cadranel J, et al. The use of tetracyclines for the treatment of sarcoidosis. Arch Dermatol 2001;137(1):69–73.

[75] Labro MT. Antibiotics as anti-inflammatory agents. Curr Opin Investig Drugs 2002;3(1):61–8.

[76] Minami J, Eishi Y, Ishige Y, et al. Pulmonary granulomas caused experimentally in mice by a recombinant trigger-factor protein of *Propionibacterium acnes*. J Med Dent Sci 2003;50(4):265–74.

[77] McCaskill JG, Chason KD, Hua X, et al. Pulmonary immune responses to *Propionibacterium acnes* in C57BL/6 and BALB/c mice. Am J Respir Cell Mol Biol 2006;35(3):347–56.

[78] Nikoskelainen J, Hannuksela M, Palva T. Antibodies to Epstein-Barr virus and some other herpes viruses in patients with sarcoidosis, pulmonary tuberculosis and erythema nodosum. Scand J Infect Dis 1974;6(3):209–16.

[79] James DG, Lipman MC. Whipple's disease: a granulomatous masquerader. Clin Chest Med 2002;23(2): 513–9, xi–xii.

[80] Schilstra A, Rottoli P, Jacobs JA, et al. Case studies to explore the pitfalls in the diagnosis of sarcoidosis. Sarcoidosis Vasc Diffuse Lung Dis 2006;23(2): 135–40.

[81] Brown ST, Brett I, Almenoff PL, et al. Recovery of cell wall-deficient organisms from blood does not distinguish between patients with sarcoidosis and control subjects. Chest 2003;123(2):413–7.

[82] Sadikot RT, Dore P, Arnold AG. Sarcoidosis and opportunistic infections. South Med J 2001;94(1): 75–7.

[83] Sapadin AN, Fleischmajer R. Tetracyclines: nonantibiotic properties and their clinical implications. J Am Acad Dermatol 2006;54(2):258–65.

[84] Heyll A, Meckenstock G, Aul C, et al. Possible transmission of sarcoidosis via allogeneic bone

marrow transplantation. Bone Marrow Transplant 1994;14(1):161–4.

[85] Sundar KM, Carveth HJ, Gosselin MV, et al. Granulomatous pneumonitis following bone marrow transplantation. Bone Marrow Transplant 2001; 28(6):627–30.

[86] Martinez FJ, Orens JB, Deeb M, et al. Recurrence of sarcoidosis following bilateral allogeneic lung transplantation. Chest 1994;106(5):1597–9.

[87] Padilla ML, Schilero GJ, Teirstein AS. Donor-acquired sarcoidosis. Sarcoidosis Vasc Diffuse Lung Dis 2002;19(1):18–24.

[88] Milman N, Andersen CB, Burton CM, et al. Recurrent sarcoid granulomas in a transplanted lung derive from recipient immune cells. Eur Respir J 2005;26(3):549–52.

[89] Klemen H, Husain AN, Cagle PT, et al. Mycobacterial DNA in recurrent sarcoidosis in the transplanted lung—a PCR-based study on four cases. Virchows Arch 2000;436(4):365–9.

[90] Cosma CL, Humbert O, Ramakrishnan L. Superinfecting mycobacteria home to established tuberculous granulomas. Nat Immunol 2004;5(8): 828–35.

[91] Rachman H, Strong M, Schaible U, et al. *Mycobacterium tuberculosis* gene expression profiling within the context of protein networks. Microbes Infect 2006;8(3):747–57.

Clin Chest Med 29 (2008) 379–390

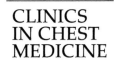

The Immunology of Sarcoidosis

Alicia K. Gerke, MD*, Gary Hunninghake, MD

*Division of Pulmonary, Critical Care, and Occupational Medicine, University of Iowa College of Medicine,
200 Hawkins Drive, Iowa City, IA 52242, USA*

Sarcoidosis is a systemic disease characterized by noncaseating granulomas in many organs, especially the lung. The immune mechanisms that cause this disease are not completely known. The process seems to begin with an antigenic stimulus, followed by T-cell and macrophage activation via a classic major histocompatibility complex (MHC) II–mediated pathway. This process has all of the features of a classic T-helper 1 (Th1) response, and in fact, sarcoidosis may be the first disorder to be clearly identified as a Th1-mediated disease. At the time of disease, there is no evidence for a defect in cellular or humoral immunity. As part of this process, cytokines and chemokines are released that recruit cells to sites of granuloma formation and trigger activation of these cells (Box 1). In some instances, there may be a disruption of the normal function of regulatory cells and/or persistence of the antigen that allows the granulomas progress instead of resolving, as they do in most patients. The local environment of the granulomas eventually may change to a more T-helper 2 (Th2)-like environment that decreases the intensity of granuloma formation but favors the development of fibrosis. Finally, the immune response seems to be compartmentalized to affected tissues, because spontaneous secretion of cytokines by lymphocytes and macrophages is seen only at sites of granuloma formation [1,2].

The methods of studying the immunologic process of sarcoidosis have evolved over time. Initial studies used blood and serum samples in attempts to identify the mechanism behind cutaneous anergy in patients who had sarcoidosis. The advent of bronchoscopy allowed more focused evaluation of granulomatous inflammation. Bronchoalveolar lavage samples are a window into the lung environment, allowing identification of cell types and of the milieu of cytokines that interact to form granulomas [3]. Most recently, immunogenetic, proteomic, and bioinformatic methods have been used to identify disease susceptibility, potential causes, and protein expression in afflicted patients.

The granuloma

Histologically, the granuloma is formed by lymphocytes, macrophages, epithelioid cells, multinucleated giant cells, mast cells, and fibroblasts. The central core of an active granuloma consists of mononuclear phagocytes in various stages of activation and differentiation. This core is surrounded by CD4+ T cells interspersed with a small number of CD8+ T cells and B cells. Miyara and colleagues [4] showed that regulatory T cells that are CD3+/CD4+/CD25+/FoxP3+ accumulate at the periphery, along with additional CD8+ T cells and fibroblasts. Fibroblasts, regulatory cells, and CD8+ cells are more prominent as the activity of the granulomas diminishes and fibrosis ensues. The granulomas seen in stage 1 sarcoidosis tend to be focused in the mediastinal lymph nodes and can be correlated with enlarged hila on chest radiographs. Extension into the bronchovascular bundles and interlobular septa, as noted by reticulonodular infiltrates on chest radiographs, is indicative of stage 2 and 3 sarcoidosis (Fig. 1). The fibrosis associated with granuloma resolution correlates with traction and scarring on the radiograph, which characterizes stage 4 sarcoidosis, an irreversible process.

---

* Corresponding author.
E-mail address: alicia-gerke@uiowa.edu
(A.K. Gerke).

Box 1. Cytokine and chemokine network in granulomatous inflammation of active sarcoidosis

Cytokines
Interferon-γ (IFNγ)
Tumor necrosis factor-α (TNFα)
Transforming growth factor-β (TGFβ)
Interleukin (IL)-1β
IL-2
IL-6
IL-12
IL-15
IL-16
IL-18
Granulocyte macrophage colony-
  stimulating factor (GM-CSF)

Chemokines
CCL2 (monocyte chemotactic protein 1,
  MCP-1)
CCL3 (macrophage inflammatory protein
  1α, MIP1α)
CCL5 (regulated on activation, normal T-
  cell expressed and selected, RANTES)
CCL20 (macrophage inflammatory
  protein 3α, MIP3α)
CXCL8 (IL-8)
CXCL10 (interferon-inducible protein 10,
  IP-10)
CXCL16

Inflammatory products
Neopterin
Osteopontin
Angiotensin-converting enzyme

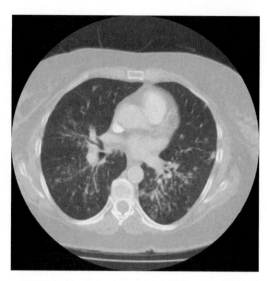

Fig. 1. Chest CT of stage 2 sarcoidosis. In stage 2 sarcoidosis the granulomatous inflammation extends along the bronchovascular bundles and pleura, forming a notable nodular pattern on the radiographic image.

Although most patients who have sarcoidosis have pulmonary and lymph node involvement, local accumulations of granulomas can present in a variety of organs. Neurologic or cardiac sarcoidosis may represent the greatest threat to life, but involvement of the eyes, skin, liver, bones, gastrointestinal tract, or kidneys also may cause significant distress and require treatment.

Comparison of granulomas in various diffuse lung diseases

Although classic to sarcoidosis, granulomas are collections of histiocytes and lymphocytes that can form in a number of infectious and noninfectious diseases (J. Weydert, personal communication, 2007). Histologically, the pattern of inflammation in each disease can be defined further by the character and distribution of the granulomas. Granulomas can be described as necrotizing or non-necrotizing, tight or loosely formed, or appearing in conjunction with a foreign body reaction. The distribution can follow the lymphatics, bronchovascular bundles, or airways or can be random. For example, granulomas caused by infections such as tuberculosis, histoplasmosis, and cryptococcal lung disease are necrotizing and well formed, often in a random distribution (Fig. 2A). Hypersensitivity pneumonitis granulomas are non-necrotizing, loosely formed, and tend to follow the airways (Fig. 2B). In contrast, sarcoidosis granulomas tend to be non-necrotizing and tightly formed, and they track along the lymphatics, interlobular septa, bronchovascular bundles, and pleura (Fig. 2D). They typically are indistinguishable from the lesions of berylliosis, requiring careful history taking to identify the correct diagnosis [5]. Similarly, foreign body reactions may mimic granulomas (Fig. 2C). These reactions form along the bronchioles and airways in response to inhaled irritants, but they can also develop in the lung through intravascular dissemination of a substance such as talc, causing perivascular inflammation. Often, refractile material can be seen with the lesions, and the fibrotic component can be increased markedly.

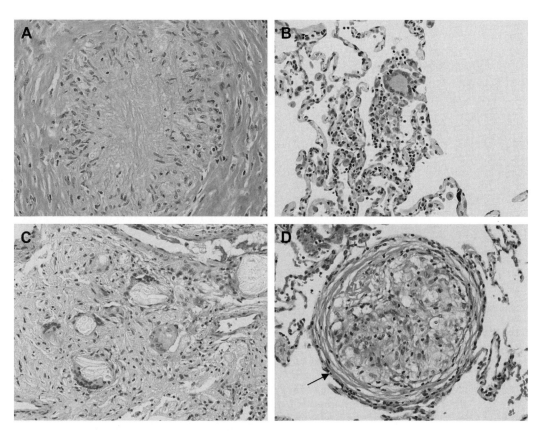

Fig. 2. A comparison of granulomas in diffuse lung diseases. (A) Infectious granulomas are necrotizing and tightly formed. (B) In hypersensitivity pneumonitis, the granuloma is non-necrotizing and loosely formed. (C) Foreign body reactions, as seen in this slide of a patient who injected talc intravenously, can resemble granulomas. (D) In sarcoidosis, the granulomas are non-necrotizing and tightly formed. In this case, the granuloma probably is resolving, as indicated by the concentric layer of fibrotic connective tissue (hematoxylin and eosin stain, original magnification ×40). (*Courtesy of* Jamie Weydert, MD, Iowa City, IA.)

The immune reaction in sarcoidosis

The T-helper 1 immune response

The CD4+ lymphocytes in the lung triggering the formation of the granuloma express a strong Th1 phenotype. The influx of these cells serves further to recruit Th1 lymphocytes and macrophages, which produce cytokines such as interferon-gamma (IFNγ), interleukin (IL-2), and IL-15 [6]. The production of IL-12 and IL-18 also is increased, which enhances IFNγ production in the lung and induces differentiation of Th0 precursors into active Th1 lymphocytes, perpetuating the response [7,8]. The increased expression of Th1 chemokine and cytokine receptors such as CXCR3, CCR5, IL-12 receptor, and IL-18 receptor in conjunction with decreased expression of the Th2 chemokine receptors CXCR4 and CCR4 provides further evidence of the Th1

predominance [9]. Interferon-inducible protein (IP-10), a chemokine induced by IFNγ and inhibited by IL-4, is enhanced in alveolar macrophages and in sarcoid granulomas [10]. The Th1 environment results in macrophage activation, communication between cells to form granulomas, production of T-cell growth factors, and inhibition of fibrosis [11].

In contrast to the Th1-dominant mechanism in the lung, the circulating cells in the periphery do not exhibit such a clear response. Although Nureki and colleagues [12] recently confirmed previous reports of high IP-10 production in the lung by lavaged cells, IP-10 production by peripheral blood mononuclear cells did not increase in sarcoidosis patients compared to controls. They also noted the Th2 chemokine, thymus and activation-regulated chemokine (TARC), was elevated, in accordance with previous data describing increased IL-13 (a Th2 cytokine) in the serum [13]. Furthermore, higher concentrations of both Th1 CXCR3 and Th2 CCR4 T cells were found in the serum of sarcoidosis patients as compared to controls, and the ratio of CXCR3 to CCR4 also was higher [12]. These findings could suggest that Th2 cytokines have a role in systemic compensation for the marked Th1 response in the lung or, alternatively, that cells mediating the Th1 response have migrated to sites of disease. In some patients, this Th1-type inflammation is replaced by a Th2 response that facilitates progression to fibrosis, because type 2 cytokines, such as IL 4 and IL-13, result in a fibroproliferative response with extracellular matrix deposition [14].

Lymphocytes

Accumulation in the lung

Recruitment of T cells to sites of inflammation involves a number of immune mechanisms, including antigen presentation to T cells by macrophages and dendritic cells and a complicated network of cytokines. Epithelial cells and the endothelium also participate in the process. The soluble adhesion molecule, vascular cell adhesion molecule 1, and beta1-integrins have been found to be elevated in lavage fluid, and serum levels of E-selectin and intercellular adhesion molecule 1 are higher in patients who have active sarcoidosis than in controls and those who have inactive disease [15]. Macrophages play an important role in the production of chemoattractants that recruit and focus lymphocytes into the tissues. These chemokines and cytokines include monocyte chemotactic protein 1 (MCP-1, CCL2), macrophage inflammatory protein-1α (MIPα, CCL3), macrophage inflammatory protein-1β (MIP1β, CCL4), regulated on activation, normal T-cell expressed and selected (RANTES, CCL5), IL-8, IL-12, and IL-15 [11,16]. IP-10 (CXCL10) interacts with the CXCR3 receptor on the T cell, which favors attraction and accumulation of the T cells [10]. Macrophages further produce IL-1, IL-15, and tumor necrosis factor-alpha (TNFα), which up-regulate adhesion molecules on the endothelium to increase interaction of the endothelial cells with T cells [17]. Airway epithelial cells produce IL-16, which seems to be involved in the migratory process [18]. CD13/aminopeptidase N, stimulated by IFNγ and found on alveolar macrophages, induces in vitro migration of

T lymphocytes [19]. T cells are recruited mainly from the periphery, but there is evidence that local proliferation occurs.

Proliferation

Once the initiating factor triggers a response, the T cells become activated through the classic MHC-antigen complex and cytokines. The initiating antigen probably is internalized by macrophages and dendritic cells and presented on the MHC site. This process allows the T cell to locate and bind to the MHC II complex, leading to clonal expansion [20,21]. Supporting this theory is that the cell-surface T-cell receptor is down-regulated in combination with increased T-cell receptor mRNA transcripts, indicating recent antigen-specific activation of the T cells in the lung [22]. T-cell markers of activation, including CD69, glycoprotein 240, and very late antigen (VLA)-1 also are expressed in T cells in the bronchoalveolar lavage fluid of certain populations [23–25]. These activated T-cell populations then expand and continue to propagate in sites of presumed continued antigenic stimulation.

After activation, the Th0 lymphocytes differentiate into Th1 lymphocytes, and a number of cytokines are produced, including IFNγ, IL-2, and IL-16, and TNFα [26–28]. IFNγ may be the most crucial, because granulomas do not develop in IFNγ knockout mice exposed to thermophilic bacteria [29]. Furthermore, a Th2 response with IL-4 and IL-5 production occurs in IFNγ-gene knockout mice exposed to mycobacteria and shistosoma [30]. Similar to IFNγ, the expression of IL-2 and its receptor has been correlated positively with T-cell alveolitis and may be a marker of extrapulmonary disease [31,32]. The production of these cytokines attracts and activates monocytes and macrophages, which in turn reciprocate lymphocyte activation.

Analysis of the T-cell receptors present in the Th1 infiltrative process suggests oligoclonal growth of the T cells, because there is decreased variability in the constant region segments and in the variable elements of lavaged cells. Certain variable regions of the alpha and beta chains of the T-cell receptor are overexpressed, particularly in the lung but also in the blood, suggesting selective usage of the T-cell receptor variable gene by the lymphocytes [33–35]. Supporting this evidence, clonal expansion of the Vβ8, Vβ5, and Vβ3 was found in T cells in the skin after injection of the Kveim reagent [36]. Clonality seems to be particularly marked in HLA-DRB1*0301+ and DRB3*0101+ patients who have expansions in the AV2S3+CD4+ T cells, and the number of AV2S3+/ CD4+ cells correlates with prognosis and clinical course [37–39]. Although clonality has been established, there also is evidence of background polyclonal T-cell expansion. This finding suggests that alveolitis in sarcoidosis is accompanied by local clonal expansion of T cells in the setting of a large, nonspecific lymphocytic response [33].

Costimulatory binding of the T cell to antigen-presenting cells also is important in the continued proliferative immune response. Normally, CD28 on the T cell binds with CD80 and CD86 on the antigen-presenting cell, leading to cytokine production. In sarcoidosis, however, CD28 expression is reduced, suggesting senescence of certain populations of T cells [25]. Also, CTLA-4–expressing T cells normally down-regulate the Th1 immune response by competing with CD28 for the CD80/86 ligand, and polymorphisms of the *CTLA-4* gene have been associated with disease severity [40]. Although the role of CD28 remains undefined, it is thought to be part of the complex interaction of antigen presentation and continued response [41].

To skew the regulatory mechanisms further toward a continued Th1 response, in patients who have active disease there is decreased expression of natural killer cell inhibitory receptors on CD8+ T cells, which may impair the ability to control the cell-mediated response [42]. CD1d-restricted natural killer T cells are reduced in the blood and lungs of patients who have sarcoidosis, perhaps reflecting a diminished regulatory mechanism because these cells protect against an exaggerated Th1 host response [43,44]. Further studies on the presence of natural killer T cells in the lymph nodes and skin have had varied results, however [45].

The role of apoptosis

Although most patients resolve granulomas spontaneously, a percentage proceed to fibrosis and irreversible injury despite immunosuppressive treatment. Several mechanisms for progression have been proposed, including disruption of the lymphocyte regulation and up-regulation of oncogenes.

Mechanisms related to disruption of the apoptotic mechanisms of the granulomas have been suggested as the cause of persistent granulomatous inflammation. TNFα, a regulator of apoptosis, and IFNγ have been implicated as major players in the persistent inflammatory response. In addition to the cytokine itself, the TNF receptor and ligand superfamilies have been found to be dysregulated in sarcoidosis and other fibrotic lung diseases and are thought to be involved in the disruption of apoptosis [46]. This supposition has not been firmly established, however.

Further dysregulation of the lymphocyte and cytokine response also may contribute to the absence of normal apoptosis. Passive apoptosis may be altered by the absence of cytokine deprivation that usually induces this phenomenon. Alveolar macrophage cytokines, such as IL-15, are enhanced and inhibit normal clearing of the lymphocytes. Also, up-regulation of nuclear factor-κβ in patients who have sarcoidosis probably has an inhibitory effect on apoptosis of activated lymphocytes and fibroblasts. Furthermore, IFNγ seems to suppress apoptosis of activated macrophages, mediated through the cyclin-dependent kinase inhibitor, p21^{wafl}, which has been found in high levels in granulomas [47]. In contrast, Th2 cytokines such as IL-4 and IL-10 that are known to induce macrophage apoptosis are lacking in the sarcoid immune response. In cutaneous lesions, IFNγ is thought to contribute to the persistent inflammation through the high expression of p21 [48].

Oncogenes have been assessed in the context of decreased apoptotic mechanisms in progressive sarcoidosis. Microarray technology has shown that the pattern of gene expression in patients who have sarcoidosis favors pro-survival genes [49]. In this context, Bcl-2 protein, one of the most important gene products involved in apoptosis, has been found to be overexpressed in alveolar lymphocytes and macrophages obtained in bronchoalveolar lavage fluid [50].

Fibrosis

The process by which the lung becomes fibrotic seems to be focused in the areas of granulomatous inflammation, but the exact immunologic mechanisms are unknown. Excessive chemokine production has been linked to progressive pulmonary fibrosis [51]. Also, a number of cytokines associated with the granulomas are thought to attract fibroblasts, and altered adhesion molecules on the fibroblasts may allow proliferation at the sites of inflammation. The exposure of these recruited fibroblasts to macrophage-produced cytokines such as insulin growth factor-1, transforming growth factor-beta, and platelet-derived growth factor results in collagen and fibronectin deposition [52,53]. A switch to Th2 cytokine predominance also may contribute to the production of cytokines such as IL-4 and IL-13, known to stimulate collagen production and fibrogenic processes. IFNγ, on the other hand, inhibits fibroblast proliferation [54].

T cells in bronchoalveolar lavage fluid

In sarcoidosis, the relative numbers of T cells in bronchoalveolar lavage fluid are more abundant as compared to T cells in the blood. An elevated CD4:CD8 ratio greater than 4:1 suggests the diagnosis with 96% specificity and 59% sensitivity [55]. It has been shown that an increased CD4:CD8 ratio is prognostically favorable in patients who have sarcoidosis [56]. The CD4:CD8 ratio and TNF levels in induced sputum seem to correlate with those in lavage fluid and to change in accordance with corticosteroid treatment [57]. The number of CD4+/HLA-DR lymphocytes also has been evaluated as a possible marker of disease activity. These cells are important, because they produce IL-2, which is partly responsible for propagation of the inflammatory response. The number of CD4+/HLA-DR lymphocytes is higher in patients who have active disease than in controls and has been inversely correlated with diffusing capacity [58]. Similarly, the AV2S3 T-cell receptor correlates with disease activity and response to treatment. Increased numbers of AV2S3 T cells are found in patients who have a shorter, more acute course of disease. These patients have a better prognosis, suggesting that these cells have a protective effect [38]. CD13/aminopeptidase N, a metalloproteinase on the surface of cells that is up-regulated by the Th1 response and may act to regulate T lymphocytes, also has been correlated with the CD4:CD8 ratio [19].

Overall, however, caution must be used with T-lymphocyte subsets in diagnosis, because the phenotypic profile can change depending on stage or in response to therapy. For diagnostic and prognostic purposes the CD4:CD8 ratio should be considered in the context of all clinical and pathologic findings.

Macrophages

Monocytes and macrophages are integral in the formation of granulomatous inflammation, and in lavage fluid the alveolar macrophage count, along with the lymphocyte count, is markedly elevated [59]. The primary roles of the macrophages are to act as antigen-presenting cells to the lymphocytes and to produce and secrete cytokines and chemokines that direct the inflammatory response. The activity probably is compartmentalized to areas of disease activity [60].

A number of macrophage-induced cytokines have been described and are important in granuloma formation. These cytokines function as chemoattractants and, as described earlier, in proliferation of inflammation. Early studies found that alveolar macrophages from bronchoalveolar lavage fluid of patients who have sarcoidosis release IL-1 and TNFα, contributing to the hypothesis that these cells are highly activated [61,62]. Alveolar macrophages spontaneously release TNFα, and the expression of TNFα mRNA is highest immediately after the fluid is removed from the lung [60]. The release of TNFα by alveolar macrophages is elevated in progressive or steroid-resistant disease, as compared with controls, and may indicate a more severe form of the disease [63]. In the serum, TNFα receptors I and II have been found to be higher in patients who have active disease and to correlate with the clinical course and radiographic findings [64,65]. TNF polymorphisms have been associated with disease severity, although it is unclear if this association is related to the actual expression of TNF [66]. Because of the importance of this cytokine in granuloma formation, agents affecting TNF such as infliximab, thalidomide, and pentoxifylline now are being studied as potential treatments.

Other macrophage cytokines involved include IL-15 and IL-12. IL-15 attracts and activates CD4+ T cells and acts as a lymphocyte growth factor [6]. IL-12 mRNA is increased in alveolar macrophages and is important in the up-regulation of IFNγ [8]. Overall, the macrophage cytokine production is largely responsible for granuloma formation and for promoting the Th1 proliferative response.

Inflammatory products of macrophages have been studied as serum markers of disease. Angiotensin-converting enzyme, produced by epithelioid cells, often is used to track disease progress if levels are elevated on diagnosis. Neopterin, a small protein released by macrophages, has been studied as a biomarker that correlates with disease severity [67].

Immune paradox

One of the notable unresolved findings in sarcoidosis is the apparent paradox of the peripheral state of anergy in the setting of an intense immune response in affected organs. This anergy has been noted by the lack of response to tuberculin and other antigens in patients who have sarcoidosis and correlates with disease activity and resolution. There also seems to be a relative lymphopenia in the peripheral blood as the activated T cells accumulate at the sites of granulomatous inflammation [68]. This lymphopenia has been suggested as a cause of the peripheral anergy, but the answer is unlikely to be simple. It also has been suggested that suppressive CD8+ T cells may be involved in the anergic response. An abundance of CD4+ T lymphocytes is seen during the acute or active phase, but as the disease becomes more chronic, CD8+ T cells become more dominant. More recently, it has been postulated that there may be disequilibrium between effector and regulatory T lymphocytes. A higher percentage of regulatory T cells, defined as CD4+/CD25 (bright) cells, was found in the blood and lavage fluid of patients who had active sarcoidosis than in controls [69]. Later data supported this finding by showing increased numbers of the T regulatory CD4+/CD25 (bright)/FoxP3+ lymphocytes at the periphery of granulomas, in bronchoalveolar lavage fluid, and in the peripheral blood of patients who had active sarcoidosis. These cells did not suppress TNFα activity fully, perhaps contributing to the overall balance of formation of granulomas, whereas the notable antiproliferative action could account for the peripheral anergy [4]. Although Grunewald and Eklund [45] reported decreased expression of the FOXP3+ marker in lavage fluid, this finding could indicate either fewer regulatory T cells or the presence of abnormal T cells that might allow the uncontrolled inflammation to occur. Although the mechanism is unclear, it is likely that the regulatory T cells do play a role.

Immunogenetics

The immunopathogenesis of sarcoidosis is undoubtedly complex, probably involving one or more antigenic stimuli in a genetically susceptible individual. Epidemiologic reports of familial and racial clustering support a possible genetic relationship [70]. Clinically, different genetic predispositions may affect the presentation and the severity of the clinical course. The predisposing gene loci could act on any number of steps in the immune process, and there may be multiple genetic susceptibilities. The human leukocyte antigens have been studied as candidate genes in the development of granulomatous inflammation because of their role in antigen presentation. For example, berylliosis, a disease almost indistinguishable from sarcoidosis, has been strongly linked to the HLA-DPB1 gene [71], suggesting that the MHC complex also may be related to other granulomatous diseases. Genes across the MHC region have been linked to sarcoidosis, although the complexity of interaction suggests that more than one gene is involved [72–75]. Further studies have focused on candidate genes thought to be related to the particular immune processes involved in granulomatous inflammation, including chemokine and cytokine polymorphisms and receptor polymorphisms such as the Toll-like receptor 4 and vitamin D receptor [76]. Gene-mapping studies to define the genomics further are under way [77]. Overall, it is likely that the etiology of sarcoidosis involves one or more of these candidate genes in the setting of an environmental interaction.

Etiology of sarcoidosis

A definitive cause of sarcoidosis has not been identified, although a number of observations suggest the presence of an unknown antigen. The immune response closely resembles that present in other granulomatous diseases caused by a known antigen, such as berylliosis and tuberculosis. Also, the immune process seems to be physiologic, and the identification of clonal populations of T cells is consistent with a normal antigenic immune response. Bacterial, viral, and environmental antigens have been suggested as the trigger, but there is no evidence to date that any one cause is associated directly with the development of sarcoidosis (Box 2). There may be multiple insults that can cause sarcoidosis in a genetically susceptible individual.

Although there is indirect evidence of an antigenic stimulus, the fundamental problem lies in the continued response of these cells once they accumulate in the tissues. It can be postulated that the continuing presence of antigen, in the form of an environmental agent or a bacterial protein, or the T-cell epitope mimicry of such an antigen could result in continued granuloma formation.

Box 2. Proposed causes of sarcoidosis

Infectious
Bacteria
    Mycobacterium tuberculosis
    Propionibacterium acnes
    Borrelia burgdorferi
    Mycoplasma
Viral
    Epstein-Barr virus
    Cytomegalovirus
    Herpes
    Hepatitis C

Environmental
Inhalants
    Aluminum
    Talc
    Zirconium
    Pollen
    Insecticides
    Mold or mildew
Occupations
    Raising birds
    Automobile manufacturing
    Teaching
    Cotton ginning
    Jobs involving radiation

Genetic
MHC genes
    BTNL2
    Human leukocyte antigens
Receptor genes
    Vitamin D receptor
    Chemokine receptor 2
    Chemokine receptor 5
    Complement receptor 1
    Toll-like receptor 4
Inflammatory genes
    Tumor necrosis factor
    Interferon α
    Transforming growth factor
    Interleukins-1 and 18
    Angiotensin-converting enzyme
    Clara cell 10-kD protein
    Heat shock proteins
    Inhibitor κB-α
    Vascular endothelial growth factor

_____

Multiple infectious, environmental [97], and genetic causes [98,99] have been studied in sarcoidosis. No single environmental antigen or genetic polymorphismhas yet been confirmed.

For example, Song and colleagues [78] identified poorly soluble antigens in tissues from patients who had sarcoidosis using mass spectrometry peptide fingerprinting and subsequent confirmation with protein immunoblotting. One of these candidate antigenic targets was derived from the mycobacterial catalase-peroxidase protein, a virulence protein that allows the tuberculous bacteria to survive inside macrophages. Supporting this premise, blood monocytes from patients who have sarcoidosis recognize mycobacterial epitopes, including catalase-peroxidase, with a Th1 response when exposed ex vivo to multiple mycobacterial antigens [79]. Although this explanation is a plausible mechanism in a set of patients, there may be a multitude of antigens that cause sarcoidosis.

The idea that sarcoidosis is caused by a persistent microbial or environmental antigen is supported by the apparent transmissibility of the antigenic response. The Kveim-Siltzbach antigen, used for diagnostic purposes, is a particulate suspension of granulomatous sarcoidal spleen tissue that induces formation of granulomas when injected intradermally in patients who have sarcoidosis. Similarly, a reaction has been noted with the autologous intradermal injection of bronchoalveolar lavage cells in patients who have sarcoidosis, with the apparent antigenic factor localized to the membrane fragments of macrophages [80]. In one sense, this finding is analogous to reports of transplant recipients developing sarcoidosis after receiving a graft from a patient who had sarcoidosis [81,82].

The persistent immune response brings up the question of whether there is an overall exaggerated response or rather a deficiency in regulatory cells resulting in an unregulated Th1 immune response. Supporting the need for an active immune system response are multiple reports of patients who have HIV who develop sarcoidosis after initiation of highly active antiretroviral therapy [83]. Patients who had a remote history of sarcoidosis and who contracted HIV infection later in life developed recurrent, progressive sarcoidosis after immune reconstitution [84]. This development suggests the necessity of functioning T-cell immunity. Given a delay in sarcoidosis onset of at least 3 to 6 months in most cases, the process is believed to be mediated by naive CD4+/IL-2r+ cells, rather than by memory T cells, which tend to appear earlier in the reconstitution [85]. Similarly, the development of sarcoidosis also has been seen in patients who are undergoing interferon therapy for hepatitis C [86], supporting the argument that a heightened Th1 immune response, potentially to a viral antigen, perpetuates sarcoidosis. The nonselective polyclonal hypergammaglobulinemia and high antibody titers in patients who have sarcoidosis also may suggest a heightened immune response before or during the onset of disease. On the other hand, patients who have a large initial immune response, as seen in Löfgren's syndrome, have better prognosis, whereas those who present with a less robust response tend to have chronic and progressive disease, a finding that argues for the role of an immunodeficiency. The deficient number of natural killer T cells and the impaired ability of these cells to produce IFNγ might play a role in the inability to clear an antigen [44].

The role of vitamin D

The link between vitamin D and the regulation of Th1 immunity in relationship to sarcoidosis is an area of intriguing study. The vitamin D receptor has been identified on multiple immune cells, including activated T lymphocytes, antigen-presenting cells, monocytes, and dendritic cells, suggesting an immunoregulatory effect. In particular, vitamin D has been shown to inhibit Th1 lymphocyte proliferation and cytokine production [87–89]. The hormone also has been shown to be a potent suppressor of IFNγ-mediated macrophage activation [90] and decreases the MHC class II antigen-presenting activity of macrophages [91]. Vitamin D inhibits monocyte differentiation as well as the differentiation of dendritic cells into antigen-presenting cells [92]. Also, vitamin D has been shown to be involved in enhancing antimicrobial peptide signaling for bacterial clearance, particularly of mycobacteria [93].

Epidemiologic evidence complements these data, suggesting that lack of vitamin D before onset of the disease could play a role in the unregulated Th1 response of sarcoidosis. The prevalence of sarcoidosis peaks in early spring, particularly in cases of erythema nodosum and Löfgren's syndrome, when vitamin D deficiency is most prevalent. Sarcoidosis is rare at the equator and increases in frequency in northern latitudes, and people who move to northern latitudes acquire that risk within 10 years [94,95]. African Americans, who are at highest risk for sarcoidosis, also are known to have an elevated risk for vitamin D deficiency because of a reduced ability to convert the hormone in the skin. Furthermore, deficiency predisposes patients to tuberculosis, a similar granulomatous reaction, and, conversely, sunshine has been used to treat patients who have tuberculosis. Last, vitamin D receptor polymorphisms have been associated with susceptibility to sarcoidosis [96].

Drawing from the epidemiologic and the laboratory findings, two links between sarcoid susceptibility and vitamin D are possible. First, deficiency could lead to impaired regulation of the Th1 immune response allowing a persistent immune response. Alternatively, low vitamin D levels could lead to delayed antigen clearance because of impaired host defense and innate immunity during the winter months, which then is overamplified with the increase in vitamin D levels and return of the Th1 response in the spring.

Summary

Sarcoidosis continues to be a disease of research interest because of its complicated immune mechanisms and elusive etiology. So far, it has been established that granulomatous inflammation in sarcoidosis is predominately a Th1 immune response mediated by a complex network of lymphocytes, macrophages, and cytokines. The reasons for progression to a chronic and potentially fibrotic form are unclear but may involve loss of apoptotic mechanisms, loss of regulatory response, or a persistent antigen that cannot be cleared. Recent genomic and proteomic technology has emphasized the importance of host susceptibility and gene–environment interaction in the expression of the disease.

References

[1] Muller-Quernheim J, Saltini C, Sondermeyer P, et al. Compartmentalized activation of the interleukin 2 gene by lung T lymphocytes in active pulmonary sarcoidosis. J Immunol 1986;137(11):3475–83.

[2] Hunninghake GW, Crystal RG. Pulmonary sarcoidosis: a disorder mediated by excess helper T-lymphocyte activity at sites of disease activity. N Engl J Med 1981;305(8):429–34.

[3] Hunninghake G, Gadek J, Weinberger S, et al. Comparison of the alveolitis of sarcoidosis and idiopathic pulmonary fibrosis. Chest 1979;75(2 Suppl):266–7.

[4] Miyara M, Amoura Z, Parizot C, et al. The immune paradox of sarcoidosis and regulatory T cells. J Exp Med 2006;203(2):359–70.

[5] Fireman E, Haimsky E, Noiderfer M, et al. Misdiagnosis of sarcoidosis in patients with chronic

beryllium disease. Sarcoidosis Vasc Diffuse Lung Dis 2003;20(2):144–8.

[6] Agostini C, Trentin L, Facco M, et al. Role of IL-15, IL-2, and their receptors in the development of T cell alveolitis in pulmonary sarcoidosis. J Immunol 1996; 157(2):910–8.

[7] Shigehara K, Shijubo N, Ohmichi M, et al. IL-12 and IL-18 are increased and stimulate IFN-gamma production in sarcoid lungs. J Immunol 2001; 166(1):642–9.

[8] Moller DR, Forman JD, Liu MC, et al. Enhanced expression of IL-12 associated with Th1 cytokine profiles in active pulmonary sarcoidosis. J Immunol 1996;156(12):4952–60.

[9] Katchar K, Eklund A, Grunewald J. Expression of Th1 markers by lung accumulated T cells in pulmonary sarcoidosis. J Intern Med 2003;254(6):564–71.

[10] Agostini C, Cassatella M, Zambello R, et al. Involvement of the IP-10 chemokine in sarcoid granulomatous reactions. J Immunol 1998;161(11): 6413–20.

[11] Agostini C, Facco M, Chilosi M, et al. Alveolar macrophage-T cell interactions during Th1-type sarcoid inflammation. Microsc Res Tech 2001;53(4):278–87.

[12] Nureki SI, Miyazaki E, Ando M, et al. Circulating levels of both Th1 and Th2 chemokines are elevated in patients with sarcoidosis. Respir Med 2007 Oct 17.

[13] Hauber HP, Gholami D, Meyer A, et al. Increased interleukin-13 expression in patients with sarcoidosis. Thorax 2003;58(6):519–24.

[14] Lukacs NW, Hogaboam C, Chensue SW, et al. Type 1/type 2 cytokine paradigm and the progression of pulmonary fibrosis. Chest 2001;120(1 Suppl):5S–8S.

[15] Berlin M, Lundahl J, Skold CM, et al. The lymphocytic alveolitis in sarcoidosis is associated with increased amounts of soluble and cell-bound adhesion molecules in bronchoalveolar lavage fluid and serum. J Intern Med 1998;244(4):333–40.

[16] Nureki SI, Miyazaki E, Ando M, et al. Circulating levels of both Th1 and Th2 chemokines are evaluated in patients with sarcoidosis. Respir Med 2008; 102(2):239–47.

[17] Agostini C, Semenzato G. Cytokines in sarcoidosis. Semin Respir Infect 1998;13(3):184–96.

[18] Center DM, Kornfeld H, Cruikshank WW. Interleukin 16 and its function as a CD4 ligand. Immunol Today 1996;17(10):476–81.

[19] Tani K, Ogushi F, Huang L, et al. CD13/aminopeptidase N, a novel chemoattractant for T lymphocytes in pulmonary sarcoidosis. Am J Respir Crit Care Med 2000;161(5):1636–42.

[20] Moller DR. T-cell receptor genes in sarcoidosis. Sarcoidosis Vasc Diffuse Lung Dis 1998;15(2):158–64.

[21] Moller DR. Involvement of T cells and alterations in T cell receptors in sarcoidosis. Semin Respir Infect 1998;13(3):174–83.

[22] Du Bois RM, Kirby M, Balbi B, et al. T-lymphocytes that accumulate in the lung in sarcoidosis have evidence of recent stimulation of the T-cell antigen receptor. Am Rev Respir Dis 1992;145(5): 1205–11.

[23] Saltini C, Hemler ME, Crystal RG. T lymphocytes compartmentalized on the epithelial surface of the lower respiratory tract express the very late activation antigen complex VLA-1. Clin Immunol Immunopathol 1988;46(2):221–33.

[24] Hol BE, Hintzen RQ, Van Lier RA, et al. Soluble and cellular markers of T cell activation in patients with pulmonary sarcoidosis. Am Rev Respir Dis 1993;148(3):643–9.

[25] Wahlstrom J, Berlin M, Skold CM, et al. Phenotypic analysis of lymphocytes and monocytes/macrophages in peripheral blood and bronchoalveolar lavage fluid from patients with pulmonary sarcoidosis. Thorax 1999;54(4):339–46.

[26] Prasse A, Georges CG, Biller H, et al. Th1 cytokine pattern in sarcoidosis is expressed by bronchoalveolar CD4+ and CD8+ T cells. Clin Exp Immunol 2000;122(2):241–8.

[27] Pinkston P, Bitterman PB, Crystal RG. Spontaneous release of interleukin-2 by lung T lymphocytes in active pulmonary sarcoidosis. N Engl J Med 1983;308(14):793–800.

[28] Robinson BW, McLemore TL, Crystal RG. Gamma interferon is spontaneously released by alveolar macrophages and lung T lymphocytes in patients with pulmonary sarcoidosis. J Clin Invest 1985; 75(5):1488–95.

[29] Gudmundsson G, Hunninghake GW. Interferon-gamma is necessary for the expression of hypersensitivity pneumonitis. J Clin Invest 1997;99(10):2386–90.

[30] Chensue SW, Warmington K, Ruth JH, et al. Mycobacterial and schistosomal antigen-elicited granuloma formation in IFN-gamma and IL-4 knockout mice: analysis of local and regional cytokine and chemokine networks. J Immunol 1997;159(7): 3565–73.

[31] Grutters JC, Fellrath JM, Mulder L, et al. Serum soluble interleukin-2 receptor measurement in patients with sarcoidosis: a clinical evaluation. Chest 2003;124(1):186–95.

[32] Muller-Quernheim J, Pfeifer S, Kienast K, et al. Spontaneous interleukin 2 release of bronchoalveolar lavage cells in sarcoidosis is a codeterminant of prognosis. Lung 1996;174(4):243–53.

[33] Bellocq A, Lecossier D, Pierre-Audigier C, et al. T cell receptor repertoire of T lymphocytes recovered from the lung and blood of patients with sarcoidosis. Am J Respir Crit Care Med 1994; 149(3 Pt 1):646–54.

[34] Grunewald J, Janson CH, Eklund A, et al. Restricted V alpha 2.3 gene usage by CD4+ T lymphocytes in bronchoalveolar lavage fluid from sarcoidosis patients correlates with HLA-DR3. Eur J Immunol 1992;22(1):129–35.

[35] Forrester JM, Wang Y, Ricalton N, et al. TCR expression of activated T cell clones in the lungs of

patients with pulmonary sarcoidosis. J Immunol 1994;153(9):4291–302.

[36] Klein JT, Horn TD, Forman JD, et al. Selection of oligoclonal V beta-specific T cells in the intradermal response to Kveim-Siltzbach reagent in individuals with sarcoidosis. J Immunol 1995;154(3):1450–60.

[37] Grunewald J, Hultman T, Bucht A, et al. Restricted usage of T cell receptor V alpha/J alpha gene segments with different nucleotide but identical amino acid sequences in HLA-DR3+ sarcoidosis patients. Mol Med 1995;1(3):287–96.

[38] Grunewald J, Berlin M, Olerup O, et al. Lung T-helper cells expressing T-cell receptor AV2S3 associate with clinical features of pulmonary sarcoidosis. Am J Respir Crit Care Med 2000;161(3 Pt 1):814–8.

[39] Katchar K, Wahlstrom J, Eklund A, et al. Highly activated T-cell receptor AV2S3(+) CD4(+) lung T-cell expansions in pulmonary sarcoidosis. Am J Respir Crit Care Med 2001;163(7):1540–5.

[40] Hattori N, Niimi T, Sato S, et al. Cytotoxic T-lymphocyte antigen 4 gene polymorphisms in sarcoidosis patients. Sarcoidosis Vasc Diffuse Lung Dis 2005;22(1):27–32.

[41] Roberts SD, Kohli LL, Wood KL, et al. CD4+CD28-T cells are expanded in sarcoidosis. Sarcoidosis Vasc Diffuse Lung Dis 2005;22(1):13–9.

[42] Mizuki M, Eklund A, Grunewald J. Altered expression of natural killer cell inhibitory receptors (KIRs) on T cells in bronchoalveolar lavage fluid and peripheral blood of sarcoidosis patients. Sarcoidosis Vasc Diffuse Lung Dis 2000;17(1):54–9.

[43] Ho LP, Urban BC, Thickett DR, et al. Deficiency of a subset of T-cells with immunoregulatory properties in sarcoidosis. Lancet 2005;365(9464):1062–72.

[44] Kobayashi S, Kaneko Y, Seino K, et al. Impaired IFN-gamma production of Valpha24 NKT cells in non-remitting sarcoidosis. Int Immunol 2004;16(2):215–22.

[45] Grunewald J, Eklund A. Role of CD4+ T cells in sarcoidosis. Proc Am Thorac Soc 2007;4(5):461–4.

[46] Kunitake R, Kuwano K, Miyazaki H, et al. Apoptosis in the course of granulomatous inflammation in pulmonary sarcoidosis. Eur Respir J 1999;13(6):1329–37.

[47] Xaus J, Cardo M, Valledor AF, et al. Interferon gamma induces the expression of p21waf-1 and arrests macrophage cell cycle, preventing induction of apoptosis. Immunity 1999;11(1):103–13.

[48] Xaus J, Besalduch N, Comalada M, et al. High expression of p21 Waf1 in sarcoid granulomas: a putative role for long-lasting inflammation. J Leukoc Biol 2003;74(2):295–301.

[49] Rutherford RM, Kehren J, Staedtler F, et al. Functional genomics in sarcoidosis–reduced or increased apoptosis? Swiss Med Wkly 2001;131(31–32):459–70.

[50] Mermigkis C, Polychronopoulos V, Mermigkis D, et al. Overexpression of bcl-2 protein in bronchoalveolar lavage lymphocytes and macrophages in sarcoidosis. Respiration 2006;73(2):221–6.

[51] Ziegenhagen MW, Schrum S, Zissel G, et al. Increased expression of proinflammatory chemokines in bronchoalveolar lavage cells of patients with progressing idiopathic pulmonary fibrosis and sarcoidosis. J Investig Med 1998;46(5):223–31.

[52] Salez F, Gosset P, Copin MC, et al. Transforming growth factor-beta1 in sarcoidosis. Eur Respir J 1998;12(4):913–9.

[53] Homma S, Nagaoka I, Abe H, et al. Localization of platelet-derived growth factor and insulin-like growth factor I in the fibrotic lung. Am J Respir Crit Care Med 1995;152(6 Pt 1):2084–9.

[54] Kunkel SL, Lukacs NW, Strieter RM, et al. Th1 and Th2 responses regulate experimental lung granuloma development. Sarcoidosis Vasc Diffuse Lung Dis 1996;13(2):120–8.

[55] Winterbauer RH, Lammert J, Selland M, et al. Bronchoalveolar lavage cell populations in the diagnosis of sarcoidosis. Chest 1993;104(2):352–61.

[56] Planck A, Eklund A, Grunewald J. Inflammatory BAL-fluid and serum parameters in HLA DR17 positive vs. DR17 negative patients with pulmonary sarcoidosis. Sarcoidosis Vasc Diffuse Lung Dis 2001;18(1):64–9.

[57] Moodley YP, Dorasamy T, Venketasamy S, et al. Correlation of CD4:CD8 ratio and tumour necrosis factor (TNF)alpha levels in induced sputum with bronchoalveolar lavage fluid in pulmonary sarcoidosis. Thorax 2000;55(8):696–9.

[58] Xaubet A, Agusti C, Roca J, et al. BAL lymphocyte activation antigens and diffusing capacity are related in mild to moderate pulmonary sarcoidosis. Eur Respir J 1993;6(5):715–8.

[59] Pforte A, Gerth C, Voss A, et al. Proliferating alveolar macrophages in BAL and lung function changes in interstitial lung disease. Eur Respir J 1993;6(7):951–5.

[60] Muller-Quernheim J, Pfeifer S, Mannel D, et al. Lung-restricted activation of the alveolar macrophage/monocyte system in pulmonary sarcoidosis. Am Rev Respir Dis 1992;145(1):187–92.

[61] Hunninghake GW. Release of interleukin-1 by alveolar macrophages of patients with active pulmonary sarcoidosis. Am Rev Respir Dis 1984;129(4):569–72.

[62] Fehrenbach H, Zissel G, Goldmann T, et al. Alveolar macrophages are the main source for tumour necrosis factor-alpha in patients with sarcoidosis. Eur Respir J 2003;21(3):421–8.

[63] Ziegenhagen MW, Rothe ME, Zissel G, et al. Exaggerated TNFalpha release of alveolar macrophages in corticosteroid resistant sarcoidosis. Sarcoidosis Vasc Diffuse Lung Dis 2002;19(3):185–90.

[64] Nakayama T, Hashimoto S, Amemiya E, et al. Elevation of plasma-soluble tumour necrosis factor receptors (TNF-R) in sarcoidosis. Clin Exp Immunol 1996;104(2):318–24.

[65] Ziegenhagen MW, Fitschen J, Martinet N, et al. Serum level of soluble tumour necrosis factor receptor II (75 kDa) indicates inflammatory activity of sarcoidosis. J Intern Med 2000;248(1):33–41.

[66] Pandey JP, Frederick M. TNF-alpha, IL1-beta, and immunoglobulin (GM and KM) gene polymorphisms in sarcoidosis. Hum Immunol 2002;63(6):485–91.

[67] Ziegenhagen MW, Rothe ME, Schlaak M, et al. Bronchoalveolar and serological parameters reflecting the severity of sarcoidosis. Eur Respir J 2003; 21(3):407–13.

[68] Hunninghake GW, Fulmer JD, Young RC Jr, et al. Localization of the immune response in sarcoidosis. Am Rev Respir Dis 1979;120(1):49–57.

[69] Planck A, Katchar K, Eklund A, et al. T-lymphocyte activity in HLA-DR17 positive patients with active and clinically recovered sarcoidosis. Sarcoidosis Vasc Diffuse Lung Dis 2003;20(2):110–7.

[70] Rybicki BA, Iannuzzi MC, Frederick MM, et al. Familial aggregation of sarcoidosis. A case-control etiologic study of sarcoidosis (ACCESS). Am J Respir Crit Care Med 2001;164(11):2085–91.

[71] Richeldi L, Sorrentino R, Saltini C. HLA-DPB1 glutamate 69: a genetic marker of beryllium disease. Science 1993;262(5131):242–4.

[72] Schurmann M, Lympany PA, Reichel P, et al. Familial sarcoidosis is linked to the major histocompatibility complex region. Am J Respir Crit Care Med 2000;162(3 Pt 1):861–4.

[73] Iannuzzi MC, Maliarik MJ, Poisson LM, et al. Sarcoidosis susceptibility and resistance HLA-DQB1 alleles in African Americans. Am J Respir Crit Care Med 2003;167(9):1225–31.

[74] Rybicki BA, Maliarik MJ, Poisson LM, et al. The major histocompatibility complex gene region and sarcoidosis susceptibility in African Americans. Am J Respir Crit Care Med 2003;167(3):444–9.

[75] Ishihara M, Ohno S, Ishida T, et al. Molecular genetic studies of HLA class II alleles in sarcoidosis. Tissue Antigens 1994;43(4):238–41.

[76] Iannuzzi MC. Advances in the genetics of sarcoidosis. Proc Am Thorac Soc 2007;4(5):457–60.

[77] Iannuzzi MC, Rybicki BA. Genetics of sarcoidosis: candidate genes and genome scans. Proc Am Thorac Soc 2007;4(1):108–16.

[78] Song Z, Marzilli L, Greenlee BM, et al. Mycobacterial catalase-peroxidase is a tissue antigen and target of the adaptive immune response in systemic sarcoidosis. J Exp Med 2005;201(5):755–67.

[79] Carlisle J, Evans W, Hajizadeh R, et al. Multiple Mycobacterium antigens induce interferon-gamma production from sarcoidosis peripheral blood mononuclear cells. Clin Exp Immunol 2007;150(3): 460–8.

[80] Holter JF, Park HK, Sjoerdsma KW, et al. Nonviable autologous bronchoalveolar lavage cell preparations induce intradermal epithelioid cell granulomas in sarcoidosis patients. Am Rev Respir Dis 1992; 145(4 Pt 1):864–71.

[81] Heyll A, Meckenstock G, Aul C, et al. Possible transmission of sarcoidosis via allogeneic bone marrow transplantation. Bone Marrow Transplant 1994;14(1):161–4.

[82] Padilla ML, Schilero GJ, Teirstein AS. Donor-acquired sarcoidosis. Sarcoidosis Vasc Diffuse Lung Dis 2002;19(1):18–24.

[83] Foulon G, Wislez M, Naccache JM, et al. Sarcoidosis in HIV-infected patients in the era of highly active antiretroviral therapy. Clin Infect Dis 2004;38(3):418–25.

[84] Lenner R, Bregman Z, Teirstein AS, et al. Recurrent pulmonary sarcoidosis in HIV-infected patients receiving highly active antiretroviral therapy. Chest 2001;119(3):978–81.

[85] Trevenzoli M, Cattelan AM, Marino F, et al. Sarcoidosis and HIV infection: a case report and a review of the literature. Postgrad Med J 2003;79(935):535–8.

[86] Tahan V, Ozseker F, Guneylioglu D, et al. Sarcoidosis after use of interferon for chronic hepatitis C: report of a case and review of the literature. Dig Dis Sci 2003;48(1):169–73.

[87] Mattner F, Smiroldo S, Galbiati F, et al. Inhibition of Th1 development and treatment of chronic-relapsing experimental allergic encephalomyelitis by a non-hypercalcemic analogue of 1,25-dihydroxyvitamin D(3). Eur J Immunol 2000;30(2):498–508.

[88] Boonstra A, Barrat FJ, Crain C, et al. 1alpha,25-dihydroxyvitamin d3 has a direct effect on naive CD4(+) T cells to enhance the development of Th2 cells. J Immunol 2001;167(9):4974–80.

[89] Imazeki I, Matsuzaki J, Tsuji K, et al. Immunomodulating effect of vitamin D3 derivatives on type-1 cellular immunity. Biomed Res 2006;27(1):1–9.

[90] Helming L, Bose J, Ehrchen J, et al. 1alpha,25-dihydroxyvitamin D3 is a potent suppressor of interferon gamma-mediated macrophage activation. Blood 2005;106(13):4351–8.

[91] Lemire JM. Immunomodulatory role of 1,25-dihydroxyvitamin D3. J Cell Biochem 1992;49(1):26–31.

[92] Piemonti L, Monti P, Sironi M, et al. Vitamin D3 affects differentiation, maturation, and function of human monocyte-derived dendritic cells. J Immunol 2000;164(9):4443–51.

[93] Liu PT, Stenger S, Li H, et al. Toll-like receptor triggering of a vitamin D-mediated human antimicrobial response. Science 2006;311(5768):1770–3.

[94] Martin WJ 2nd, Iannuzzi MC, Gail DB, et al. Future directions in sarcoidosis research: summary of an NHLBI working group. Am J Respir Crit Care Med 2004;170(5):567–71.

[95] Kitaichi M. Prevalence of sarcoidosis around the world. Sarcoidosis Vasc Diffuse Lung Dis 1998;15(1):16–8.

[96] Niimi T, Tomita H, Sato S, et al. Vitamin D receptor gene polymorphism in patients with sarcoidosis. Am J Respir Crit Care Med 1999;160(4):1107–9.

[97] Newman LS, Rose CS, Bresnitz EA, et al. A case control etiologic study of sarcoidosis: environmental and occupational risk factors. Am J Respir Crit Care Med 2004;170(12):1324–30.

[98] Iannuzzi MC. Genetics of sarcoidosis. Semin Respir Crit Care Med 2007;28(1):15–21.

[99] Spagnolo P, du Bois RM. Genetics of sarcoidosis. Clin Dermatol 2007;25(3):242–9.

**ELSEVIER
SAUNDERS**

Clin Chest Med 29 (2008) 391–414

**CLINICS
IN CHEST
MEDICINE**

Genetics of Sarcoidosis

Joachim Müller-Quernheim, MD[a,*], Manfred Schürmann, MD[b],
Sylvia Hofmann, PhD[c], Karoline I. Gaede, PhD[d],
Annegret Fischer, MSc[c], Antje Prasse, MD[a],
Gernot Zissel, PhD[a], Stefan Schreiber, MD[c,e]

[a]*Department of Pneumology, University Medical Center, Killianstraße 5, D 79106 Freiburg, Germany*
[b]*Institute of Human Genetics, Medical University of Schleswig-Holstein, University of Lübeck,
Ratzeburger Allee 160, D 23538 Lübeck, Germany*
[c]*Institute of Clinical Molecular Biology, Christian-Albrechts-University, Schittenhelmstrasse 12,
D 24105 Kiel, Germany*
[d]*Department of Clinical Medicine, Research Center Borstel, Parkallee 35, D 23845 Borstel, Germany*
[e]*Department of General Internal Medicine, Christian-Albrechts-University, Schittenhelmstrasse 12, Kiel, Germany*

Sarcoidosis is a systemic granulomatous disease of unknown etiology in which environmental exposures are believed to interact with genetic factors in determining the pattern of sarcoidosis presentation, progression, and prognosis [1–3]. Based on numerous immunologic studies the current understanding of its pathogenesis is that several sequential immunologic events eventually resulting in granuloma formation are involved:

1. Exposure to one or more still elusive antigen(s)
2. Acquiring T cell immunity against the putative antigen(s) mediated by antigen processing and presentation by macrophages
3. Generation of specific T effector cells
4. Activation of macrophages
5. Induction of granuloma formation [4]

These events, however, depend on a predisposing genetic background.

The assumption of a genetic contribution to the etiology of sarcoidosis is based mainly on two observations: prevalence and incidence rates of sarcoidosis are different between ethnic groups and races, and the disease tends to cluster in families. The frequency of sarcoidosis varies widely between ethnicities and populations from different geographic regions around the world [5,6]. The lifetime risk of sarcoidosis was calculated to be 2.4% for African Americans and 0.85% for Caucasians in the United States [7]. A study of a Swedish urban population reported a lifetime risk of 1.0% and 1.3% for men and women, respectively [6]. Incidence rates of 1.5 cases per 100,000 population for Caucasians, 16.8 cases per 100,000 population for Asians and 19.8 cases per 100,000 for people of African extraction have been reported from London [8]. In addition to differences in the incidence, the average clinical picture of sarcoidosis shows characteristic variability between ethnic groups. The acute form of sarcoidosis with a favorable prognosis is more common in Caucasian populations, while chronic disease and extrapulmonary manifestations are more frequent in African Americans and patients of Caribbean origin [9,10].

In general, the quality of genetic studies depends on precise definitions of the phenotypes of their cohorts. Although detailed concepts of the immunopathogenesis of sarcoidosis do exist, it is often difficult to allocate a given patient to a distinct phenotype using clinical or immunologic

This work was supported by a Grant No. 01GS0426 of the National Genome Research Network Germany and Grant No. Mu 692/7-1 of the Deutsche Forschungsgemeinschaft, Bonn, Germany.

* Corresponding author.

E-mail address: jmq@medizin.ukl.uni-freiburg.de (J. Müller-Quernheim).

criteria, because there is a broad variability of phenotypes beyond acute and chronic disease. In addition, phenotyping of patients requires long-term follow-up, because a considerable percentage of patients presenting initially with acute disease and good prognosis might develop chronic sarcoidosis with severe organ damage later on [11,12]. Moreover, the fact that environmental [13] and occupational phenocopies of sarcoidosis exist complicates its genetic analysis. Chronic beryllium disease (CBD), an occupational disorder seen in up to 16% of beryllium-exposed workers [14], is a complete phenocopy of sarcoidosis [15] but is associated with a distinct susceptibility locus in the major histocompatibility complex (MHC) II gene region (ie, glutamine-69 positive HLA [human leukocyte antigen]-DPB1 alleles) [16]. Other anorganic and organic compounds such as zirconium, aluminum [17], cristobalite [18] or even bioaerosols [13] might cause the manifestation of granulomatous disorders presenting as phenocopies of sarcoidosis [19]. These considerations support the notion that non-necrotizing granuloma, the hallmark of sarcoidosis, represent a final overlapping, immunologic pathway induced by different agents. Thus, sarcoidosis needs to be addressed as a group of related disorders rather than a clear-cut entity, which makes genetic analysis even more complex.

Thus, at present one is left with the problems that two pivotal components of sarcoid pathogenesis (ie, genetic susceptibility and etiologic agent) are elusive and that phenotyping of patients is not as reliable as desired for genetic studies. In this context one must consider the recent accumulation of genetic knowledge on sarcoidosis and put it in perspective with findings of other granulomatous disorders. Numerous candidate genes have been delineated from the pathogenesis of sarcoidosis or from other granulomatous diseases and scrutinized. A comprehensive discussion of all candidate genes studied is beyond the scope of this article and a selection based on pathophysiological considerations in regard of chronic inflammatory processes had to be made. More complete discussions of sarcoidosis candidate genes have been published very recently [20,21].

Familial sarcoidosis and linkage studies

The contribution of an inherited predisposition to the etiology of sarcoidosis is documented by an increased risk of sarcoidosis in close relatives of patients. Based on information from a nationwide chest radiograph screening program performed in the 1960s in Germany, Jörgensen identified among 2471 patients' 40 families with two or more close relatives suffering from sarcoidosis [22]. He calculated a recurrence risk of 0.9% in siblings and 0.5% in parents of patients. Kirsten and Wirnsberger questioned the members of large national patients' organizations in Germany and the Netherlands [23,24]. They found that 49 of 651 (7.5%) responders of the German study and 170 of 1026 (16.6%) responders of the Dutch study had close relatives who had sarcoidosis. McGrath and colleagues [25] asked 406 patients with sarcoidosis attending the Royal Brompton Hospital, London, and found 24 (5.9%) who had a family history of sarcoidosis. The same group compiled and reviewed published information concerning familial aggregation of sarcoidosis and found that the percentage of patients who had a positive family history ranged from 2.7% in Spain to 17% in African Americans [26–28]. A Case-Control Etiologic Study in Sarcoidosis (ACCESS) including 706 index cases plus 706 matched controls and information on more than 10,000 first-degree (parents, full siblings, and children) and 17,000 second-degree relatives (avuncular and grandparents) revealed a familial relative risk of 4.7, which was higher in Caucasians in the United States than in African Americans [29].

In all of these surveys, most of the families with repeated occurrence of sarcoidosis include two patients, and affected parent and offspring pairs are roughly as common as affected sibling pairs. This constellation is indicative of multiple small-or-moderate genetic effects, as known from more common complex inflammatory diseases like Crohn's disease (CD) or rheumatoid arthritis. More extended multicase pedigrees that can help to pinpoint a single causative gene effect are rare in sarcoidosis. A pedigree with five siblings suffering from cutaneous sarcoid affections has been communicated in an early report from Hungary [30]. Jörgensen found one family with eight affected members among 2471 patients [22]. The most impressive multicase pedigree of a complex family with 18 patients, who lived in a remote area of Northern Sweden close to the polar circle, was published by Wiman [31]. The distribution of sarcoidosis cases in these families resembles autosomal dominant inheritance of a single gene mutation. Unfortunately, these families are lost from follow-up, and today the local prevalence of sarcoidosis is with four cases in a community of 4000 inhabitants in the upper normal range of Sweden, which is one of the highest in the world. Interestingly, two of the four patients are brothers (Manfred Schürman, unpublished data, 1999).

Based on available information, it is adequate to communicate a sarcoidosis recurrence risk of approximately 1 in 100 for siblings and offspring of patients of European extraction. In the context of genetic family counseling, this generally is perceived as a small risk by the clients and should lead to enhanced awareness but does not justify specific medical investigations in the absence of complaints. On the other hand, the approximately 20-fold increased recurrence risk in close relatives has stimulated numerous attempts to identify the genetic cause of this phenomenon.

Two principal strategies to detect predisposing gene variations have been employed: genetic linkage analyses and case–control association studies. Genetic linkage analysis is based on the degree of cosegregation of the disease and neutral DNA variations (highly informative microsatellite markers or ubiquitous single nucleotide polymorphisms) of known chromosomal position in the pedigree of multiplex families. In the affected sibling pair analysis, the most basic form of linkage analysis, this cosegregation is documented by the quantification of marker alleles that are identical by descent in the two affected siblings. Association analysis is a population-based approach that follows the "common variant, common disease" hypothesis, which means that in a general population, the frequency of a disease relevant mutation is expected to be different between affected subjects and healthy controls. The potential of both linkage and association analysis increases with a growing sample and the selection of adequate markers.

Both study designs have specific advantages and limitations; the major advantage of linkage analysis is that the linkage score increases gradually with decreasing distance between markers and a predisposing gene locus. The position of a major susceptibility gene can be detected with flanking markers that are located far outside the gene of interest. Therefore, one can achieve striking results with a relatively small number of markers selected for optimal informativity. Analyzing a complex disease like sarcoidosis with a family-based approach, however, might point to variants that confer susceptibility only in this special subset of families, and even a high-resolution linkage map is not sufficient to identify a predisposing gene variation directly.

By contrast, an association study resembles a borehole. It is a necessary prerequisite to know a promising candidate gene to probe, but even than the target can be missed, even on a short distance. Linkage analyses and association studies are complementary strategies. Usually a relatively large region of interest defined by linkage analysis is tested for association in a case–control comparison, subsequently narrowing down the disease susceptibility to one or a few causative variants. The recent development of extremely high-density genotyping chips allows genome-wide association studies based on hundreds of thousands of single nucleotide polymorphisms in several thousand of cases and controls. This offers the possibility to create an extensive genetic map and to identify previously unsuspected predisposing genes without the need to gather and genotype extended series of multiplex families. The example of CD, with comparable epidemiology and complexity as sarcoidosis, shows that at this level of resolution, major linkage peaks and association signals largely coincide [32].

Genetic linkage analysis is straightforward in monogenic diseases with Mendelian inheritance if only extended families are available. This has been the case in Blau syndrome, a monogenic autosomal dominant disease addressed as familial granulomatosis and characterized by arthritis, skin rush, iritis that will be discussed because of its similarity with sarcoidosis. The gene locus of Blau syndrome has been mapped to the centromeric region of chromosome 16 by linkage analysis of a single three-generation family [33]. A major susceptibility gene locus in CD, IBD1, has been assigned to the same chromosomal position [34]. Therefore, this part of the genome could be considered to be a promising candidate region of a sarcoidosis susceptibility gene. Rybicki and colleagues [35] tested 35 pairs of siblings (sibling pairs) affected by sarcoidosis for eight polymorphisms and excluded cosegregation of sarcoidosis and markers of the Blau syndrome and IBD1 locus. It turned out in 2001 that Blau syndrome and predisposition to CD are caused by the same gene, CARD15 or NOD2, and that sarcoidosis is not [36–38].

An early example of family genotyping to understand the genetics of sarcoidosis has been preformed on the previously mentioned Swedish families described by Wiman [39]. Ten affected members of two families together with unaffected relatives have been typed for HLA by microcyto-toxicity assays. The authors concluded from the results that "it is obvious from these studies that there is no correlation between HLA genotypes and disease." Nevertheless a high degree of HLA-A identity by descent was reported for the more extended family of seven affected siblings and cousins This is compatible with inheritance of a sarcoidosis susceptibility gene in this family that is located within or in close vicinity of the extended MHC gene cluster on the short arm of chromosome 6.

Numerous reports were published in the following years that emphasized a meaning of the MHC genes in sarcoidosis. In addition, Richeldi and colleagues [16] showed that HLA-DP alleles with glutamine at amino acid position 69 of the gene product are major risk factors for CBD, a phenocopy of sarcoidosis. This prompted the authors to start collecting sarcoidosis families from Germany for linkage analyses in the search for predisposing genes. The focus of a pilot study was on the MHC region on the short arm of chromosome 6 [40]. One hundred and twenty-two affected siblings from 55 German families were genotyped for seven microsatellite markers within and around the MHC and for HLA-DPB1 alleles. There was a suggestive linkage signal all over the MHC with a peak (nonparametric linkage [NPL] score 3.2; $P = .0008$) at marker D6S1666 in the MHC III gene cluster. A closer look at haplotypes shared by affected siblings, however, did not reveal any overrepresentation of distinct HLA-DPB1 alleles. Consecutively, the linkage scan was expanded to cover all chromosomes with 225 microsatellite markers tested in 63 families. Again, the most prominent peak was at marker D6S1666 in the MHC gene region with an NPL score of 2.99; $P = .001$, but it decreased after inclusion of 10 additional families [38]. There were six minor peaks at a significance level of $P < .05$ on chromosomes 1, 3, 7, 9, and the X chromosome. A three- stage fine mapping approach focused on a chromosome 6 segment of approximately 16,000 nucleotides around the D6S1666 peak. It turned out that two genes contributed independently to the linkage peak, HLA-DR and a new gene, BTNL2 [41]; both will be discussed in detail.

A multicenter sarcoidosis linkage study of the Sarcoidosis Genetic Analysis (SAGA) Consortium in the United States was based on the investigation of African American families, because patients of African extraction have a higher risk of sarcoidosis, and familial aggregation is more easily found because of larger progeny than in United States Caucasian families [28,42]. The consortium enrolled members of 229 families with two or more siblings suffering from sarcoidosis. The study population included a total of 519 sibling pairs and was genotyped for 380 microsatellites evenly distributed over all 22 autosomes. Eight linkage peaks with a p-value less than .05 were found on the long and on the short arm of chromosome 5, and on chromosomes 1, 2, 9, 11, and 20, with the most prominent peak labeled by marker D5S2500 at chromosomal position 5q11. Two of the peaks, on the short arm of chromosome 1 and on the long arm of chromosome 9, coincided with peaks found in German families, although different marker sets were used in both scans. No significant linkage was found in African American families at the at MHC gene locus. Interestingly, in the German study a small subset of nine more complex families with three or more patients contributed only little to the peak at marker D6S1666 [43]. Possibly a more pronounced heritability of sarcoidosis leading to a higher recurrence risk in African Americans and in some German families is linked to genes outside the MHC. Subsequent fine mapping of the candidate linkage regions of the SAGA genome scan mapped the major peak more precisely to chromosome 5q11.2 (D5S407), revealed a gene locus linked to protection against sarcoidosis on the short arm of chromosome 5 (*5p15.2*), and found suggestive evidence of joint action between two loci (3p14-11 and 5p15.2) to confer susceptibility to sarcoidosis [44]. Further investigation concerned linkage of specific features or symptoms of sarcoidosis, the disease phenotype, to chromosome segments shared by affected siblings [45]. As to prognosis, chest radiographic resolution was the feature with the most significant linkage to D1S3720 on chromosome 1p36. Single organ involvement was not as informative as affection of organ clusters, as known from clinical praxis. The authors stressed that linkage to the disease phenotype did not coincide with linkage to susceptibility and assumed that different genes were influencing the beginning and the progress of sarcoidosis.

Large amounts of genotype data are accumulated in the course of a genome-wide linkage scan. Thompson and colleagues of the SAGA consortium used this resource to stratify their study population of 229 African American families according to diverse ancestry [46]. Subpopulations were formed as clusters of families on the basis of subpopulation-specific patterns of linkage marker allele frequencies. Even though only a minor portion of 10 families (six families with very similar and unique allele pattern and four families with below average similarity) were separated, there was evidence that the small subpopulation of six very similar families were solely responsible for two of the previously found linkage peaks and did not contribute to most of the remaining peaks. A new susceptibility locus on chromosome 2q37 only was found in the six families.

Another spin-off of the collection of sarcoidosis families for genetic linkage analyses is the value of this resource to study the similarity of disease phenotypes in affected siblings, as demonstrated by Judson and colleagues [47]. They evaluated the information on disease characteristics of the participants of the SAGA study in respect to 15 parameters including different patterns of organ involvement and clinical outcomes. They found only minimally increased concordance of affected pairs of siblings with the exception of ocular and liver involvement, which was found to be significantly more likely to be present in either both or none of them. Sibling pair information concerning the question of a comparable course of disease in sarcoidosis has been communicated by the authors' group [48]. The authors studied the distribution of acute sarcoidosis with early and complete recovery versus chronic disease in 75 affected sibling pairs. In 24 and 26 sibling pairs both siblings were concordant for acute and chronic sarcoidosis, respectively, and the remaining 25 pairs showed discordance. These figures document a considerable tendency toward recurrence of a comparable course of disease, but there are obviously many exceptions.

Association studies—candidate genes

Major histocompatibility complex genes

As discussed previously, familial occurrence and different disease prevalences in different ethnic groups support the hypothesis of a genetic predisposition for sarcoidosis. Because of the importance of human leukocyte antigens (HLA) in antigen presentation and immunoregulation, the highly polymorphic MHC locus has been investigated intensively. The MHC III genes also are involved in the regulation of the immune response and are located between the HLA class I and II genes on the short arm of chromosome 6.

Reports examining MHC III genes did not find conclusive associations with susceptibility for sarcoidosis. No associations of complement proteins C4A, C4B, and complement factor B could be found in Caucasians [49]. The same is reported in Japanese for the transporter associated with antigen processing 2 (TAP2) gene and for the latent membrane protein 1 gene [50,51]. However, a second investigation on TAP1 and TAP2 in Caucasians from the United Kingdom and Poland, however, found significant differences in TAP2 when comparing the respective ethnic case–control groups. Another interesting aspect of this study was a significant difference in TAP1 on comparing the United Kingdom and Polish control groups [52]. This indicates that the use of multiple ethnic-defined patient cohorts complicates the analyses but will help defining the role of genetic factors in sarcoidosis.

Early studies on MHC in sarcoidosis in 1977 revealed an association of the class I gene HLA-B8 with acute sarcoidosis [39,53]. This finding was reproduced [54,55] and extended to a susceptibility haplotype composed of HLA-B8/DR3 [54,56]. Most interestingly, this haplotype is found frequently in Caucasians suffering from autoimmune disorders [57]. Numerous studies on HLA class II genes have been performed and have revealed different alleles segregating with susceptibility and protection. A recent study by Grunewald and colleagues demonstrated an interplay of class I and II genes. A class I effect such as disease persistence or resolution is superimposed on a disease risk mediated by class II alleles [58].

Studies on HLA-DRB1 associations with sarcoidosis predominate the literature, reporting gene variations affecting susceptibility, phenotype, and prognosis. An HLA-DRB1*03 association with spontaneous resolution and mild disease was demonstrated in Swedish [11] and Polish cohorts [59]. In Swedish sarcoidosis patients, chronicity is associated with HLA-DRB1*14 and *15 [11], while in Irish patients, it is associated with HLA-DRB1*15 [60]. In Japanese patients, it is associated with HLA-DRB1*11 and *14 [61], and in Germans, it is associated with HLA-DRB1*09, *11, *14, and *15 [41,62]. Moreover, an association of different MHC variants or haplotypes with different radiographic types, disease severity, and clinical phenotypes of sarcoidosis has been demonstrated [63–65].

Strong linkage disequilibrium is observed within the MHC, which couples HLA-DR and HLA-DQ alleles. Consequently also, HLA-DQB1 alleles have been found to be associated with sarcoidosis in Japanese (*0601), in Swedish, British, Dutch (*0201/0202), and German (*0603/0604) patient cohorts [11,61,62,66]. Moreover, the Swedish study demonstrated that HLA-DQB1*0602 is associated with persistent and *0201 with resolving disease [11], a result that was expected from their strong linkages with the respective HLA-DRB1 alleles. For HLA-DQB1*0201, this finding could be reproduced in British and Dutch cohorts [66]. In several other studies, the Swedish group could demonstrate that T cells expressing the T cell antigen receptor chain AV2S3 are accumulating in the lungs of HLA-DRB1*0301-positive patients [67,68]. This leads to the hypothesis that in these patients with good prognosis, efficient sarcoid-antigen presentation takes place in the context of HLA-DRB1*0301, generating an efficient AV2S3 T cell immune response that eliminates the antigen and induces spontaneous resolution.

Most interestingly, the products encoded by the protective HLA-DRB1*01 and *04 alleles, which consequently are under-represented in sarcoidosis cohorts, share hydrophobic residues at their only variable position (ie, position 11). The remaining nonprotective alleles (HLA-DRB1*08, *09, * 12, *14, *15 and *17) shared a hydrophilic residue at this position [69]. Position 11 is located within the pocket of the antigen-presenting groove of the HLA-DR molecule and might determine peptide-binding characteristics, which in turn determine the efficiency of antigen presentation. This leads to the hypothesis that the protective alleles initiate a highly efficient immune response, which eliminates the sarcoid antigen and by this prevents the manifestation of disease. This notion is supported by a Dutch study that could demonstrate an association of variants of pocket nine in DQ and pocket 5 in DR with different radiographic stages [70]. In this context, it is worth mentioning that in CBD HLA-DPB1 alleles with a glutamate at position 69 allow the sensitization against beryllium [16,71]. The amino acid at this position determines the shape of the antigen-presenting groove [72] and thus influences the structure of the peptides to be presented to T cells. Although in familial sarcoidosis position 69 glutamate-positive HLA-DPB1 alleles are over-represented among HLA-DPB1 alleles that were shared by affected relatives, most data suggest that this residue is not involved directly in sarcoidosis susceptibility [62,73]. Maliarik and colleagues [73] studied African American cases and controls

and found association with other hypervariable positions of HLA-DPB1 such as Val 36 and Asp 55 but not with Glu 69.

Genes regulating inflammatory responses

Costimulatory molecules

CD4 T helper (TH) lymphocytes are essential regulators of immune activation in inflammatory diseases. Members of the costimulatory B7 receptor family play major roles in the pathways of T cell activation and tolerance (eg, CD28, CD80, and CD86). The butyrophilin-like 2 gene (BTNL2, BTL-II), which has been identified as a sarcoidosis susceptibility gene [41] in a genome-wide single nucleotide polymorphism association study and replicated in independent studies [40,41], belongs to the same immunoglobulin superfamily. Because of its sequence homology to CD80 and CD86, BTNL2 probably functions as a costimulatory molecule in the T cell activation pathway [32]. Indeed, the authors could demonstrate that the lead SNP rs2076530 alters the splicing pattern of BTNL2, and a premature stop codon is inserted. The resulting truncated protein product encoded by this splice form lacks the transmembrane helix and the IgC domain. The protein product therefore has lost its ability to insert in the cell membrane. Under the assumption of a role of BTNL2 in costimulation, the truncating polymorphism could result in an impairment of T cell down-regulation, leading to dysregulated TH cell activation in autoimmune responses [41]. Recently it has been shown in mice that a putative receptor for BTNL2 is expressed on activated T and B cells and that BTNL2 inhibits T cell proliferation [74], supporting the idea that BTNL2 has a potential role as a costimulatory molecule in sarcoidosis immunopathogenesis.

BTNL2 is located on 6p21.3 in close proximity to the HLA-DRB1 locus. Based on regression models, BTNL2 appears to be a risk locus that is independent of the neighboring HLA loci [41]. In African Americans, however, where the BTNL2 association with sarcoidosis is much weaker than in Caucasians, a negative association with HLA-DR seems to overlay the genetic signal [75]. To assess the independence of the BTNL2 conferred risk for sarcoidosis from the known HLA class II risk alleles, Spagnolo and colleagues [76] analyzed data of British and Dutch sarcoidosis patients, stratifying by the distinct disease subset

Löfgren's syndrome (LS). They replicated association with rs2076530 and closely flanking SNPs of the BTNL2 gene. In the complete cohort, sarcoidosis risk was associated with rs2076530 A and the more common allele C of rs2294878, the next marker upstream. After exclusion of patients who had LS, both SNPs remained significant. In the LS cohort, the most significantly associated risk allele was rs3117099 T, the next marker downstream, which resided mainly on the most common haplotype 2, together with rs2294878 C and rs2076530 A. In the larger group of sarcoidosis patients without LS, the most significantly associated haplotype 4 included the complementary allele rs2076530 G and was under-represented in cases. Generally, in the complete cohort, haplotypes with rs2076530 A were more common in cases as compared with controls, and haplotypes with rs2076530 G were less common, in agreement with previous findings [48]. HLA-DRB1 alleles showed the well-known association of HLA-DRB1*03 with LS and under-representation of this allele, together with DRB1*01, in sarcoidosis without LS. HLA-DRB1*12, DRB1*14, and DRB1*15 were over-represented in the latter group. The authors concluded that despite apparently convincing evidences, the issue of how much the BTNL2 associations are independent of the known HLA-DBR1 alleles has not been resolved satisfactorily.

Because of the complex and long-range linkage disequilibrium within the HLA area, the exact resolution of the arrangements of putative susceptibility loci and the question of whether BTNL2 associations are independent of the known HLA-DRB1 alleles have not been resolved. Future work is needed to evaluate the exact function of BTNL2 in the costimulatory system and to assess how it interacts with other genes in sarcoidosis.

The hypothesis of a missing control of T cell activation by BTNL2 in sarcoidosis is underlined by the importance of the costimulatory molecules and the costimulatory capacity of alveolar macrophages in sarcoidosis. Alveolar macrophages from healthy volunteers do not support or block T cell activation [77]. In contrast, alveolar macrophages from patients who have sarcoidosis effectively stimulate antigen- and lectin-driven stimulation of T cells [78]. This increased accessory function is mediated by increased expression of costimulatory molecules like CD86, CD40, CD54, and CD58 on the surface of the alveolar macrophages [79]. Thus, the potent capability of alveolar macrophages from sarcoidosis patients to deliver accessory signals without an effective counterbalance by inhibitory signals like BTNL2 reveal an exaggerated state of T cell activation as it is seen in active sarcoidosis.

Cytokine network

Analyses of the cytokines released by activated immune cells of the lower respiratory tract demonstrate a predominance of TH1 cytokines, and cytokine patterns heralding spontaneous resolution or progressing disease have been identified [80]. Many of these cytokines disclose functional polymorphisms, which suggest a genetic basis for their release in health and disease.

Transforming growth factor β (TGFβ) is a pluripotent immune-modulating cytokine involved in down-regulation of inflammation [81] and in fibrogenesis (eg, functional polymorphisms associate with pulmonary allograft fibrosis) [82]. Its action depends on extracellular activation in the micromilieu and on the status of its target cells [83]. In sarcoidosis, elevated TGFβ production is associated with spontaneous resolution [81]. A functional polymorphism in codon 25 of the $TGF\beta_1$ gene influences its release by immune cells, opening the possibility that genetically defined high producers encounter spontaneous resolutions more frequently. Neither a German nor a recent United States study, however, found a disease association in Caucasian patients who had sarcoidosis [84,85]. Also a coinvestigated -1082 polymorphism of the immunosuppressive cytokine interleukin (IL)-10 gene did not show any association with the phenotype of sarcoidosis [84]. Polymorphisms of all three isoforms of TGFβ have been associated with variations in protein expression [86]. Kruit and colleagues reported that the alleles $TGF\beta_2$ 59941G, $TGF\beta_3$ 4875A, and $TGF\beta_3$ 17369C were found more frequently in patients who had chest radiographic evidence of fibrosis [87].

IL-4 and its receptor (IL-4R) represent another system involved in the down-regulation of TH1 responses. The role of polymorphisms of IL-4R in sarcoidosis has been studied by genotyping 241 members of 62 families with 136 affected siblings and 304 healthy individuals for three functional SNPs within the IL-4R gene (ie, I50V, S478S, and Q551R) [88]. Genotypes of two flanking microsatellite markers were included to enhance the power of the study. Linkage analysis under different models of inheritance and tests of equal transmission of parental haplotypes showed no significant results. There were no different allele frequencies in patients and founders of the families and independent healthy controls. Overall, a significant role of IL-4R polymorphisms in the etiology of sarcoidosis was excluded.

IL-18 is a mediator released by sarcoid alveolar macrophages generating increased levels in alveolar lining fluid and serum-driving TH1 responses. An association between the functional polymorphism IL-18-607A/C polymorphism has been reported in an Irish [89] cohort and refuted in a Dutch [90], and equivocal results are reported from Japan [91,92].

Alveolar macrophages but not peripheral blood monocytes of patients who have active sarcoidosis release large amounts of tumor necrosis factor α (TNF-α) that is not seen in inactive disease and after successful treatment or after spontaneous resolution [93,94]. Variation in TNF-α production level is an innate host characteristic that was shown to vary between individuals and to be associated with certain HLA-DR alleles [95,96]. The TNF gene locus, comprising the TNF-α, lymphotoxin-α (formerly TNF-β) and lymphotoxin-β genes, is located in the class III region of the MHC, telomeric to the class II region and centromeric to the class I region. Genetic analysis has revealed several polymorphisms in these genes, and new polymorphisms with potential functional consequences continue to be discovered. The MHC III region contains more genes than TNF-α but the most extensive data have accumulated studying functional polymorphisms of this gene. One of these has been identified at position -308 in the promoter region of the TNF-α gene as a biallelic polymorphism (TNFA1/TNFA2) and is associated with variation of TNF-α production in health and disease. The rare TNFA2 allele confers susceptibility to severe disease phenotypes of cerebral malaria [97], mucocutaneous leishmaniasis [98], and chronic bronchitis [99]. Moreover, as shown in a recent meta-analysis, this rare phenotype is associated with the susceptibility for rheumatoid arthritis in Latin Americans but not in Caucasians, and another meta-analysis demonstrated that the A allele confers poor responsiveness to anti-TNF-α therapy [100,101].

Motivated by these results, the authors studied the TNFA1/TNFA2 (-308) polymorphism in 101 patients with sarcoidosis and 216 controls and discovered a significant shift to the TNFA2 allele in LS (TNFA1/TNFA2 = 0.59/0.41 versus

0.81/0.19 in controls, $P > .01$). Comparing LS with nonacute sarcoidosis also revealed a significant shift toward the less common TNFA2 allele in LS. The entire sarcoidosis cohort, however, did not differ in their TNFA1/TNFA2 allele frequency from control (0.77/0.23). Thus, in contrast to the diseases cited for patients with sarcoidosis, the rare TNFA2 allele seems to be linked with a good prognosis [102], which leads to the conclusion that exaggerated TNF-α release should correlate with LS. To test this hypothesis, the authors investigated spontaneous TNF-α release of bronchoalveolar cells from their patients with sarcoidosis in correlation to their TNFA1/TNFA2 genotype. Most interestingly, contrary to what the authors expected, no exaggerated spontaneous TNF-α release of BAL-cells of patients with TNFA2 allele was observed [103]. This finding demonstrates that it is impossible to conclude from other disorders or even from in vitro data to the phenotypical or pathophysiological influence of a given genotype. In the case of sarcoidosis, the TNFA2 allele is not associated with an exaggerated TNF-α release, what affirms the demand to analyze genotype–phenotype relationships in any disease separately. Moreover, the good prognosis of TNFA2-positive sarcoidosis is not in conflict with the elevated risk for disease progression of patients who have elevated spontaneous TNF-α release of BAL cells [104], because in sarcoidosis the release of this cytokine is not influenced by the named polymorphism [103]. This notion is supported further by the recent finding of Idali and colleagues who demonstrated a reduced expression of proinflammatory cytokines, including TNF-α in HLA-DRB1*0301-positive patients [105], which is not explained by the linkage disequilibrium between TNFA2 and the named HLA-DR allele. Supplementary statistical analysis of these patient data [106] was performed to resolve which allele confers the greater risk (TNFA or HLA-DR) for expression of either disease phenotype and to determine whether disease haplotypes in correlation to the different disease courses can be defined [107]. The results demonstrated that the risk for developing or not developing LS is conferred not by these two genetic traits alone, but that other elements possibly in linkage disequilibrium should contribute to the development of these different disease phenotypes. In addition, the construction of virtual haplotypes by means of a statistical calculation [107] showed that the DR3.TNFA2 haplotype was associated with LS and that the

DR2.TNFA1 haplotype was associated with the non-LS patients, giving substance to the hypothesis that haplotypes, rather than single genes interacting with each other, are the most likely explanation for these correlations.

Grutters and colleagues studied a series of different TNF promoter polymorphisms, at position -1031, -863, -857, -307, and -237 in 96 British and 100 Dutch patients who had sarcoidosis, and 354 British and 222 Dutch control subjects [108]. The results reproduced the previously mentioned on the -308 polymorphism in a German population and showed a significant increase in the rarer TNF–857T allele in the British and Dutch sarcoidosis populations. Haplotype reconstruction revealed that a -307A-containing haplotype was associated with good prognosis and a -857T-containing one with persistent disease. Both reside on separate and unique haplotypes. In summary, these reports demonstrate that the genes conferring good or poor prognosis within a given MHC haplotype cannot be identified unequivocally, and informative meta-analyses are lacking for sarcoidosis.

Chemokine receptors

One of the linkage peaks detected in a German cohort is located on the short arm of chromosome 3, in a region that encompasses a cluster of chemokine receptor genes [43]. The cluster contains, among others, the genes encoding the C-C chemokine receptor 2 (CCR2) and the C-C chemokine receptor 5 (CCR5). In a Dutch and a British cohort, a CCR5 haplotype could be identified that was associated with chronic disease but not with susceptibility of sarcoidosis [109]. The CCR2 gene has been investigated in various association studies as a candidate for sarcoidosis susceptibility, showing an association with LS or some protective effect [110–112]. In a Dutch population, association of a specific four-SNP haplotype in the CCR2 gene region was observed with LS [112]. This finding, however, could not be confirmed in German sarcoidosis patients suffering from LS or non-LS [48].

Toll-like receptors

Toll-like receptors (TLRs) play a crucial role in activation of the innate and adaptive immune response. TLR4 recognizes pathogen-associated molecular patterns as found in bacterial LPS. The functional mutations Asp299Gly and Thr399Ile of the TLR 4 gene are more prevalent in German sarcoidosis patients studied by Pabst and colleagues than in healthy control subjects. A significant association between TLR4 mutations and sarcoidosis, however, only could be found in the chronic but not in the acute phenotype, suggesting a role of this receptor in disease-modifying processes [113]. Veltkamp and colleagues could not reproduce this finding in a larger Dutch cohort. Allele frequencies, however, differed considerably between the Dutch and the German controls [114]. In addition, the Dutch group looked at a TLR2 polymorphism but did not obtain unequivocal results. Interestingly, this polymorphism influenced ex vivo cytokine release [115]. Recent data of the authors' groups demonstrate a linkage between sarcoidosis and TLR4 variants using transmission desequilibrium test (TDT), but a case–control study largely excludes an influence of functional TLR4 gene polymorphisms [116]. This distorted transmission could be explained by an extended haplotype that carries the real risk allele and is only labeled by a TLR4 variant. In the vicinity of TLR4, there are at least three reasonable candidate genes (ie, ORM1, TNFSF15, and TRAF1). For the acute-phase protein orsomucoid 1 (ORM1), an association with sarcoidosis has been reported in a Swedish study [117]. TNFSF15 is a member of the TNF superfamily and confers a risk for CD in Japanese and European cohorts [118], and TRAF1 (TNF receptor-associated factor 1) is involved in the regulation of NF-kappa B activity, which plays a crucial role in sarcoidosis [119]. These facts illustrate the difficulties in compiling a list of sarcoid candidate genes, because good reasons for and against the inclusion of TLR4 cannot be balanced on the basis of current knowledge.

Other candidate genes

Prostaglandin—endoperoxide synthase 2

Prostaglandin–endoperoxide synthase 2 (PTGS2) is a key regulatory enzyme in the synthesis of the antifibrotic agent prostaglandin E2 and is reduced in sarcoidosis lung [120]. A promoter polymorphism in PTGS2, $-765G > C$, is reported to reduce its expression. Polymorphisms in this gene have been demonstrated to associate with inflammatory, noninflammatory, and fibrotic disorders. Hill and colleagues tested whether the named polymorphism might define susceptibility for progressive sarcoidosis developing pulmonary fibrosis. Carriage of the -765C allele was associated with susceptibility to sarcoidosis (odds ratio, 2.50; 95% confidence interval, 1.51 to 4.13; $P = .006$) and, within this disease, with poorer outcome (odds ratio, 3.11; 95% confidence interval, 1.35 to 7.13; $P = .008$). The association was replicated in a second Austrian population. The -765G > C polymorphism is functional, with the -765C allele having lower promoter activity than the -765G allele. These data demonstrate that the expected functional variation takes place in sarcoidosis [121].

Natural resistance-associated macrophage protein 1

Natural resistance-associated macrophage protein 1 (NRAMP-1), now named SLC11A1, is found in human macrophages and polymorphnuclear leukocytes, and it plays a role in macrophage activation. NRAMP-1 polymorphisms have been associated with the susceptibility for the granulomatous disorders leprosy and tuberculosis in endemic areas [122,123]. In marked contrast, Maliarik and colleagues [124] found a protective effect of a (CA) (n) repeat in the immediate 5′ region of the gene. In a Polish study, other functional polymorphisms not involved in tuberculosis have been analyzed, and an association with sarcoidosis was noted. The identified haplotype also is found in autoimmune disorders [125].

Angiotensin-converting enzyme

A molecule with relevance in another physiologic context, angiotensin-converting enzyme (ACE), has attracted much interest in sarcoidosis. ACE is produced primarily by vascular and renal epithelial cells and plays an important role in blood pressure regulation. The enzyme is secreted by the epithelioid cells of sarcoid granulomas as well, and variable percentages of patients who have clinically active sarcoidosis exhibit elevated serum ACE levels [126,127]. The extent of serum ACE increase appears to reflect the total body granuloma load [128]. The ACE gene carries a polymorphism generated by the insertion of 287 base pairs into intron 16 that does not alter the enzyme structure but affects its production. Average serum ACE levels are decreased in individuals homozygous for the insertion (allele I, genotype II) and increased in persons without the insertion (homozygous for the deletion allele D, genotype DD). The same pattern, on a higher level, consistently has been found in patients who have sarcoidosis [126,129]. In an early report from

Japan, an association of the D allele with the risk of sarcoidosis has been found in females [130]. Most investigations, however—including a recent meta-analysis—could not confirm this finding [131–135], and reports on an association with poor prognosis or complication by coincident autoimmune disorders [136,137] have been refuted by more recent publications [131,132,138]. The ACE DD genotype has been found to be over-represented in African American and in German patients with a family history of sarcoidosis [139,140], consistent with the hypothesis that this constitution could be a promoter to clinical manifestation in patients with a yet unknown inherited predisposition.

Besides the ACE gene deletion/insertion (D/I) polymorphism, there is also a polymorphism in the angiotensin II receptor type 1 (AT2R1) at position 1166 ($A^{1166} \rightarrow C$) that also might influence the contribution of angiotensin to the pathogenesis of sarcoidosis. Genotyping for the AT2R1 $A^{1166} \rightarrow C$ polymorphism revealed an increase in homozygous genotypes CC and AA in male patients who had sarcoidosis. This gene polymorphism, however, did not disclose an impact on sarcoidosis disease progression as determined by radiological type, medication, or loss of lung function. Interestingly, although located on different chromosomes, the co-incidence of the heterocygotes DI and AC was less frequent in patients who had sarcoidosis, suggesting a protective role of the combination of DI and AC against the manifestation of the disease [141].

Levels of serum ACE (sACE) are used widely to determine disease activity in sarcoidosis. Because sACE levels are influenced by the D/I polymorphism, however, the sensitivity and specificity of this test for disease monitoring are limited. Therefore genotype-adjusted reference values for sACE were established [126]. The necessity to deal with three different reference values can be circumvented by the usage of Z scores, a statistical method of normalization [142]. The application of these genotype-adjusted reference values to gauge sACE levels in sarcoidosis patients who have known D/I genotype increases the sensitivity and specificity of the sACE test.

Recently, a second ACE (ACE2) was described. ACE2 catalyzes angiotensin I to angiotensin [1–9], which is cleaved by ACE into angiotensin [1–7]. Unlike angiotensin II, resulting from angiotensin I by ACE-cleavage, angiotensin [1–7] exerts anti-inflammatory, antiproliferative, and vasodilatatory activity. Kruit and colleagues investigated haplotypes of seven SNPs in the ACE2 gene located on the X chromosome. They found a significantly higher frequency of one of those haplotypes in males without lung parenchyma involvement compared with male patients who had lung parenchyma involvement [143]. No difference was found in females. Because protein data are lacking, however, the significance of this report is difficult to evaluate.

Phenotyping sarcoidosis

Only a small number of the genetic variants associated with sarcoidosis segregate with an overall phenotype, because it has been demonstrated for the MHC genes. For the newly described susceptibility gene, BTNL2 genotype–phenotype relationships are unclear because of the lack in depth in the subphenotype definition and the small genetic effect size [144]. For studying genotype–phenotype relationships with the aim to identify risk profiles, however, in-depth phenotyping would be required. This is hampered by the broad clinical variability of the disease, which is recognized [145] and complicates the diagnosis, and the lack of clear subphenotype descriptions [146]. For phenotyping, three aspects are of importance:

1. There is a high variability in organ involvement, and any organ of the human body can be affected.
2. Some patients suffer from systemic disease with an elevated acute phase response and acute onset, while others present with only minor constitutional complaints without any symptoms of a systemic disease.
3. There is a wide variety in the course of the disease including response to treatment.

Moreover, differences in organ involvement and course of the disease between Caucasians, African Americans, and other ethnicities are well-described. For instance, the acute form of sarcoidosis with a favourable prognosis is more common in Caucasian populations, while the frequency of extrapulmonary manifestations and recalcitrant disease is elevated in African Americans and subjects of Caribbean origin [9,10]. In addition, to complicate the matter, gender-related differences of the phenotype have been observed [68]. An improved phenotyping is therefore subject of current research and consensus protocols.

Organ involvement is highly variable, and there are no typical clusters of organ involvement.

The only exception might be LS and some rare syndromes as Heerfordt-Waldenström's syndrome and lupus pernio. Establishing a system that is able to classify all sarcoidosis patients unequivocally with regard to the pattern of organ involvement and course is a tremendous challenge. Nevertheless, the phenotyping data of the ACCESS study can be used for field testing of newly designed protocols. It has been demonstrated that half of the patients suffer from mono organ involvement, being most often the lung, including adjacent lymph nodes. Thirty percent of the patients suffer from the involvement of two organs, and in only 13% of patients, is multiorgan involvement observed [10].

As far back as 1953, Sven and Löfgren [147] already showed that there was a distinct form of sarcoidosis with an acute onset, bihiliar lymphadenopathy, and bilateral arthritis, which differed from the remaining cohort. It is described, that patients who have LS have a better prognosis than patients who have other manifestations of the disease [1]. Only 10% of all patients who have LS will suffer from recalcitrant disease with a need for immunosuppressive treatment strategies. Unfortunately, it is impossible to identify these patients at time of diagnosis, and there is no generally accepted definition of LS. Some authors tend to classify all patients who have an acute onset of disease, weight loss, and fatigue as suffering from LS, while others only include patients with the full picture of the disease as described by Sven Löfgren, including bihiliar lymphadenopathy, arthritis, and erythema nodosum (EN). Future genetic studies might be able to show if there is a genetic difference in patients who have LS, patients who have sole EN, and patients who have just acute onset without the full picture of LS, and whether these patients differ from patients who have nonacute disease. The usefulness of those studies recently was demonstrated, showing gender-specific differences of acute-onset sarcoidosis and different clinical outcomes in dependence of the MHC genotype [68]. The term reverse phenotyping has been coined for this approach [148].

As mentioned previously, the authors could identify 75 sibling pairs with sarcoidosis. In 50 sibling pairs, the disease was concordant in respect to either acute or chronic disease. Only 26 sibling pairs had a discordant disease, suggesting a genetic influence on the phenotype [48] and raising the question of the stability of the phenotype. In this regard it has to be noted that acute-phase serum markers can be observed in any phenotype of sarcoidosis [149]. In a recent study, the authors showed that patients who have acute disease have a higher acute phase response with elevated serum markers than patients who have nonacute disease. Furthermore, patients who have acute disease and recalcitrant course have had the highest acute phase response and signs of a systemic disease including multiorgan involvement [150]. Thus, a sophisticated clinical and immunologic phenotyping will allow one to categorize patients according to disease risk, and a reverse phenotyping will be the approach to identify genes defining the genetic background of a given disease course.

From the clinical perspective, the most important issue would be the availability of a genetic marker predicting disease outcome and response to therapy. Studies analyzing outcome published so far used the occurrence of spontaneous resolution of the disease or changes in chest radiograph types. It has to be kept in mind, however, that the definition of spontaneous solution differs. Some authors demand a complete resolution of any chest radiograph findings, while others only consider clinical symptoms. Furthermore, there is some controversy regarding the length of the required observational period to clearly detect spontaneous resolution. Sugisaki and colleagues [151] suggest that a observational period of 5 years might be a good time period, but for practical reasons most studies used a 2-year follow-up [150,152]. In fact, this definition of resolution will detect mainly patients who have LS, because they represent the largest group with complete resolution of symptoms and chest radiograph findings within 2 years. Nevertheless, in a genotype–phenotype relationship study in an African American cohort, chest radiograph resolution could be correlated with a high linkage score to a marker on chromosome 1 [45]. Another phenotyping approach consists of a severity score employing a panel of reviewers who use a visual scale to score severity of symptoms of multiple organ manifestations [153]. The usefulness of these new instruments needs to be established in genotype–phenotype relationship studies. These considerations show that the categories of disease course and severity need to be defined f specifically or the questions to be asked in a particular study.

Up to now, genetic markers that predict the need for treatment are elusive, and any study will be complicated by the high clinical variability of the disease and the manifold reasons of treatment implementation. In this context, the authors feel that it is essential to subdivide patient cohorts into two major categories regarding disease onset, (ie, acute and nonacute). There are fundamental differences between these two categories in the spontaneous and also in the treatment-modified course of the disease. Therefore, the authors recently proposed to use a system that additionally classifies each of the categories acute and nonacute in three groups with regard to treatment indication over a course of 2 years. These three groups are

1. Patients who have no need for treatment
2. Patients who have the need for immunosuppressive treatment for one period shorter than 1 year
3. Patients who have the need for immunosuppressive treatment more often than one period or of longer duration than 1 year.

The authors compared this protocol named sarcoid clinical activity classification (SCAC) with the widely used radiologic classification system introduced by Scadding in 1967 [154] and demonstrated that the patient stratification according to disease severity is superior in the SCAC protocol [150]. Thus, new instruments to stratify patient cohorts for genotype–phenotype relationship studies are available, and their results will allow early treatment of unfortunate courses and help to prevent severe organ damage.

Other granulomatous disorders

Chronic beryllium disease

Current concepts of the pathogenesis of sarcoidosis postulate an exogenous trigger and a genetic susceptibility to allow the manifestation of sarcoidosis [2,145]. Both prerequisites, however, are elusive. CBD elicited by occupational beryllium exposure can be used to study this pathogenetic concept, because CBD is a perfect phenocopy of sarcoidosis, which only can be distinguished by demonstrating hypersensitivity to beryllium [15,155]. Approximately 2% to 16% of exposed workers become sensitized, possibly dependent on the severity of exposure. In about 50% of sensitized individuals, the immune response proceeds to chronic granulomatous lung disease [156]. In a study of 33 cases and 44 exposed persons without CBD (controls), Richeldi and colleagues [16] found particular HLA-DP alleles with a glutamic acid residue at position 69 of the beta chain (DPB1 Glu69+) in 97% of cases and in 30% of controls. Subsequent investigations confirmed this association and added more details in that different HLA-DPB1 Glu69+ alleles and their copy number have been shown to predispose to hypersensitivity and CBD, while other HLA-DR and HLA-DQ alleles seem to confer susceptibility to hypersensitivity or to progression to chronic disease selectively [71,157–161]. In addition it could be verified that beryllium binds preferentially to the HLA-DPB1 Glu69+ epitope, enabling antigen-presenting cells to stimulate beryllium-specific T cells [162]. As mentioned previously, however, the HLA-DPB1 associations seen in CBD seem not to confer sarcoidosis susceptibility [62,73].

In susceptible individuals, inhaled beryllium induces an alveolitis with antigen-specific T cells [163,164] and exaggerated proinflammatory cytokine release as seen in sarcoidosis [165]. The observation that beryllium stimulates TNF-α production by bronchoalveolar lavage cells in CBD patients [166,167] initiated several genetic studies. It was found that high TNF-α production is associated with the presence of the rare A allele of the TNFA (-308) gene polymorphism [168]. An early molecular epidemiologic study reported that this rare allele is more frequent in beryllium-sensitized individuals [158]. Recent studies investigating greater cohorts or differing ethnicities, however, did not find any associations between the rare A allele of the functional TNFA (-308) gene polymorphism or other TNFA polymorphisms and CBD or beryllium sensitization [169–171].

The immune-modulating capacities of TGFβ in granulomatous disorders qualified the TGFβ gene as candidate gene in CBD. There have been two genetic studies on functional polymorphisms in the TGFβ gene in Caucasian CBD patients originating from Europe and the United States [85,169]. The first case–control study investigating the functional TGFβ$_1$ (codon 25) polymorphism in two different Caucasian cohorts revealed a significantly higher frequency of low-producing non-GG genotypes in European and Israeli CBD patients but not in CBD patients from the United States [169]. The second study confirmed the data on CBD patients from the United States. Additionally, the authors investigated further TGFβ variants and haplotypes and found haplotypes including -509C and codon 10T to be associated with severe disease [85]. As in sarcoidosis, elevated serum levels of ACE also can be observed in CBD [172]. Interestingly, the analysis of the functional insertion/deletion polymorphism in intron 16 of the ACE gene revealed a trend that the DD genotype predisposes for more rapid disease manifestation [173] that is not seen in sarcoidosis [132].

Blau syndrome and early onset sarcoid arthritis

Both Blau syndrome and early onset sarcoid arthritis (EOS) are granulomatous disorders of juvenile onset, and their genetic background recently was elucidated. Blau syndrome is characterized by a classical symptomatic triad of granulomatous lesions in skin, joints, and eyes [174]. It is a very rare condition, with about 15 families reported worldwide. The mode of inheritance is autosomal dominant, with full penetrance and variable expression (ie, all carriers of the mutation show symptoms, but the range and the severity may be different within families). The disease occurs in consecutive generations, with a recurrence risk of 0.5 for the offspring of patients. CARD15 (caspase-activating recruitment domain 15) on chromosome 16 is a peptidoglycan sensing, intracellular molecule, also called NOD2, which activates NFkB. A mutation in its nucleotide-binding site leads to a constitutive activation and is responsible for Blau syndrome [37]. Cases with sporadic juvenile sarcoid arthritis (EOS) have been observed lacking a disease history in parents. In EOS, the classical triad is observed in combination with additional manifestations such as fever, hypertension, and cranial nerve lesions. In contrast to sarcoidosis, pulmonary manifestations are seen only in later stages of these syndromes [175]. In 9 out of 10 patients who have EOS, miss-sense mutations of CARD15 were found that also showed increased basal NFkB activity [176]. This demonstrates that Blau syndrome and EOS share a common genetic etiology with inherited (Blau syndrome) and sporadic (EOS) mutations of CARD15. Clinically, these syndromes have to be separated from adult sarcoidosis in childhood [175,177].

Because malfunctions of CARD15 can induce granulomatous diseases, the authors have studied the meaning of this gene in 138 families with two or more patients with sarcoidosis and in 127 patients without a family history of sarcoidosis who participated with both parents (trios) [38]. Sarcoidosis families, trios, and a suitable control group of healthy individuals were genotyped for four SNPs that are associated with CD. Linkage analyses, transmission tests, and association studies showed—with the exception of suggestive transmission disequilibrium of one of the SNPs in the trios—no evidence of a risk factor in sarcoidosis. In addition, 39 patients from the families, who shared at least one extended CARD15 haplotype with the affected relative, were selected for sequence analysis of the critical Blau syndrome and EOS mutation region. No mutations were found in patients who had sarcoidosis. In summary, a major effect of the CARD15 gene could be excluded in sarcoidosis, thus confirming that sarcoidosis in adults and EOS are strictly different diseases.

Crohn's disease

CD, a subphenotype of inflammatory bowel disease (IBD), is a complex and chronic inflammatory barrier disease that shares several clinical and immunologic features with sarcoidosis, like the formation of noncaseating granulomas. The understanding of the pathogenesis of CD remains limited. The present body of evidence, however, supports the hypothesis that ubiquitous, intestinal bacteria trigger a hyperactive and ongoing mucosal immune response that leads to intestinal tissue damage in genetically susceptible individuals.

Genome-wide linkage and association studies have established more than 10 susceptibility loci and convincing causative mutations on different chromosomes for CD (eg, NOD2, 5q31, DLG5, and TNFSF15 [178,179]). Most recently, IL23R, ATG16L1, 5p13.1, IRGM, NKX2-3, PTPN2, and NELL1 have been identified as additional risk genes and loci in CD [180].

The identification of the first CD disease gene NOD2 was responsible for a broad interest in the innate immune response in complex inflammatory diseases. NOD2 seems to have a crucial function in the activation of the nuclear regulatory factor NF-kB pathway in response to stimulation with microbial lipopolysaccharides. The disease-associated variants result in a premature truncation of the NOD2 protein, leading to a reduced ability of NOD2 to activate NF-kB in human cells, and subsequently an impaired host defense against bacteria [181].

The discovery of the association between ILR23 and CD is consistent with the key function of IL23 in mucosal inflammation, as IL23 activates Th17T cells that enhance chronic inflammation. It is suggested that a loss of function of IL23 could suppress this effect and may protect against the development of the disease [182].

Alternatively, IL23R exerts a clear mechanism to protect epithelial cells against microbacterial infection, and a lack of function results in impaired host defense.

A novel link between autophagy and CD has been given attention because of the association of ATG16L1 [183] and IRGM [182]. ATG16L1 encodes a protein in the autophagosome biological pathway that processes intracellular bacteria. Autophagy induced by *Salmonella typhimurium* is reduced significantly in ATG16L1 knockdown HeLa cells, suggesting that ATG16L1 is required for the autophagy trafficking pathway. Human IRGM seems also to be implicated in the handling of intracellular bacteria, as it is required for the formation of macrophages and thereby the control of intracellular *Mycobacterium tuberculosis* in people [184]. In addition to degradation of bacterial products, autophagy is involved in degradation of misfolded proteins and other protein degradation products.

Several other genes that were identified by the association and linkage studies in CD are potential candidates with plausible functional relevance in the development and regulation of bowel inflammation. Detailed recent reviews of the pathogenesis of IBD are available [178–180].

Given the phenotypic overlap of CD and sarcoidosis, it is not surprising that several sarcoidosis-associated loci seem to play also key roles in the pathogenesis of CD and vice versa, such as IL-18 or TNF-α [185]. Therefore, a combined analysis of both diseases may render common etiologic pathways in such complex inflammatory diseases by the identification of novel susceptibility loci.

Wegener's granulomatosis

Wegener's granulomatosis (WG) is a further multisystemic disorder of unknown etiology, characterized by granulomatous lesions in the respiratory tract and systemic necrotizing vasculitis. It belongs to the heterogeneous group of systemic antineutrophil cytoplasmatic antibody (ANCA)-associated vasculitides. WG specifically is associated with antibodies against proteinase 3 (PR3), which is present in the azurophil granules of the neutrophils and lysosomes of monocytes and involved in their activation [186]. Genotyping of polymorphisms within the obvious candidate gene of PR3 revealed an association only for the A564G polymorphism [187]. Functional studies, however, revealed that this association is not responsible for the increased PR3 expression seen in patients who have WG [188]. Investigating a number of microsatellite markers in the 6p21.3 region for their association with WG included also the sarcoidosis risk factor BTNL2, but the results showed that BTNL2 is not associated with WG in the German cohort [189]. Another candidate suspected to be involved in the regulation of the T cell activation is the intracellular tyrosine phosphatase encoded by the PTPN22 gene. Interestingly, significant differences in the allele frequency indicate that the functional 620W allele appears to be involved in the pathogenesis of WG [190]. Another player crucial for balanced T cell activation is the cytotoxic T lymphocyte-associated antigen-4 (CTLA-4). Two independent studies on a Scandinavian and a United States cohort resulted both in a significant association between the longer allele and WG [191,192].

There are several studies investigating gene polymorphisms that have been analyzed in sarcoidosis also. As in sarcoidosis, also in WG genotyping for the ACE insertion/deletion polymorphism excluded this gene variant as a genetic factor of influence [193]. In contrast, the immunoregulatory cytokines $TGF\beta_1$ and IL-10 showed a shift toward low-producing alleles of functional polymorphisms in WG that were not found in sarcoidosis [84,193]. In an independent study, a role for the functional gene polymorphism located in codon 25 of the $TGF\beta_1$ gene could be excluded for WG, but a significant elevation of the frequency of the homozygous AA genotype of the IL-10 (-1082) polymorphism was found in WG [194]. An association of a second IL-10 gene polymorphism was found in another study, giving rise to the hypothesis that the IL-10 gene may influence the disease by influencing the production of autoantibodies [195]. Thus, analyzing gene variants of the cytokine network demonstrates marked differences between WG and sarcoidosis.

Search for risk profiles

Genetic risk profiles are individual predictors to manifest a certain disease. They are developed from a molecular epidemiologic understanding of a given genotype and a clinical phenotype. Risk prediction is clear in Blau syndrome, where one dominant CARD15 mutation causes the manifestation of a granulomatous disorder with striking similarities with sarcoidosis. Carriers of the mutation will suffer from Blau syndrome and will pass the mutation to 50% of their offspring.

Noncarriers have no risk at all to entail the disease. The time point and severity of the affection, however, tend to vary considerably between mutation carriers within Blau syndrome families as a consequence of modifying effects of other genes or environmental triggers [174,175]. In sarcoidosis, a dominant gene effect of comparable penetrance could not be observed until now [38]. From experience with other complex diseases and the broad phenotypic variations, it appears unlikely that only a few genes predispose to sarcoidosis. Rather, it can be expected that a mix of gene effects, or even several distinct and different interacting etiologies lead to the disease.

Several degrees of complexity have been observed in association studies in sarcoidosis. At a single highly polymorphic gene as HLA-DRB1, not only one mutation but several different alleles can confer protection against sarcoidosis as demonstrated by Foley and colleagues [69]. A common feature of protective alleles is a codon at position 11 that codes for hydrophobic amino acids. Susceptibility also can be associated with a risk haplotype (ie, a series of alleles of neighboring genes along a chromosome). This is especially true with respect to the highly polymorphic HLA gene cluster as discussed previously. At present, it is not possible to model the contribution of each allele of the risk haplotype in one affected individual. Finally, an additive effect of two distant gene loci can be observed, as noted by Spagnolo and colleagues [112] in the case of CCR2 on the short arm of chromosome 3 and the HLA gene cluster on chromosome 6 in the genetic etiology of LS. For sarcoidosis, some evidence for complex MHC-haplotypes on chromosome 6 has been obtained as discussed for TNF-α spanning haplotypes [107,108,135,196]. HLA class II spanning haplotypes [63] and haplotypes also covering BTNL2 have been described, which further supports this concept [58,75,144]. Reclassifying HLA class II in two categories of susceptible and protective as reported by Grutters and colleagues [197] demonstrates the importance of the MHC, because about at third of the patients carried at least one HLA susceptibility allele. In consequence, this means that the causative variants most likely have not been identified yet and probably cannot be resolved by further positional genetic work.

One must assume that as in most multifactorial and polygenic disorders including sarcoidosis, (unknown) causative agents from the environment act on a genetically susceptible host and elicit disease-initiating events. The response spectrum of the host is defined genetically, which results both in susceptibility and in a disease-modifying process influencing the (sub)phenotype of the disease (Fig. 1). At the present finesse (ie, the shallow depth) of the phenotyping of sarcoidosis, this aspect cannot be explored further in the material published thus far. From CBD, it can be learned that the physical characteristics of these molecules decide whether an eliciting agent will be able to activate T cells [72], and beyond doubt, glutamate 69-positive HLA-DPB alleles are susceptibility alleles for CBD. After inhalation, beryllium will modify HLA II-dependent macrophage–T cell interaction, and numerous genes will be activated in the host response [165,198], which is thought to be influenced by the genetic background and ethnicity as shown for the functional TGFβ₁ (codon 25) polymorphism. The frequency of low-producing non-GG genotypes was significantly higher in European and Israeli CBD patients as compared with matched controls, which was not the case in CBD patients from the United States [85,169]. Equivocal results have been reported for gene variants influencing TNF-α release [158,160,168,169] and the ACE D/I polymorphism [173], which seems to influence clinical outcome. This indicates that multiple haplotypes on two or more chromosomes are involved as genetic disease modifiers (Fig. 2). Most interestingly, the newly discovered susceptibility gene for sarcoidosis BTNL2 seems not to be involved in the genetic background predisposing for CBD [199].

These considerations demonstrate that for the elucidation of the genetics of sarcoidosis one needs a more precise phenotyping to be used in large association studies employing high-throughput genotyping technologies. Fortunately, new phenotyping instruments for the stratification of patient cohorts in those studies are emerging [150,153] and can be compared with traditional ones [45,154]. On the molecular side, the complete knowledge of sequence (ie, through next-generation sequencing technologies) will open a new level of genetic understanding. The genetic risk profiles developed, however, will most likely only be applicable to the (sub)ethnicity investigated. Only few gene variations (eg, some HLA-DRB1 alleles categorized as susceptible or protective) disclose these characteristics in several populations of different ethnicities [69,197]. Moreover, HLA-DRB1*03 could be demonstrated to enable the host for an effective T cell response using identical T cell receptor variable regions independently of racial background [200]. In marked contrast, the rare TNFA2 allele associated with LS and a good prognosis in Caucasian cohorts [107,197] predisposes for cardiac disease with poor prognosis in Japanese patients [201]. Vice versa, haplotypes including BTNL2 have been identified to confer an increased sarcoidosis risk in white Americans but act antagonistically in AfricanAmericans [75]. Thus, a far aim achievable with the available high-throughput genotyping technologies is the definition of genetic risk profiles for different sarcoidosis phenotypes such as spontaneous resolution, recalcitrant disease, or heart disease for

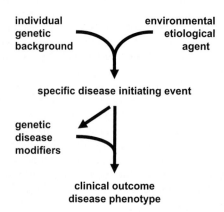

Fig. 1. Schematic depiction of the interplay between genetic background, environmental events, and genetic disease modifiers in multifactorial and multigenic disorders that determine the clinical outcome.

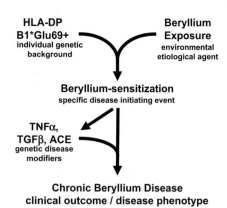

Fig. 2. Schematic depiction of the interplay between genetic background, environmental events, and genetic disease modifiers in chronic beryllium disease that determine the clinical outcome. Genes allocated to the categories genetic background and genetic disease modifier have been added.

different racial backgrounds. In addition, this knowledge will lead to the improvement of therapies, because genetically identical study cohorts will be stratified to test new therapeutic approaches.

Although the etiology of sarcoidosis remains obscure, there is increasing evidence that this highly variable inflammatory disorder represents not only one disease, but rather a spectrum of more or less related dysbalanced states of T cell immunity. It seems that the highly complex process of immune activation and deactivation can be disturbed at different levels, leading to deviations toward very different pathophysiological endpoints or clinical phenotypes. Most probably all the components of the network show some degree of inherited variability, and therefore it appears possible that knowledge of the genetic conformation at pivotal switches can help to predict the clinical outcome.

Perspective

So far the results in the attempt to understand the genetic background of sarcoidosis primarily have corroborated the initial presumption of a complex condition, and thus repeated the lessons learned from other multifactorial diseases. Large study cohorts, including detailed information on occupational and private exposures as collected in the course of the ACCESS survey [10], in combination with automated methods of mass genotype analysis, provide the prerequisites for future, systematic gene–gene and gene environment investigations. On the other hand, the application of gene expression profile analysis by DNA microarrays [202,203], in combination with proteomic techniques as already applied in sarcoidosis by several authors [204–206], offers an additional new and promising approach to uncover the genomics of sarcoidosis and its consequences on the gene expression level. Employing a combination of genetic and proteomic techniques, Wahlström and coworkers demonstrated amino acid sequences of self-antigens in the peptide-binding groove of MHC II molecules. Some of these molecules are known autoantigens and might play a role in eliciting the sarcoid inflammatory response [207]. These findings, together with the mounting knowledge on genetics, open a new field of sarcoidosis research.

References

[1] American Thoracic Society. Statement on sarcoidosis. Joint Statement of the American Thoracic Society (ATS), the European Respiratory Society (ERS), and the World Association of Sarcoidosis and Other Granulomatous Disorders (WASOG) adopted by the ATS Board of Directors and by the ERS Executive Committee, February 1999. Am J Respir Crit Care Med 1999;160(2):736–55.

[2] Müller-Quernheim J. Sarcoidosis: immunopathogenetic concepts and their clinical application. Eur Respir J 1998;12(3):716–38.

[3] Iannuzzi MC, Rybicki BA, Teirstein AS. Sarcoidosis. N Engl J Med 2007;357(21):2153–65.

[4] Zissel G, Prasse A, Muller-Quernheim J. Sarcoidosis—immunopathogenetic concepts. Semin Respir Crit Care Med 2007;28(1):3–14.

[5] Teirstein AS, Lesser M. Worldwide distribution and epidemiology of sarcoidosis. In: Fanburg B, editor. Sarcoidosis and other granulomatous diseases of the lung. Basel (Switzerland): Dekker; 1983. p. 101–34.

[6] Hillerdal G, Nöu E, Osterman K, et al. Sarcoidosis: epidemiology and prognosis. A 15-year European study. Am Rev Respir Dis 1984;130:29–32.

[7] Rybicki BA, Major M, Popovich J Jr, et al. Racial differences in sarcoidosis incidence: a 5-year study in health maintenance organization. Am J Epidemiol 1997;145:234–41.

[8] Edmondstone WM, Wilson AG. Sarcoidosis in Caucasians, blacks and Asians in London. Br J Dis Chest 1985;79(1):27–36.

[9] James DG, Neville E, Siltzbach LE. A worldwide review of sarcoidosis. Ann N Y Acad Sci 1976; 278:321–34.

[10] Baughman RP, Teirstein AS, Judson MA, et al. Clinical characteristics of patients in a case–control study of sarcoidosis. Am J Respir Crit Care Med 2001;164(10 Pt 1):1885–9.

[11] Berlin M, Fogdell-Hahn A, Olerup O, et al. HLA-DR predicts the prognosis in Scandinavian patients with pulmonary sarcoidosis. Am J Respir Crit Care Med 1997;156(5):1601–5.

[12] Maná J, Gomez-Vaquero C, Montero A, et al. Löfgren's syndrome revisited: a study of 186 patients. Am J Med 1999;107(3):240–5.

[13] Rose CS, Martyny JW, Newman LS, et al. Lifeguard lung: endemic granulomatous pneumonitis in an indoor swimming pool. Am J Public Health 1998;88(12):1795–800.

[14] Newman LS, Mroz MM, Balkissoon R, et al. Beryllium sensitization progresses to chronic beryllium disease: a longitudinal study of disease risk. Am J Respir Crit Care Med 2005;171(1): 54–60.

[15] Müller-Quernheim J, Gaede KI, Fireman E, et al. Diagnoses of chronic beryllium disease within cohorts of sarcoidosis patients. Eur Respir J 2006; 27:1190–5.

[16] Richeldi L, Sorrentino R, Saltini C. HLA-DPB 1 glutamate 69: a genetic marker of beryllium disease. Science 1993;262:242–4.

[17] Newman LS. Metals that cause sarcoidosis. Semin Respir Infect 1998;13(3):212–20.

[18] Rafnsson V, Ingimarsson O, Hjalmarsson I, et al. Association between exposure to crystalline silica and risk of sarcoidosis. Occup Environ Med 1998; 55(10):657–60.

[19] Newman LS. Beryllium disease and sarcoidosis: clinical and laboratory links. Sarcoidosis 1995;12: 7–19.

[20] Iannuzzi MC, Rybicki BA. Genetics of sarcoidosis: candidate genes and genome scans. Proc Am Thorac Soc 2007;4(1):108–16.

[21] Spagnolo P, du Bois RM. Genetics of sarcoidosis. Clin Dermatol 2007;25(3):242–9.

[22] Jörgensen G. Die Genetik der Sarkoidose. Acta Medica Scandinavica 1964;425(Suppl):209–12.

[23] Kirsten D. [Sarcoidosis in Germany. Analysis of a questionnaire survey in 1992 of patients of the German Sarcoidosis Group]. Pneumologie 1995; 49(6):378–82 [in German].

[24] Wirnsberger RM, de Vries J, Wouters EF, et al. Clinical presentation of sarcoidosis in the Netherlands: an epidemiological study. Neth J Med 1998;53(2):53–60.

[25] McGrath DS, Daniil Z, Foley P, et al. Epidemiology of familial sarcoidosis in the UK. Thorax 2000;55(9):751–4.

[26] McGrath DS, Goh N, Foley PJ, et al. Sarcoidosis: genes and microbes—soil or seed? Sarcoidosis Vasc Diffuse Lung Dis 2001;18(2):149–64.

[27] Fite E, Alsina JM, Anto JM, et al. Sarcoidosis: family contact study. Respiration 1998;65(1): 34–9.

[28] Rybicki BA, Harrington D, Major M, et al. Heterogeneity of familial risk in sarcoidosis. Genet Epidemiol 1996;13(1):23–33.

[29] Rybicki BA, Iannuzzi MC, Frederick MM, et al. Familial aggregation of sarcoidosis. A case–control etiologic study of sarcoidosis (ACCESS). Am J Respir Crit Care Med 2001;164(11):2085–91.

[30] Sellei J, Berger M. Sarkoidos Geschwülste in einer Falmilie. Archiv für Dermatologie und Syphilis (Wien) 1926;150:47–51.

[31] Wiman LG. Familial occurrence of sarcoidosis. Scand J Respir Dis Suppl 1972;80:115–9.

[32] Wellcome Trust Case Control Consortium. Genome-wide association study of 14,000 cases of seven common diseases and 3000 shared controls. Nature 2007;447(7145):661–78.

[33] Tromp G, Kuivaniemi H, Raphael S, et al. Genetic linkage of familial granulomatous inflammatory arthritis, skin rash, and uveitis to chromosome 16. Am J Hum Genet 1996;59(5):1097–107.

[34] Hugot JP, Laurent-Puig P, Gower-Rousseau C, et al. Mapping of a susceptibility locus for Crohn's disease on chromosome 16. Nature 1996;379(6568): 821–3.

[35] Rybicki BA, Maliarik MJ, Bock CH, et al. The Blau syndrome gene is not a major risk factor for sarcoidosis. Sarcoidosis Vasc Diffuse Lung Dis 1999;16(2):203–8.

[36] Hampe J, Cuthbert A, Croucher PJ, et al. Association between insertion mutation in NOD2 gene and Crohn's disease in German and British populations. Lancet 2001;357(9272):1925–8.

[37] Miceli-Richard C, Lesage S, Rybojad M, et al. CARD15 mutations in Blau syndrome. Nat Genet 2001;29(1):19–20.

[38] Schürmann M, Valentonyte R, Hampe J, et al. CARD15 gene mutations in sarcoidosis. Eur Respir J 2003;22(5):748–54.

[39] Moller E, Hedfors E, Wiman LG. HL-A genotypes and MLR in familial sarcoidosis. Tissue Antigens 1974;4(4):299–305.

[40] Schürmann M, Lympany PA, Reichel P, et al. Familial sarcoidosis is linked to the major histocompatibility complex region. Am J Respir Crit Care Med 2000;162(3 Pt 1):861–4.

[41] Valentonyte R, Hampe J, Huse K, et al. Sarcoidosis is associated with a truncating splice site mutation in BTNL2. Nat Genet 2005;37(4):357–64.

[42] Iannuzzi MC, Iyengar SK, Gray-McGuire C, et al. Genome-wide search for sarcoidosis susceptibility genes in African Americans. Genes Immun 2005; 6(6):509–18.

[43] Schürmann M, Reichel P, Müller-Myhsok B, et al. Results from a genome-wide search for predisposing genes in sarcoidosis. Am J Respir Crit Care Med 2001;164(5):840–6.

[44] Gray-McGuire C, Sinha R, Iyengar S, et al. Genetic characterization and fine mapping of susceptibility loci for sarcoidosis in African Americans on chromosome 5. Hum Genet 2006;120(3): 420–30.

[45] Rybicki BA, Sinha R, Iyengar S, et al. Genetic linkage analysis of sarcoidosis phenotypes: the sarcoidosis genetic analysis (SAGA) study. Genes Immun 2007;8(5):379–86.

[46] Thompson CL, Rybicki BA, Iannuzzi MC, et al. Reduction of sample heterogeneity through use of population substructure: an example from a population of African American families with sarcoidosis. Am J Hum Genet 2006;79(4):606–13.

[47] Judson MA, Hirst K, Iyengar SK, et al. Comparison of sarcoidosis phenotypes among affected African American siblings. Chest 2006;130(3): 855–62.

[48] Valentonyte R, Hampe J, Croucher PJ, et al. Study of C-C chemokine receptor 2 alleles in sarcoidosis, with emphasis on family-based analysis. Am J Respir Crit Care Med 2005;171(10):1136–41.

[49] Pasturenzi L, Martinetti M, Cuccia M, et al, Group tP-PSS. HLA class I, II, and III polymorphism in Italian patients with sarcoidosis. Chest 1993;104: 1170–5.

[50] Ishihara M, Ohno S, Ishida T, et al. Analysis of allelic variation of the TAP2 gene in sarcoidosis. Tissue Antigens 1997;49(2):107–10.

[51] Ishihara M, Ohno S, Mizuki N, et al. Genetic polymorphisms of the major histocompatibility complex-encoded antigen-processing genes TAP and LMP in sarcoidosis. Hum Immunol 1996; 45(2):105–10.

[52] Foley PJ, Lympany PA, Puscinska E, et al. Analysis of MHC encoded antigen-processing genes TAP1 and TAP2 polymorphisms in sarcoidosis. Am J Respir Crit Care Med 1999;160(3): 1009–14.

[53] Brewerton DA, Cockburn C, James DC, et al. HLA antigens in sarcoidosis. Clin Exp Immunol 1977;27(2):227–9.

[54] Smith MJ, Turton CW, Mitchell DN, et al. Association of HLA B8 with spontaneous resolution in sarcoidosis. Thorax 1981;36(4):296–8.

[55] Dubaniewicz A, Szczerkowska Z, Hoppe A. Comparative analysis of HLA class I antigens in pulmonary sarcoidosis and tuberculosis in the same ethnic group. Mayo Clin Proc 2003;78(4):436–42.

[56] Hedfors E, Lindstrom F. HLA-B8/DR3 in sarcoidosis. Correlation to acute-onset disease with arthritis. Tissue Antigens 1983;22(3):200–3.

[57] Lio D, Candore G, Romano GC, et al. Modification of cytokine patterns in subjects bearing the HLA-B8,DR3 phenotype: implications for autoimmunity. Cytokines Cell Mol Ther 1997; 3(4):217–24.

[58] Grunewald J, Eklund A, Olerup O. Human leukocyte antigen class I alleles and the disease course in sarcoidosis patients. Am J Respir Crit Care Med 2004;169(6):696–702.

[59] Bogunia-Kubik K, Tomeczko J, Suchnicki K, et al. DRB1*11 or DRB1*12 and their respective DRB3 specificities in clinical variants of sarcoidosis. Tissue Antigens 2001;57(1):87–90.

[60] Rutherford RM, Brutsche MH, Kearns M, et al. HLA-DR2 predicts susceptibility and disease chronicity in Irish sarcoidosis patients. Sarcoidosis Vasc Diffuse Lung Dis 2004;21(3):191–8.

[61] Naruse TK, Matsuzawa Y, Ota M, et al. HLA-DQB1*0601 is primarily associated with the susceptibility to cardiac sarcoidosis. Tissue Antigens 2000;56(1):52–7.

[62] Schürmann M, Bein G, Kirsten D, et al. HLA-DQB1 and HLA-DPB1 genotypes in familial sarcoidosis. Respir Med 1998;92:649–52.

[63] Voorter CE, Drent M, van den Berg-Loonen EM. Severe pulmonary sarcoidosis is strongly associated with the haplotype HLA-DQB1*0602-DRB1*150101. Hum Immunol 2005;66(7):826–35.

[64] Rossman MD, Thompson B, Frederick M, et al. HLA-DRB1*1101: a significant risk factor for sarcoidosis in blacks and whites. Am J Hum Genet 2003;73(4):720–35.

[65] Voorter CE, Drent M, Hoitsma E, et al. Association of HLA DQB1 0602 in sarcoidosis patients with small fiber neuropathy. Sarcoidosis Vasc Diffuse Lung Dis 2005;22(2):129–32.

[66] Sato H, Grutters JC, Pantelidis P, et al. HLA-DQB1*0201: a marker for good prognosis in British and Dutch patients with sarcoidosis. Am J Respir Cell Mol Biol 2002;27(4):406–12.

[67] Grunewald J, Olerup O, Persson U, et al. T-cell receptor variable region gene usage by CD4+ and CD8+ T cells in bronchoalveolar lavage fluid and peripheral blood of sarcoidosis patients. Proc Natl Acad Sci USA 1994;91(11):4965–9.

[68] Grunewald J, Eklund A. Sex-specific manifestations of Löfgren's syndrome. Am J Respir Crit Care Med 2007;175(1):40–4.

[69] Foley PJ, McGrath DS, Puscinska E, et al. Human leukocyte antigen-DRB1 position 11 residues are a common protective marker for sarcoidosis. Am J Respir Cell Mol Biol 2001;25(3):272–7.

[70] Voorter CE, Amicosante M, Berretta F, et al. HLA class II amino acid epitopes as susceptibility markers of sarcoidosis. Tissue Antigens 2007;70(1):18–27.

[71] Wang Z, White PS, Petrovic M, et al. Differential susceptibilities to chronic beryllium disease contributed by different Glu69 HLA-DPB1 and -DPA1 alleles. J Immunol 1999;163(3):1647–53.

[72] Lombardi G, Germain C, Uren J, et al. HLA-DP allele-specific T cell responses to beryllium account for DP-associated susceptibility to chronic beryllium disease. J Immunol 2001;166(5):3549–55.

[73] Maliarik MJ, Chen KM, Major ML, et al. Analysis of HLA-DPB1 polymorphisms in African Americans with sarcoidosis. Am J Respir Crit Care Med 1998;158(1):111–4.

[74] Nguyen T, Liu XK, Zhang Y, et al. BTNL2, a butyrophilin-like molecule that functions to inhibit T cell activation. J Immunol 2006;176(12): 7354–60.

[75] Rybicki BA, Walewski JL, Maliarik MJ, et al. The BTNL2 gene and sarcoidosis susceptibility in African Americans and whites. Am J Hum Genet 2005;77(3):491–9.

[76] Spagnolo P, Sato H, Grutters JC, et al. Analysis of BTNL2 genetic polymorphisms in British and Dutch patients with sarcoidosis. Tissue Antigens 2007;70(3):219–27.

[77] Toews GB, Vial WC, Dunn MM, et al. The accessory cell function of human alveolar macrophages in specific T cell proliferation. J Immunol 1984; 132(1):181–6.

[78] Zissel G, Ernst M, Schlaak M, et al. Accessory function of alveolar macrophages from patients with sarcoidosis and other granulomatous and nongranulomatous lung diseases. J Investig Med 1997;45(2):75–86.

[79] Nicod LP, Isler P. Alveolar macrophages in sarcoidosis coexpress high levels of CD86 (B7.2), CD40, and CD30L. Am J Respir Cell Mol Biol 1997;17(1):91–6.

[80] Ziegenhagen MW, Muller-Quernheim J. The cytokine network in sarcoidosis and its clinical relevance. J Intern Med 2003;253(1):18–30.

[81] Zissel G, Homolka J, Schlaak J, et al. Anti-inflam-matory cytokine release by alveolar macrophages in pulmonary sarcoidosis. Am J Respir Crit Care Med 1996;154:713–9.

[82] El-Gamel A, Awad MR, Hasleton PS, et al. Trans-forming growth factor-beta (TGF-beta1) genotype and lung allograft fibrosis. J Heart Lung Trans-plant 1999;18(6):517–23.

[83] Ludviksson BR, Gunnlaugsdottir B. Transforming growth factor-beta as a regulator of site-specific T-cell inflammatory response. Scand J Immunol 2003;58(2):129–38.

[84] Muraközy G, Gaede KI, Zissel G, et al. Analysis of gene polymorphisms in interleukin-10 and trans-forming growth factor-beta 1 in sarcoidosis. Sar-coidosis Vasc Diffuse Lung Dis 2001;18(2):165–9.

[85] Jonth AC, Silveira L, Fingerlin TE, et al. TGF-beta1 variants in chronic beryllium disease and sarcoidosis. J Immunol 2007;179(6):4255–62.

[86] Awad MR, El-Gamel A, Hasleton P, et al. Geno-typic variation in the transforming growth factor-beta1 gene: association with transforming growth factor-beta1 production, fibrotic lung disease, and graft fibrosis after lung Transplantation. Trans-plantation 1998;66(8):1014–20.

[87] Kruit A, Grutters JC, Ruven HJ, et al. Transform-ing growth factor-beta gene polymorphisms in sarcoidosis patients with and without fibrosis. Chest 2006;129(6):1584–91.

[88] Bohnert A, Schurmann M, Hartung A, et al. No linkage of the interleukin-4 receptor locus on chromosome 16p11.2-12.1 with sarcoidosis in German multiplex families. Eur J Immunogenet 2002;29(3):269–72.

[89] Kelly DM, Greene CM, Meachery G, et al. Endo-toxin up-regulates interleukin-18: potential role for gram-negative colonization in sarcoidosis. Am J Respir Crit Care Med 2005;172(10):1299–307.

[90] Janssen R, Grutters JC, Ruven HJ, et al. No association between interleukin-18 gene polymor-phisms and haplotypes in Dutch sarcoidosis patients. Tissue Antigens 2004;63(6):578–83.

[91] Takada T, Suzuki E, Morohashi K, et al. Associa-tion of single nucleotide polymorphisms in the IL-18 gene with sarcoidosis in a Japanese popula-tion. Tissue Antigens 2002;60(1):36–42.

[92] Zhou Y, Yamaguchi E, Hizawa N, et al. Roles of functional polymorphisms in the interleukin-18 gene promoter in sarcoidosis. Sarcoidosis Vasc Diffuse Lung Dis 2005;22(2):105–13.

[93] Müller-Quernheim J, Pfeifer S, Mannel D, et al. Lung-restricted activation of the alveolar macro-phage/monocyte system in pulmonary sarcoidosis. Am Rev Respir Dis 1992;145(1):187–92.

[94] Ziegenhagen MW, Rothe ME, Zissel G, et al. Exag-gerated TNF-alpha release of alveolar macro-phages in corticosteroid resistant sarcoidosis. Sarcoidosis Vasc Diffuse Lung Dis 2002;19(3):185–90.

[95] Bendtzen K, Morling N, Fomsgaard A, et al. Association between HLA-DR2 and production of tumour necrosis factor alpha and interleukin 1 by mononuclear cells activated by lipopoly-saccharide. Scand J Immunol 1988;28(5):599–606.

[96] Jacob CO, Fronek Z, Lewis GD, et al. Heritable major histocompatibility complex class II-associ-ated differences in production of tumor necrosis factor alpha: relevance to genetic predisposition to systemic lupus erythematosus. Proc Natl Acad Sci USA 1990;87(3):1233–7.

[97] McGuire W, Hill A, Allsopp C, et al. Variation in the TNF-α promoter region associated with suscep-tibility to cerebral malaria. Nature 1994;371:508–11.

[98] Cabrera M, Shaw MA, Sharples C, et al. Polymor-phism in tumor necrosis factor genes associated with mucocutaneous leishmaniasis. J Exp Med 1995;182(5):1259–64.

[99] Huang SL, Su CH, Chang SC. Tumor necrosis factor-alpha gene polymorphism in chronic bron-chitis. Am J Respir Crit Care Med 1997;156(5):1436–9.

[100] Lee YH, Ji JD, Song GG. Tumor necrosis factor-alpha promoter -308 A/G polymorphism and rheumatoid arthritis susceptibility: a meta-analysis. J Rheumatol 2007;34(1):43–9.

[101] Lee YH, Rho YH, Choi SJ, et al. Association of TNF-alpha -308 G/A polymorphism with respon-siveness to TNF-alpha blockers in rheumatoid arthritis: a meta-analysis. Rheumatol Int 2006;27(2):157–61.

[102] Seitzer U, Swider C, Stüber F, et al. Tumour necro-sis factor alpha promoter gene polymorphism in sarcoidosis. Cytokines 1997;9(10):787–90.

[103] Somoskövi A, Zissel G, Seitzer U, et al. Polymor-phism at position -308 in the promotor region of the TNF-alpha and in the first intron o the TNF-beta genes and spontaneous and lipopolysaccha-ride-induced TNF-alpha release in sarcoidosis. Cytokines 1999;11(11):882–7.

[104] Ziegenhagen MW, Benner UK, Zissel G, et al. Sar-coidosis: TNF-alpha release from alveolar macro-phages and serum level of sIL-2R are prognostic markers. Am J Respir Crit Care Med 1997;156(5):1586–92.

[105] Idali F, Wiken M, Wahlstrom J, et al. Reduced Th1 response in the lungs of HLA-DRB1*0301 patients with pulmonary sarcoidosis. Eur Respir J 2006;27(3):451–9.

[106] Swider C, Schnittger L, Bogunia-Kubik K, et al. TNF-alpha and HLA-DR genotyping as potential prognostic markers in pulmonary sarcoidosis. Eur Cytokine Netw 1999;10(2):143–6.

[107] Seitzer U, Gerdes J, Müller-Quernheim J. Evidence for disease phenotype associated haplotypes (DR. TNF) in sarcoidosis. Sarcoidosis Vasc Diffuse Lung Dis 2001;18(3):279–83.

[108] Grutters JC, Sato H, Pantelidis P, et al. Increased frequency of the uncommon tumor necrosis factor -857T allele in British and Dutch patients with sarcoidosis. Am J Respir Crit Care Med 2002;165(8):1119–24.

[109] Spagnolo P, Renzoni EA, Wells AU, et al. C-C chemokine receptor 5 gene variants in relation to lung disease in sarcoidosis. Am J Respir Crit Care Med 2005;172(6):721–8.

[110] Petrek M, Drabek J, Kolek V, et al. CC chemokine receptor gene polymorphisms in Czech patients with pulmonary sarcoidosis. Am J Respir Crit Care Med 2000;162(3 Pt 1):1000–3.

[111] Hizawa N, Yamaguchi E, Furuya K, et al. The role of the C-C chemokine receptor 2 gene polymorphism V64I (CCR2-64I) in sarcoidosis in a Japanese population. Am J Respir Crit Care Med 1999; 159(6):2021–3.

[112] Spagnolo P, Renzoni EA, Wells AU, et al. C-C chemokine receptor 2 and sarcoidosis: association with Lofgren's syndrome. Am J Respir Crit Care Med 2003;168(10):1162–6.

[113] Pabst S, Baumgarten G, Stremmel A, et al. Toll-like receptor (TLR) 4 polymorphisms are associated with a chronic course of sarcoidosis. Clin Exp Immunol 2006;143(3):420–6.

[114] Veltkamp M, Grutters JC, van Moorsel CH, et al. Toll-like receptor (TLR) 4 polymorphism Asp299Gly is not associated with disease course in Dutch sarcoidosis patients. Clin Exp Immunol 2006;145(2):215–8.

[115] Veltkamp M, Wijnen PA, van Moorsel CH, et al. Linkage between Toll-like receptor (TLR) 2 promotor and intron polymorphisms: functional effects and relevance to sarcoidosis. Clin Exp Immunol 2007;149(3):453–62.

[116] Schürmann M, Kwiatkowski R, Albrecht M, et al. Study of Toll-like receptor gene loci in sarcoidosis. Clin Exp Immunol 2008; submitted for publication.

[117] Fan C, Nylander PO, Sikstrom C, et al. Orosomucoid and haptoglobin types in patients with sarcoidosis. Exp Clin Immunogenet 1995;12(1): 31–5.

[118] Yamazaki K, McGovern D, Ragoussis J, et al. Single nucleotide polymorphisms in TNFSF15 confer susceptibility to Crohn's disease. Hum Mol Genet 2005;14(22):3499–506.

[119] Drent M, van den Berg R, Haenen GR, et al. NF-kappaB activation in sarcoidosis. Sarcoidosis Vasc Diffuse Lung Dis 2001;18(1):50–6.

[120] Petkova DK, Clelland CA, Ronan JE, et al. Reduced expression of cyclooxygenase (COX) in idiopathic pulmonary fibrosis and sarcoidosis. Histopathology 2003;43(4):381–6.

[121] Hill MR, Papafili A, Booth H, et al. Functional prostaglandin–endoperoxide synthase 2 polymorphism predicts poor outcome in sarcoidosis. Am J Respir Crit Care Med 2006;174(8): 915–22.

[122] Abel L, Sanchez FO, Oberti J, et al. Susceptibility to leprosy is linked to the human NRAMP1 gene. J Infect Dis 1998;177(1):133–45.

[123] Bellamy R. Identifying genetic susceptibility factors for tuberculosis in Africans: a combined approach using a candidate gene study and a genome-wide screen. Clin Sci (Lond) 2000;98(3): 245–50.

[124] Maliarik MJ, Chen KM, Sheffer RG, et al. The natural resistance-associated macrophage protein gene in African Americans with sarcoidosis. Am J Respir Cell Mol Biol 2000;22(6):672–5.

[125] Dubaniewicz A, Jamieson SE, Dubaniewicz-Wybieralska M, et al. Association between SLC11A1 (formerly NRAMP1) and the risk of sarcoidosis in Poland. Eur J Hum Genet 2005; 13(7):829–34.

[126] Biller H, Zissel G, Ruprecht B, et al. Genotype-corrected reference values for serum angiotensin-converting enzyme. Eur Respir J 2006;28(6): 1085–90.

[127] Ziegenhagen MW, Rothe ME, Schlaak M, et al. Bronchoalveolar and serological parameters reflecting the severity of sarcoidosis. Eur Respir J 2003;21(3):407–13.

[128] Gilbert S, Steinbrech DS, Landas SK, et al. Amounts of angiotensin-converting enzyme mRNA reflect the burden of granulomas in granulomatous lung disease. Am Rev Respir Dis 1993; 148:483–6.

[129] Sharma P, Smith I, Maguire G, et al. Clinical value of ACE genotyping in diagnosis of sarcoidosis. Lancet 1997;349:1602–3.

[130] Furuya K, Yamaguchi E, Itoh A, et al. Deletion polymorphism in the angiotensin I converting enzyme (ACE) gene as a genetic risk factor for sarcoidosis. Thorax 1996;51(8):777–80.

[131] Planck A, Eklund A, Yamaguchi E, et al. Angiotensin-converting enzyme gene polymorphism in relation to HLA-DR in sarcoidosis. J Intern Med 2002;251(3):217–22.

[132] McGrath DS, Foley PJ, Petrek M, et al. Ace gene I/D polymorphism and sarcoidosis pulmonary disease severity. Am J Respir Crit Care Med 2001; 164(2):197–201.

[133] Tomita H, Ina Y, Sugiura Y, et al. Polymorphism in the angiotensin-converting enzyme (ACE) gene and sarcoidosis. Am J Respir Crit Care Med 1997;156:255–9.

[134] Arbustini E, Grasso M, Leo G, et al. Polymorphism of angiotensin-converting enzyme gene in sarcoidosis. Am J Respir Crit Care Med 1996;153: 851–4.

[135] Medica I, Kastrin A, Maver A, et al. Role of genetic polymorphisms in ACE and TNF-alpha gene in sarcoidosis: a meta-analysis. J Hum Genet 2007; 52(10):836–47.

[136] Pietinalho A, Furuya K, Yamaguchi E, et al. The angiotensin-converting enzyme DD gene is

associated with poor prognosis in Finnish sarcoidosis patients. Eur Respir J 1999;13(4):723–6.

[137] Papadopoulos KI, Melander O, Orho-Melander M, et al. Angiotensin-converting enzyme (ACE) gene polymorphism in sarcoidosis in relation to associated autoimmune diseases. J Intern Med 2000;247(1):71–7.

[138] Alia P, Mana J, Capdevila O, et al. Association between ACE gene I/D polymorphism and clinical presentation and prognosis of sarcoidosis. Scand J Clin Lab Invest 2005;65(8):691–7.

[139] Schürmann M, Reichel P, Müller-Myhsok B, et al. Angiotensin-converting enzyme (ACE) gene polymorphisms and familial occurrence of sarcoidosis. J Intern Med 2001;249(1):77–83.

[140] Maliarik MJ, Rybicki BA, Malvitz E, et al. Angiotensin-converting enzyme gene polymorphism and risk of sarcoidosis. Am J Respir Crit Care Med 1998;158(5 Pt 1):1566–70.

[141] Biller H, Gaede KI, Ruprecht B, et al. Genepolymorphisms of ACE and the angiotensin receptor AT2R1 influence serum ACE levels in sarcoidosis. Mol Med, Submitted for publication.

[142] Kruit A, Grutters JC, Gerritsen WB, et al. ACE I/D-corrected Z-scores to identify normal and elevated ACE activity in sarcoidosis. Respir Med 2007;101(3):510–5.

[143] Kruit A, Ruven HJ, Grutters JC, et al. Angiotensin-converting enzyme 2 (ACE2) haplotypes are associated with pulmonary disease phenotypes in sarcoidosis patients. Sarcoidosis Vasc Diffuse Lung Dis 2005;22(3):195–203.

[144] Li Y, Wollnik B, Pabst S, et al. BTNL2 gene variant and sarcoidosis. Thorax 2006;61(3):273–4.

[145] Baughman RP, Lower EE, du Bois RM. Sarcoidosis. Lancet 2003;361(9363):1111–8.

[146] Judson MA, Thompson BW, Rabin DL, et al. The diagnostic pathway to sarcoidosis. Chest 2003; 123(2):406–12.

[147] Löfgren S. Primary pulmonary sarcoidosis. Acta Med Scand 1953;145:424–65.

[148] Iannuzzi MC, Baughman RP. Reverse phenotyping in sarcoidosis. Am J Respir Crit Care Med 2007;175(1):4–5.

[149] Drent M, Wirnsberger RM, de Vries J, et al. Association of fatigue with an acute-phase response in sarcoidosis. Eur Respir J 1999;13(4):718–22.

[150] Prasse A, Katic C, Germann M, et al. Phenotyping sarcoidosis from the pulmonary perspective. Am J Respir Crit Care Med 2008;177(3):330–6.

[151] Sugisaki K, Yamaguchi T, Nagai S, et al. Clinical characteristics of 195 Japanese sarcoidosis patients treated with oral corticosteroids. Sarcoidosis Vasc Diffuse Lung Dis 2003;20(3):222–6.

[152] Judson MA, Baughman RP, Thompson BW, et al. Two-year prognosis of sarcoidosis: the ACCESS experience. Sarcoidosis Vasc Diffuse Lung Dis 2003;20(3):204–11.

[153] Wasfi YS, Rose CS, Murphy JR, et al. A new tool to assess sarcoidosis severity. Chest 2006;129(5): 1234–45.

[154] Scadding J. Sarcoidosis. London: Eyre & Spottiswoode; 1967.

[155] Maier L, Martyny J, Mroz M, et al. Genetic and environmental risk factors in beryllium sensitization and chronic beryllium disease. Chest 2002;121 (3 Suppl):81S.

[156] Newman LS, Lloyd J, Daniloff E. The natural history of beryllium sensitization and chronic beryllium disease. Environ Health Perspect 1996; 104S(5):937–43.

[157] Rossman MD, Stubbs J, Lee CW, et al. Human leukocyte antigen class II amino acid epitopes: susceptibility and progression markers for beryllium hypersensitivity. Am J Respir Crit Care Med 2002;165(6):788–94.

[158] Saltini C, Richeldi L, Losi M, et al. Major histocompatibility locus genetic markers of beryllium sensitization and disease. Eur Respir J 2001;18(4): 677–84.

[159] Richeldi L, Kreiss K, Mroz MM, et al. Interaction of genetic and exposure factors in the prevalence of berylliosis. Am J Ind Med 1997;32(4):337–40.

[160] McCanlies EC, Ensey JS, Schuler CR, et al. The association between HLA-DPB1Glu69 and chronic beryllium disease and beryllium sensitization. Am J Ind Med 2004;46(2):95–103.

[161] Maier LA, McGrath DS, Sato H, et al. Influence of MHC class II in susceptibility to beryllium sensitization and chronic beryllium disease. J Immunol 2003;171(12):6910–8.

[162] Amicosante M, Sanarico N, Berretta F, et al. Beryllium binding to HLA-DP molecule carrying the marker of susceptibility to berylliosis glutamate beta69. Hum Immunol 2001;62(7):686–93.

[163] Saltini C, Winestock K, Kirby M, et al. Maintenance of alveolitis in patients with chronic beryllium disease by beryllium-specific helper T cells. N Engl J Med 1989;320:1103–9.

[164] Fontenot AP, Canavera SJ, Gharavi L, et al. Target organ localization of memory CD4(+) T cells in patients with chronic beryllium disease. J Clin Invest 2002;110(10):1473–82.

[165] Amicosante M, Berretta F, Franchi A, et al. HLA-DP-unrestricted TNF-alpha release in beryllium-stimulated peripheral blood mononuclear cells. Eur Respir J 2002;20(5):1174–8.

[166] Tinkle SS, Newman LS. Beryllium-stimulated release of tumor necrosis factor-alpha, interleukin-6, and their soluble receptors in chronic beryllium disease. Am J Respir Crit Care Med 1997;156(6): 1884–91.

[167] Bost T, Newman L, Riches D. Increased TNF-alpha and IL6 mRNA expression by alveolar macrophages in chronic beryllium disease. Chest 1993;103(2 Suppl):138S.

[168] Maier LA, Sawyer RT, Bauer RA, et al. High beryllium-stimulated TNF-alpha is associated with the -308 TNF-alpha promoter polymorphism and with clinical severity in chronic beryllium disease. Am J Respir Crit Care Med 2001;164(7):1192–9.

[169] Gaede KI, Amicosante M, Schurmann M, et al. Function-associated transforming growth factor-beta gene polymorphism in chronic beryllium disease. J Mol Med 2005;83(5):397–405.

[170] Sato H, Silveira L, Fingerlin T, et al. TNF polymorphism and bronchoalveolar lavage cell TNF-alpha levels in chronic beryllium disease and beryllium sensitization. J Allergy Clin Immunol 2007;119(3):687–96.

[171] McCanlies EC, Schuler CR, Kreiss K, et al. TNF-alpha polymorphisms in chronic beryllium disease and beryllium sensitization. J Occup Environ Med 2007;49(4):446–52.

[172] Newman LS, Orton R, Kreiss K. Serum angiotensin-converting enzyme activity in chronic beryllium disease. Am Rev Respir Dis 1992;146(1):39–42.

[173] Maier LA, Raynolds MV, Young DA, et al. Angiotensin-1 converting enzyme polymorphisms in chronic beryllium disease. Am J Respir Crit Care Med 1999;159(4 Pt 1):1342–50.

[174] Blau EB. Familial granulomatous arthritis, iritis, and rash. J Pediatr 1985;107(5):689–93.

[175] Becker ML, Rose CD. Blau syndrome and related genetic disorders causing childhood arthritis. Curr Rheumatol Rep 2005;7(6):427–33.

[176] Kanazawa N, Okafuji I, Kambe N, et al. Early onset sarcoidosis and CARD15 mutations with constitutive nuclear factor-kappaB activation: common genetic etiology with Blau syndrome. Blood 2005;105(3):1195–7.

[177] Milman N, Hoffmann AL, Byg KE. Sarcoidosis in children. Epidemiology in Danes, clinical features, diagnosis, treatment, and prognosis. Acta Paediatr 1998;87(8):871–8.

[178] Duerr RH. Genome-wide association studies herald a new era of rapid discoveries in inflammatory bowel disease research. Gastroenterology 2007; 132(5):2045–9.

[179] Van Limbergen J, Russell RK, Nimmo ER, et al. The genetics of inflammatory bowel disease. Am J Gastroenterol 2007;102(12):2820–31.

[180] Mathew CG. New links to the pathogenesis of Crohn's disease provided by genome-wide association scans. Nat Rev Genet 2008;9(1):9–14.

[181] Schreiber S, Rosenstiel P, Albrecht M, et al. Genetics of Crohn's disease, an archetypal inflammatory barrier disease. Nat Rev Genet 2005;6(5):376–88.

[182] Neurath MF. IL-23: a master regulator in Crohn's disease. Nat Med 2007;13(1):26–8.

[183] Hampe J, Franke A, Rosenstiel P, et al. A genome-wide association scan of nonsynonymous SNPs identifies a susceptibility variant for Crohn's disease in ATG16L1. Nat Genet 2007;39(2):207–11.

[184] Parkes M, Barrett JC, Prescott NJ, et al. Sequence variants in the autophagy gene IRGM and multiple other replicating loci contribute to Crohn's disease susceptibility. Nat Genet 2007;39(7):830–2.

[185] Xavier RJ, Podolsky DK. Unraveling the pathogenesis of inflammatory bowel disease. Nature 2007;448(7152):427–34.

[186] Rarok AA, van der Geld YM, Stegeman CA, et al. Diversity of PR3-ANCA epitope specificity in Wegener's granulomatosis. Analysis using the biosensor technology. J Clin Immunol 2003;23(6): 460–8.

[187] Gencik M, Meller S, Borgmann S, et al. Proteinase 3 gene polymorphisms and Wegener's granulomatosis. Kidney Int 2000;58(6):2473–7.

[188] Pieters K, Pettersson A, Gullberg U, et al. The - 564 A/G polymorphism in the promoter region of the proteinase 3 gene associated with Wegener's granulomatosis does not increase the promoter activity. Clin Exp Immunol 2004;138(2):266–70.

[189] Szyld P, Jagiello P, Csernok E, et al. On the Wegener's granulomatosis-associated region on chromosome 6p21.3. BMC Med Genet 2006;7:21–32.

[190] Jagiello P, Aries P, Arning L, et al. The PTPN22 620W allele is a risk factor for Wegener's granulomatosis. Arthritis Rheum 2005;52(12):4039–43.

[191] Huang D, Giscombe R, Zhou Y, et al. Polymorphisms in CTLA-4 but not tumor necrosis factor-alpha or interleukin 1beta genes are associated with Wegener's granulomatosis. J Rheumatol 2000;27(2):397–401.

[192] Zhou Y, Huang D, Paris PL, et al. An analysis of CTLA-4 and proinflammatory cytokine genes in Wegener's granulomatosis. Arthritis Rheum 2004; 50(8):2645–50.

[193] Muraközy G, Gaede KI, Ruprecht B, et al. Gene polymorphisms of immunoregulatory cytokines and angiotensin-converting enzyme in Wegener's granulomatosis. J Mol Med 2001;79(11):665–70.

[194] Bartfai Z, Gaede KI, Russell KA, et al. Different gender-associated genotype risks of Wegener's granulomatosis and microscopic polyangiitis. Clin Immunol 2003;109(3):330–7.

[195] Zhou Y, Giscombe R, Huang D, et al. Novel genetic association of Wegener's granulomatosis with the interleukin 10 gene. J Rheumatol 2002; 29(2):317–20.

[196] Seitzer U, Gerdes J, Müller-Quernheim J. Genotyping in the MHC locus: potential for defining predictive markers in sarcoidosis. Respir Res 2002;3(1):6–12.

[197] Grutters JC, Sato H, Welsh KI, et al. The importance of sarcoidosis genotype to lung phenotype. Am J Respir Cell Mol Biol 2003;29(3 Suppl): S59–62.

[198] Gaede KI, Kataria YP, Mamat U, et al. Analysis of differentially regulated mRNAs in monocytic cells induced by in vitro stimulation with

Kveim-Siltzbach test reagent. Exp Lung Res 2004;
30(3):181–92.

[199] Sato H, Spagnolo P, Silveira L, et al. BTNL2 allele
associations with chronic beryllium disease in
HLA-DPB1*Glu69-negative individuals. Tissue
Antigens 2007;70(6):480–6.

[200] Grunewald J, Eklund A. Human leukocyte antigen
genes may outweigh racial background when
generating a specific immune response in sarcoidosis. Eur Respir J 2001;17(5):1046–8.

[201] Takashige N, Naruse TK, Matsumori A, et al.
Genetic polymorphisms at the tumour necrosis
factor loci (TNFA and TNFB) in cardiac sarcoidosis. Tissue Antigens 1999;54(2):191–3.

[202] Rutherford RM, Kehren J, Staedtler F, et al. Functional genomics in sarcoidosis-reduced or increased
apoptosis? Swiss Med Wkly 2001;131(31–32):
459–70.

[203] Thonhofer R, Maercker C, Popper HH. Expression of sarcoidosis related genes in lung lavage

cells. Sarcoidosis Vasc Diffuse Lung Dis 2002;
19(1):59–65.

[204] Sabounchi-Schutt F, Astrom J, Hellman U, et al.
Changes in bronchoalveolar lavage fluid proteins
in sarcoidosis: a proteomics approach. Eur Respir
J 2003;21(3):414–20.

[205] Magi B, Bini L, Perari MG, et al. Bronchoalveolar
lavage fluid protein composition in patients with
sarcoidosis and idiopathic pulmonary fibrosis:
a two-dimensional electrophoretic study. Electrophoresis 2002;23(19):3434–44.

[206] Rottoli P, Magi B, Perari MG, et al. Cytokine profile
and proteome analysis in bronchoalveolar lavage of
patients with sarcoidosis, pulmonary fibrosis associated with systemic sclerosis and idiopathic pulmonary fibrosis. Proteomics 2005;5(5):1423–30.

[207] Wahlstrom J, Dengjel J, Persson B, et al. Identification of HLA-DR-bound peptides presented by
human bronchoalveolar lavage cells in sarcoidosis.
J Clin Invest 2007;117(11):3576–82.

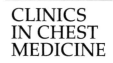

CLINICS
IN CHEST
MEDICINE

Clin Chest Med 29 (2008) 415–427

The Diagnosis of Sarcoidosis

Marc A. Judson, MD

Division of Pulmonary and Critical Care Medicine, CSB-812, Medical University of South Carolina,
96 Jonathan Lucas Street, Charleston, SC 29466, USA

Although it has been claimed that the method of diagnosis of sarcoidosis has been established [1], the reality is that the diagnosis can never be assured completely. There are certain clinical features that are typical of sarcoidosis but there are none that are specific for the diagnosis. Thus, sarcoidosis is a diagnosis of exclusion and it is impossible to fully exclude alternative diagnoses. This article outlines the current diagnostic criteria, diagnostic strategies, and pitfalls in making the diagnosis of sarcoidosis.

Definition

Sarcoidosis has been defined as a multisystem disorder of unknown cause [1]. Clinicoradiologic findings alone are inadequate to make a diagnosis of sarcoidosis, although in special situations a presumptive diagnosis may be made (vide infra). Likewise, the presence of granulomas on tissue biopsy alone is also inadequate for the diagnosis of sarcoidosis. Even finding the histologic evidence in a patient with clinical and radiographic features of sarcoidosis is not definitive. The diagnosis is established when clinicoradiologic findings are supported by histologic evidence of noncaseating epitheliod cell granulomas, and other causes of granulomas and local sarcoid reactions must be excluded [1]. It is prudent to maintain a healthy degree of skepticism at all times that an alternative diagnosis has been overlooked.

Diagnostic approach

Fig. 1 outlines the diagnostic approach to sarcoidosis. This is a multistep process that usually involves collecting clinical information, histologic examination of tissue for the presence of granulomatous inflammation, exclusion of other known causes of granuloma formation, and documentation that the granulomatous inflammation is present in at least two organs. Establishing a diagnosis of sarcoidosis without following this algorithm is suspect and should be done with caution. In subsequent sections of this article, each aspect of this algorithm is described in detail.

Clinical findings

As with most diseases, establishing the diagnosis of sarcoidosis begins with collecting clinical data. Certain clinical findings suggest the diagnosis of sarcoidosis, although none of them is pathopneumonic. The process involves judging the clinical data that support the diagnosis of sarcoidosis and weighing it against data that refute it. If sufficient clinical evidence accumulates to suggest the diagnosis of sarcoidosis, a tissue biopsy is normally indicated. Table 1 outlines clinical data often used to gauge the likelihood of the diagnosis of sarcoidosis.

Demographics

Sarcoidosis is rare before adulthood and in the elderly. The disease usually presents before 40 years of age, peaking in those aged 20 to 29 [2]. There is a second smaller peak in women over age 50 [3]. The disease is more prevalent in certain ethnicities, such as African Americans [4] and Northern Europeans [3].

Medical history

Patients with sarcoidosis often have no symptoms, and therefore the diagnosis should be

E-mail address: judsonma@musc.edu

0272-5231/08/$ - see front matter © 2008 Elsevier Inc. All rights reserved.
doi:10.1016/j.ccm.2008.03.009

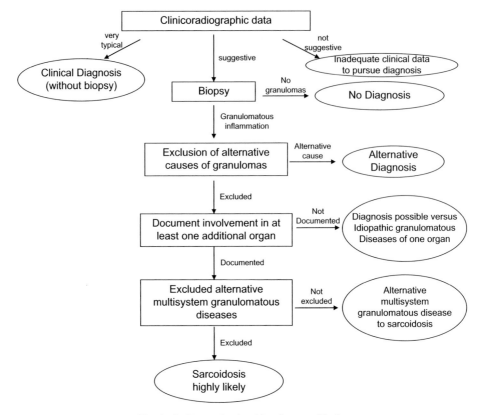

Fig. 1. A diagnostic algorithm for sarcoidosis.

considered in asymptomatic patients with mediastinal or hilar adenopathy or diffuse parenchymal ifiltrates on a chest radiograph [5,6]. A family history should be obtained because first degree relatives of sarcoidosis patients have a much higher prevalence rate of sarcoidosis than that found in the general population [7]. A smoking history should be elucidated because sarcoidosis is more common in nonsmokers [8].

Evidence of extrapulmonary involvement

Because sarcoidosis is a systemic disease, evidence that a disorder is present in two or more organ systems supports the diagnosis of sarcoidosis. At presentation, 95% of patients have clinical evidence of pulmonary sarcoidosis, and more than 40% of sarcoidosis patients have evidence of involvement of the skin, peripheral lymph node, eye, or liver [9]. Therefore, sarcoidosis should be considered in patients who present with pulmonary disease and concomitant disease in one of these organs.

Serum angiotensin converting enzyme

Serum angiotensin-converting enzyme (SACE) is produced in the epithelioid cell of the sarcoid granuloma [10], and SACE levels reflect the total granuloma burden in sarcoidosis [11]. Although an elevated SACE was initially thought to be diagnostic of sarcoidosis [12], it is neither sensitive nor specific enough to be diagnostic for the disease. In a study of 1,941 sarcoidosis patients, 1,575 control subjects, and 1,355 patients with other diseases, the sensitivity of SACE for sarcoidosis was 57%, the specificity 90%, the positive predictive value 90%, and the negative predictive value 60% [13].

Radiographic findings

Bilateral hilar adenopathy on chest radiograph suggests the diagnosis of sarcoidosis, especially if the patient has no fever, night sweats, or weight loss [5,6]. Findings on chest high-resolution computed tomography (HRCT) may be more specific for the diagnosis of sarcoidosis than the chest

Table 1
Clinicoradiographic data supporting or weakening the likelihood of sarcoidosis

	Supports	Weakens
Demographics	United States African American	Age <18 years
	Northern European	Age >50 years in males
Medical history	Nonsmoking	Exposure to tuberculosis
	No symptoms (in patients with CXR findings)	Exposure to organic bioaerosol
	Positive family history of sarcoidosis	Exposure to beryllium
	Symptoms involving >2 organs commonly involved with sarcoidosis (eg, lung and eyes)	Intravenous drug abuse
Laboratory data	Elevated SACE	
Radiographic findings	Bilateral hilar adenopathy (especially if without symptoms)	
	HRCT: Disease along the bronchovascular bundle	

Abbreviations: CXR, chest radiograph; HRCT, high-resolution computer tomography; SACE, serum angiotensin converting enzyme.

radiograph, although inadequate for the diagnosis to be made without histologic confirmation. Pulmonary sarcoidosis has a predilection for the bronchovascular bundle and subpleural locations (Fig. 2) [14]. Thoracic adenopathy is also more often detected on HRCT than chest radiograph.

Making a diagnosis of sarcoidosis based on clinical findings alone

On rare occasions, the constellation of presenting clinical findings is so typical of sarcoidosis that the diagnosis can be assumed without a tissue biopsy (see Fig. 1). Even in these situations, the clinician often must exclude alternative diagnoses before assuming that the patent has sarcoidosis (eg, Lofgren's syndrome, which is bilateral hilar adenopathy on chest radiograph and erythema nodosum skin lesions, requires the exclusion of coccidiodomycosis). Box 1 lists clinical presentations that may be assumed to be sarcoidosis without tissue confirmation.

Selection of the biopsy site

With the exception of the rare instance where the clinical findings are very specific for sarcoidosis, the diagnosis will require a tissue biopsy (see Fig. 1). Even when the patient has evidence of pulmonary or other visceral organs involved with sarcoidosis, it is in the patient's interest to select a biopsy site associated with least morbidity. For example, a skin biopsy is at lower risk of complications than a biopsy of other organs.

Therefore, a careful skin examination should be performed in a patient with suspected sarcoidosis. The patient should be questioned about the presence of scars and tattoos because nodules that develop on these are usually granulomatous reactions. Other biopsy sites that should be considered include enlarged peripheral lymph nodes and the conjunctiva if nodules are seen [15].

Transbronchial lung biopsy (TLB) has a diagnostic yield for pulmonary sarcoidosis in 40% to more than 90% of cases. It is recommended that four to five lung biopsies be performed to maximize the diagnostic yield. TLB is more likely to be diagnostic in patients with parenchymal disease on chest radiograph (radiographic stage II or III) than in those with a normal lung parenchyma (radiographic stage 0 or I) [16].

Endobronchial biopsy has a diagnostic yield of 40% to 60% for sarcoidosis. Furthermore, endobronchial biopsy can be performed with the TLB procedure and has been shown to increase the diagnostic yield for sarcoidosis above that by using TLB alone [17].

The conditions associated with bilateral hilar adenopathy may have to be reevaluated. The yield of TLB for the diagnosis of sarcoidosis is approximately 50% in patients with hilar adenopathy alone [18,19]. In the past, the alternative diagnostic approach was mediastinoscopy, which is associated with significant cost and morbidity [6]. Recently, the diagnostic yield from endobronchial needle aspiration has approached 90% when ultrasound guidance has been used [20,21]. Therefore, many cases of bilateral hilar adenopathy that were assumed to be sarcoidosis because of

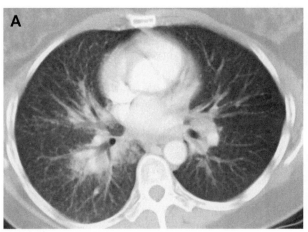
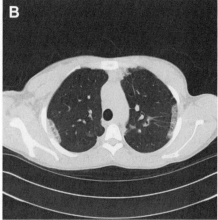

Fig. 2. (*A*) Chest CT scan of a patient with pulmonary sarcoidosis showing disease primarily along the brochovascular bundles, a common location. (*B*) Chest CT scan of a patient with pulmonary sarcoidosis showing subpleural parenchymal disease, another common location.

the risks of mediastinoscopy can now be diagnosed with lower risk, at lower cost, and as an outpatient procedure.

Bronchoalveolar lavage (BAL) with examination of lymphocyte populations (CD4/CD8 ratio) is sometimes used as a complementary test for the diagnosis of sarcoidosis. Greater than 15% lymphocytes in BAL fluid has a sensitivity of 90% for the diagnosis of sarcoidosis [22], although the specificity is low. In one study [22], a lymphocyte CD4/CD8 ratio of greater than 3.5 had a sensitivity of 53%, specificity of 94%, a positive predictive value of 76%, and a negative predictive value of 85% for the diagnosis of sarcoidosis.

Pathology

Although in almost all cases granulomas are necessary to establish a diagnosis of sarcoidosis, it is important to recognize that granulomas are nonspecific inflammatory reactions, and they are not diagnostic of sarcoidosis or any other granulomatous disease [23]. Every biopsy should be searched for causes of granulomatous inflammation, such as mycobacteria, fungi, parasites, and foreign bodies (eg, talc) [24].

Although there are no specific diagnostic features of sarcoid granulomas, there may be certain typical characteristics that suggest the diagnosis. The sarcoid granuloma usually consists of a compact (organized) collection of mononuclear phagocytes (macrophages or epitheliod cells) [25]. There is typically no necrosis, but on occasion there is a small to moderate amount.

Usually there is fusion of giant cells within the sarcoid granuloma to form multinucleated giant cells. These granulomas are usually surrounded by a peripheral mantle of lymphocytes. A variety of inclusions may be present, such as Schaumann's bodies, asteroid bodies, birefringent crystals, and Hamazaki-Wesenberg bodies; however, these inclusions are nonspecific and not diagnostic of sarcoidosis [23].

Box 1. Clinical presentations that may be assumed to be sarcoidosis without tissue comformation, provided additional data does not suggest an alternative diagnosis

Lofgren's syndrome
   Bilateral hilar adenopathy on chest
     radiograph
   Erythema nodosum skin lesions
   Fever (often)
   (ankle) arthralgias/arthritis (often)
Herfort's syndrome
   Uveitis
   Parotidis
   Fever (often)
Bilateral hilar adenopathy on chest
   radiograph without symptoms
Positive Panda sign (parotid and lacrimal
   gland uptake) and Lambda sign
   (bilateral hilar and right paratracheal
   lymph node uptake) on gallium −67
   scan

Box 2. Major pathologic differential diagnosis of sarcoidosis at biopsy

Lung
  Tuberculosis
  Atypical mycobacteriosis
  Fungi
  Pneumocystis carinii
  Mycoplasma
  Hypersensitivity pneumonitis
  Pneumoconiosis: beryllium (chronic beryllium disease), titanium, aluminum
  Drug reactions
  Aspiration of foreign materials
  Wegener's granulomatosis (sarcoid-type granulomas are rare)
  Necrotizing sarcoid granulomatosis
Lymph node
  Tuberculosis
  Atypical mycobacteriosis
  Brucellosis
  Toxoplasmosis
  Granulomatous histiocytic necrotizing lymphademitis (Kikuchi's disease)
  Cat-scratch disease
  Sarcoid reaction in regional lymph nodes to carcinoma
  Hodgkin's disease
  Non-Hodgkin's lymphomas
  Granulomatous lesions of unknown significance (GLUS syndrome)
Skin
  Tuberculosis
  Atypical mycobacteriosis
  Fungi
  Reaction to foreign bodies: beryllium, zirconium, tattooing, paraffin, and others
  Rheumatoid nodules
Liver
  Tuberculosis
  Brucellosis
  Schistosomiasis
  Primary biliary cirrhosis
  Crohn's disease
  Hodgkin's disease
  Non-Hodgkin's lymphomas
  GLUS syndrome
Bone marrow
  Tuberculosis
  Histoplasmosis

  Infectious mononucleosis
  Cytomegalovirus
  Hodgkin's disease
  Non-Hodgkin's lymphomas
  Drugs
  GLUS syndrome
Other biopsy sites
  Tuberculosis
  Brucellosis
  Other infections
  Crohn's disease
  Giant cell myocarditis
  GLUS syndrome

Exclusion of alternative causes of granulomatous inflammation

Box 2 lists the differential diagnosis for granulomata based on the organ system involved. The diagnosis of sarcoidosis requires that all of these diseases be excluded to a reasonable degree.

The exclusion of alternative causes of granulomatous inflammation requires a multifaceted approach. The histologic specimen must be examined for infectious agents and foreign bodies capable of inducing a granulomatous reaction. This requires staining the specimen for mycobacteria and fungi at a minimum. Cultures for these organisms should usually be performed.

A detailed medical history is essential to exclude potential occupational exposures (eg, beryllium), environmental exposures (eg, an organic bioaerosol, such as significant bird or hot tub exposure causing hypersensitivity pneumonitis), and potential exposure to infectious agents (eg, tuberculosis). A recent study found that 40% of patients diagnosed with sarcoidosis demonstrated hypersensitivity to beryllium and had significant beryllium exposure [26].

If the medical history suggests a possible alternative diagnosis, additional tests may need to be performed. Examples include a beryllium lymphocyte proliferation test for chronic beryllium disease and antibody testing for hypersensitivity pneumonitis.

Verifying multiple organ involvement

The presence of noncaseating granulomata in a single organ does not conclusively establish the diagnosis of sarcoidosis because sarcoidosis, by definition, is a systemic disease that should involve multiple organs. There are idiopathic granulomatous diseases of individual organs that are distinguished from sarcoidosis. For example, idiopathic granulomatous hepatitis, where non-caseating granulomas of unknown cause are found solely in the liver, is rarely found to be sarcoidosis (extrahepatic granulomata usually do not develop over time) [27]. Another example is idiopathic panuveitis, a granulomatous uveitis without additional organ involvement that is common in the southeastern United States [28].

Even though granulomatous inflammation documented in only one organ is not diagnostic of sarcoidosis, treatment is usually identical to that for sarcoidosis provided that alternative causes of granulomatous inflammation can be excluded. Therefore, it is usually unnecessary to search for involvement of a second organ if it is not clinically obvious. Box 3 lists the extent of the workup that should be performed to evaluate for a second organ involved with granulomatous inflammation.

Although the diagnosis of sarcoidosis requires proof of granulomatous involvement in at least two separate organs, histologic confirmation is not necessarily required in the second organ. For example, noncaseating granulomata in the skin alone is inadequate for the diagnosis of sarcoidosis, but the presence of concomitant bilateral hilar adenopathy on chest radiograph is thought to be sufficient evidence of second organ involvement such that a hilar lymph node or lung is not required [29]. A consensus panel of sarcoidosis experts has developed clinical criteria for when a second organ can be considered involved with sarcoidosis without biopsy (this presumes that noncaseating granulomas have been detected in the "first" organ) (Table 2) [29].

Box 3. Extent of workup for second organ involvement if a biopsy has revealed granulomatous inflammation consistent with sarcoidosis

Chest radiograph
Liver function tests
Complete blood count
Ophthalmologic examination
Electrocardiogram
Serum calcium
Urinalysis

The Kveim test

An old diagnostic test for sarcoidosis is the Kveim test, where a splenic suspension from a spleen involved with sarcoidosis is innoculated intradermally [30]. If after 4 to 6 weeks a skin nodule appears at the inoculation site, is biopsied, and reveals noncaseating granulomas, this is highly specific for the diagnosis of sarcoidosis. Unfortunately, the test is not extremely sensitive: both the sensitivity and specificity vary depending upon the spleen that is used, and the suspension is not Food and Drug Administration approved. Therefore the Kveim test is not a standard diagnostic test for sarcoidosis.

Examples of diagnostic dilemmas

This section describes some examples of applying the diagnostic sarcoidosis algorithm to specific cases.

Case 1

The patient was a 66-year-old Caucasian man referred for the evaluation of dyspnea. He had a clinical diagnosis of sarcoidosis made 20 years earlier, based upon chest radiographic findings without a confirmatory tissue biopsy. He was short of breath both walking on level ground and climbing stairs. He also developed dyspnea when he visited Colorado and went to high altitudes. Further history revealed that he worked at a Cruise missile factory and specifically worked with beryllium in the 1960s. His job was to mix beryllium into wet clay to make a porcelain cone for the missile. He used sealed sacks of beryllium and wore a respirator. The air was filtered before it was exhaled from the mixing box. He was also assigned to changing and cleaning this filter, which he also performed wearing a respirator.

His physical examination was essentially normal. Pulmonary function tests revealed a forced vital capacity (FVC) 2.54 L (55% predicted), forced expiratory volume in 1 second (FEV_1) 1.08 L (30% predicted), FEV_1/FVC equaling 0.43, and diffusing capacity (DLCO) 13.1 mL/ mm Hg per minute (39% predicted).

Chest HRCT revealed bilateral hilar adenopathy (Fig. 3A) and scattered parenchymal opacities most prominent in subpleural locations (see Fig. 3B). A beryllium lymphocyte proliferation test of lymphocytes obtained from peripheral blood showed abnormally high stimulation to beryllium sulfate (mean stimulation index for 10^{-4}M beryllium sulfate: 7.5 at day 4, 5.2 at day 6; for 10^{-5}M beryllium sulfate: 8.3 at day 4, 11.7 at day 6; abnormal is two or more values >2.5).

Final diagnosis
Chronic beryllium disease.

Comment
Chronic beryllium disease (CBD) can mimic pulmonary sarcoidosis radiographically by demonstrating bilateral hilar adenopathy and pulmonary infiltrates [31]. Although CBD is usually confined to the lung, extrapulmonary manifestations can sometimes occur [32]. CBD has been misdiagnosed as sarcoidosis in up to 40% of cases [26]. For these reasons it is mandatory to take an adequate occupational history concerning possible beryllium exposure in all patients with a potential diagnosis of sarcoidosis. Beryllium lymphocyte proliferation testing is the diagnostic test for CBD [33]. Usually lymphocytes obtained from peripheral blood are adequate, but the sensitivity and specificity of the test are nearly 100% when lymphocytes obtained from BAL are used [34].

Case 2

The patient was a 65-year-old Caucasian woman who presented with neutropenic fever. She had been treated for 1 week for pneumonia. She complained of a productive cough and fevers for months. She also had nausea and abdominal pain. Splenomegaly had been detected 9 months earlier. Monospot and Epstein Barr virus titers had been negative. Her physical examination revealed a temperature of 99.7°F and a spleen edge 4 cm below the left costal margin. Her admission white blood cell count was 1,730/cu mm with an absolute neutrophil count of 560/cu mm. A chest HRCT showed significant mediastinal adenopathy (Fig. 4A) and scattered bilateral ground glass infiltrates. Her marked splenomegaly was confirmed on abdominal CT scan (see Fig. 4B). A transbronchial needle aspiration of a mediastinal lymph node under ultrasound guidance (TBNA-EBUS) revealed noncaseating granulomatous inflammation consistent with sarcoidosis. BAL showed 184 red blood cells, 387 nucleated cells, with 85% lymphocytes. CD markers were not obtained. Although a bone marrow biopsy had been planned to evaluate her neutropenia, it was cancelled once a diagnosis of sarcoidosis had been made.

The patient was started on a prednisone at a dose of 20 mg daily, which was tapered to 10 mg per day over the subsequent 3 months. However, her neutropenia, abdominal pain, and splenomegaly failed to resolve. She again developed neutropenic fevers and was admitted to the hospital. Because of her failure to respond to corticosteroid therapy, a bone marrow biopsy was performed that revealed a B-cell lymphoma.

Final diagnosis
B-cell lymphoma.

Comment
Lymphoma needs to be considered when lymph node tissue shows granulomatous inflammation (see Box 2). One clue that sarcoidosis was the incorrect diagnosis was the patient's failure to respond to corticosteroid therapy. Another important clue concerned the appearance of the spleen on the abdominal CT scan. Splenic sarcoidosis usually appears as low attenuation nodules that may coalesce into mass-like lesions [35]. This patient's spleen appeared quite enlarged but without evidence of low attenuation lesions.

Case 3

The patient was a 62-year-old Caucasian female who was referred for an abnormal chest radiograph. She had a history of pneumonia 8 months previously. She smoked more than one pack of cigarettes daily for the previous 45 years and carried a diagnosis of chronic obstructive pulmonary disease. She had chronic dyspnea, with difficulty climbing stairs and doing household chores. She had no symptoms of cough, chest pain, fever, or weight loss. She had a history of several episodes of depression, including previous suicide attempts.

Her physical examination was normal except for diffusely diminished breath sounds. Pulmonary function tests showed FVC 1.80 L (67% predicted), FEV_1 0.95 L (49% predicted), FEV_1/FVC equaling 0.53. A chest radiograph revealed a left hilar mass that was confirmed on a chest CT scan (Fig. 5A). Given the patient's significant smoking history, a lung carcinoma was suspected. The patient underwent total body 18F-fluorodeoxyglucose PET scanning that showed intense uptake in the left hilum, corresponding to the lesion seen on the chest CT scan. A TBNA-EBUS biopsy of the enlarged left hilar lymph node showed granulomatous inflammation without any evidence of malignancy (see Fig. 5B).

Table 2
Clinical criteria for extrapulmonary sarcoidosis organ involvement in patients with biopsy-confirmed sarcoidosis in another organ

Organ	Definite	Probable	Possible
Lungs	Chest roentgenogram with one or more of the following: Bilateral hilar adenopathy Diffuse infiltrates Upper lobe fibrosis Restriction on pulmonary function tests	Lymphocytic alveolitis by BAL Any pulmonary infiltrates Isolated reduced diffusing capacity for carbon monoxide	Any other adenopathy Obstructive pulmonary function tests
Skin	Lupus pernio Annular lesion Erythema nodosum	Macular/palular New nodules	Keloids Hypopigmentation
Eyes	Lacrimal gland swelling Uveitis Optic neuritis	Blindness Positive in vivo confocal microscopy	Glaucoma Cataract
Liver	Liver function tests > three times the upper limit of normal	Compatible CT scan Elevated alkaline phosphate	
Hypercalcemia/hypercalciuria/ nephrolithiasis	Increased serum calcium with no other cause	Increased urine calcium Nephrolithiasis analysis showing calcium	Nephrolithiasis—no stone analysis Nephrolithiasis with negative family history for stones
Neurologic	Positive MRI with uptake in meninges or brainstem Cerebrospinal fluid with increased lymphocytes or protein Diabetes insipidus Bell's palsy Cranial nerve dysfunction Peripheral nerve biopsy PET scan of central nervous system or spinal cord	Other abnormalities on MR imaging Unexpected neuropathy Positive electromyogram	Unexplained headaches Peripheral nerve radiculopathy
Renal	Treatment responsive renal failure	Steroid responsive diabetes failure in patient who has diatetes or hypertension	Renal failure in absence of other disease

Organ			
Cardiac	Treatment responsive cardiomyopathy Electrocardiogram showing intraventricular conduction defect or nodal block Positive gallium scan of heart PET scan of the heart	No other cardiac problem and either: Ventricular arrhythmias Cardiomyuopathy Positive thallium scan	In patient with diabetes or hypertension: Cardiomyopathy Ventricular arrhythmias
Nonthoracic lymph node		New palpable node above waist Lymph node > 2 cm by CT scan	New palpable femoral lymph node
Bone marrow	Unexplained anemia Leukopenia Thrombocytopenia		Anemia with low mean corpuscular volume
Spleen		Enlargement by: Exam CT scan Radioisotope scan	
Bone/joints	Cystic changes on hand or feet radiographs	Asymmetric, painful clubbing	Arthritis with no other cause
Ear/nose/throat		Unexplained hoarseness with examination consistent with granulomatous involvement	New onset sinusitis New onset dizziness
Parotid/salivary glands	Symmetric parotitis with syndrome of mumps Positive gallium scan (Panda sign)		Dry mouth
Muscles	Increased creatine phosphokinase (CK)/aldolase which decreases with treatment	Increased CK/aldolase	Myalgias responding to treatment
Other organs			

There can be no other explanation for the clinical findings in this table for these criteria to be valid. In addition, biopsy of each of these organs would constitute "definite" involvement.

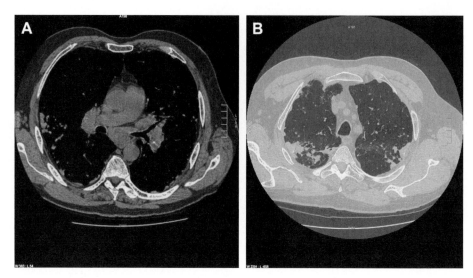

Fig. 3. (*A*) Chest CT scan of case #1 showing bilateral hilar adenopathy with some calcium in the lymph nodes. (*B*) Chest CT scan of case #1 showing peripheral/subleural parenchymal opacities.

Corticosteroid therapy was considered as a treatment and a diagnostic test, because if the mass would decrease in size, this would favor sarcoidosis as the diagnosis. However, this was rejected because of the potential effect of corticosteroids upon the patient's psychologic disorder. A plan was devised to inject decadron into the left hilar mass via a transbronchial needle under ultrasound guidance. This procedure was arranged 3 months after the first TBNA. However, in the interim, numerous pulmonary nodules had developed (see

Fig. 5C). The left hilar mass also decreased somewhat in size. The patient underwent a bronchoscopy with BAL and transbrochial lung biopsy. The BAL revealed 500 nucleated cells with 5% lymphocytes and 87% macrophages. The TLB showed an acute lung injury pattern with no granulomas seen.

Final diagnosis

Indeterminate. This is probably sarcoidosis but lung carcinoma cannot be excluded.

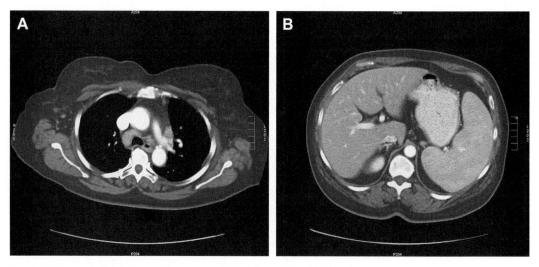

Fig. 4. (*A*) Chest CT scan of case #2 showing mediastinal adenopathy. (*B*) Lower cut of chest CT scan of case #2 showing an enlarged spleen.

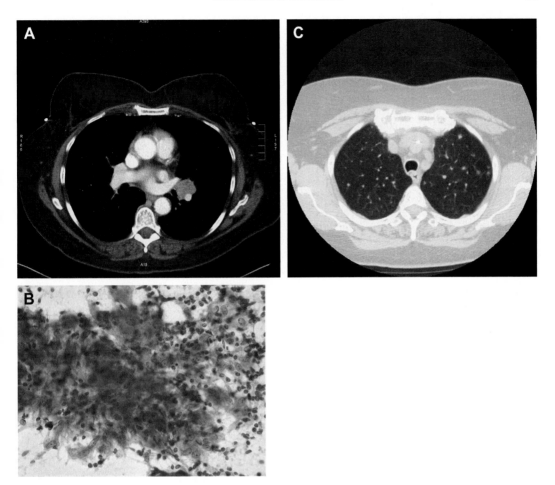

Fig. 5. (*A*) Chest CT scan of case #3 revealing a left hilar mass. (*B*) Transbrochial needle aspiration biopsy under ultrasound guidance of case #3 revealed this specimen, showing granulomatous inflammation (hematoxylin and eosin stain, original magnification x20). (*C*) Chest CT scan of case #3 taken 3 months after the first scan. Numerous pulmonary nodules are seen, mostly on the left side in this particular cut. The left hilar mass has shrunk in size (not shown).

Comment

The patient has a unilateral hilar mass and an extensive smoking history. Both of these facts are suggestive of lung carcinoma and make the diagnosis of sarcoidosis less likely. The 18F-fluorodeoxyglucose PET scan may reveal uptake both in malignant and sarcoidosis lesions, so this test cannot differentiate the two [36]. Fluorine-18-alpha-methyltyrosine PET scanning may be better than 18F-fluorodeoxyglucose to distinguish sarcoidosis from malignancy, as it is only positive in the latter [37]. The subsequent HRCT showed the development of numerous pulmonary nodules. This would be more likely seen with sarcoidosis than lung cancer, although both conditions remain possible. This case illustrates that on

occasion the diagnosis of sarcoidosis cannot be distinguished from alternative diagnoses.

Other idiopathic systemic granulomatous diseases

To confuse matters further, there are other multiorgan idiopathic granulomatous syndromes that are clinically disparate from sarcoidosis, such that they are thought to be separate entities (see Fig. 1). Blau's Syndrome consists of granulomatous arthritis, iritis, and skin rash. It is autosomal dominant with variable penetrance, and the age of onset is usually before age 12 years. It is considered a separate entity from childhood sarcoidosis on the basis of a lack of visceral (including pulmonary) involvement and mode of inheritance [38].

Recently, the Blau's syndrome gene has been identified [39].

In 1989, Brinker described a syndrome with: prolonged fever; epithelioid granulomata in the liver, bone marrow, spleen, and lymph nodes; a benign course; and a tendency for recurrence. This entity has been labeled the GLUS syndrome: granulomatous lesions of unknown significance. Although it has been argued that the GLUS syndrome is a form of extrapulmonary sarcoidosis, differences include the following: (1) elevated SACE levels have never been found with the GLUS syndrome, (2) hypercalcemia is never found with the GLUS syndrome, (3) the Kveim test has always been negative in the GLUS syndrome, and (4) immunotyping of T cells in the granulomata of GLUS syndrome patients is distinctly different from that of the granulomata of sarcoidosis patients [40].

Necrotizing sarcoid granulomatosis is a disease characterized by a granulomatous vasculitis. Because vessels are involved, necrosis is a prominent feature unlike most cases of sarcoidosis [41]. It is a systemic disease and may involve extrapulmonary organs [42]. It is debated whether it is a separate disease entity or a form of sarcoidosis [43].

The future

Obviously sarcoidosis has causes. A half century ago, chronic beryllium disease was diagnosed as sarcoidosis as the metal was not known to cause a granulomatous reaction. In the future, it is likely that other "sarcoidoses" of known cause will be identified that can be pared off from what is now diagnosed as sarcoidosis.

In addition, the future diagnosis of sarcoidosis will probably couple genetics with exposure. It is thought that sarcoidosis results from the exposure of genetically susceptible hosts to specific environmental agents. As more is understood about the immune response, it may be possible to identify individuals who mount a granulomatous response to specific exposures causing sarcoidosis. In this way, sarcoidosis may move from a disease of unknown cause to disease where the etiology is known.

Summary

The diagnosis of sarcoidosis is never definitive. The process of diagnosis begins with the collection of clinical data. If enough data accumulate so that sarcoidosis is a reasonable possibility, a search is made for a possible organ to biopsy, selecting the least invasive biopsy location (eg, the skin). The biopsy should reveal granulomatous inflammation. Histologic examination should exclude other known causes of granulomatous inflammation, such as infectious agents and foreign bodies. Medical history should be carefully reviewed to be certain that it included exposures that are associated with known granulomatous diseases, as these may have been omitted at the initial evaluation. The features of the biopsy should be examined for the compactness of the granulomas and the degree of necrosis. Although these characteristics are not specific for or against the diagnosis of sarcoidosis, they can contribute to the degree of certainty of the diagnosis. If sarcoidosis remains a reasonable consideration, a second organ involved with sarcoidosis should be identified. This can often be accomplished without the need of a second biopsy. The net result of this algorithm is not a definite diagnosis of sarcoidosis but a statistical likelihood of the diagnosis.

Acknowledgments

The author would like to thank Dr. Beth Baker for supplying the chronic beryllium disease case.

References

[1] Hunninghake GW, Costabel U, Ando M, et al. ATS/ERS/WASOG statement on sarcoidosis. American Thoracic Society/European Respiratory Society/World Association of Sarcoidosis and other Granulomatous Disorders. Sarcoidosis Vasc Diffuse Lung Dis 1999;16:149–73.

[2] Gordis L. Sarcoidosis. Epidemiology of chronic lung diseases in children. Baltimore (MD): Johns Hopkins University Press; 1973. p. 53–78.

[3] Milman N, Selroos O. Pulmonary sarcoidosis in the Nordic countries 1950–1982. Epidemiology and clinical picture. Sarcoidosis 1990;7:50–7.

[4] Rybicki BA, Major M, Popovich J Jr, et al. Racial differences in sarcoidosis incidence: a 5-year study in a health maintenance organization. Am J Epidemiol 1997;145:234–41.

[5] Winterbauer RH, Belic N, Moores KD. Clinical interpretation of bilateral hilar adenopathy. Ann Intern Med 1973;78:65–71.

[6] Reich JM, Brouns MC, O'Connor EA, et al. Mediastinoscopy in patients with presumptive stage I sarcoidosis: a risk/benefit, cost/benefit analysis. Chest 1998;113:147–53.

[7] Rybicki BA, Iannuzzi MC, Frederick MM, et al. Familial aggregation of sarcoidosis. A case-control

etiologic study of sarcoidosis (ACCESS). Am J Respir Crit Care Med 2001;164:2085–91.

[8] Newman LS, Rose CS, Bresnitz EA, et al. A case control etiologic study of sarcoidosis: environmental and occupational risk factors. Am J Respir Crit Care Med 2004;170:1324–30.

[9] Baughman RP, Teirstein AS, Judson MA, et al. Clinical characteristics of patients in a case control study of sarcoidosis. Am J Respir Crit Care Med 2001;164:1885–9.

[10] Sheffield EA. Pathology of sarcoidosis. Clin Chest Med 1997;18:741–54.

[11] Lynch JP 3rd, Kazerooni EA, Gay SE. Pulmonary sarcoidosis. Clin Chest Med 1997;18:755–85.

[12] Lieberman J. Elevation of serum angiotensin-converting-enzyme (ACE) level in sarcoidosis. Am J Med 1975;59:365–72.

[13] Studdy PR, James DG, editors. The specificity and sensitivity of serum angiotensin-converting enzyme in sarcoidosis and other diseases. Paris: Pergamon Press; 1983.

[14] Dawson WB, Muller NL. High-resolution computed tomography in pulmonary sarcoidosis. Semin Ultrasound CT MR 1990;11:423–9.

[15] Spaide RF, Ward DL. Conjunctival biopsy in the diagnosis of sarcoidosis. Br J Ophthalmol 1990;74:469–71.

[16] Gilman MJ, Wang KP. Transbronchial lung biopsy in sarcoidosis. An approach to determine the optimal number of biopsies. Am Rev Respir Dis 1980; 122:721–4.

[17] Shorr AF, Torrington KG, Hnatiuk OW. Endobronchial biopsy for sarcoidosis: a prospective study. Chest 2001;120:109–14.

[18] Poe RH, Israel RH, Utell MJ, et al. Probability of a positive transbronchial lung biopsy result in sarcoidosis. Arch Intern Med 1979;139:761–3.

[19] Koonitz CH, Joyner LR, Nelson RA. Transbronchial lung biopsy via the fiberoptic bronchoscope in sarcoidosis. Ann Intern Med 1976;85:64–6.

[20] Garwood S, Judson MA, Silvestri G, et al. Endobronchial ultrasound for the diagnosis of pulmonary sarcoidosis. Chest 2007;132:1298–304.

[21] Wong M, Yasufuku K, Nakajima T, et al. Endobronchial ultrasound: new insight for the diagnosis of sarcoidosis. Eur Respir J 2007;29:1182–6.

[22] Nagai S, Izumi T. Bronchoalveolar lavage. Still useful in diagnosing sarcoidosis? Clin Chest Med 1997; 18:787–97.

[23] Rosen Y. Pathology of sarcoidosis. Semin Respir Crit Care Med 2007;28:36–52.

[24] Schilstra A, Rottoli P, Jacobs JA, et al. Case studies to explore the pitfalls in the diagnosis of sarcoidosis. Sarcoidosis Vasc Diffuse Lung Dis 2006;23:135–40.

[25] Adams DO. The biology of the granuloma. In: Ioachim HL, editor. Pathology of granulomas. New York: Raven; 1983. p. 1–20.

[26] Muller-Quernheim J, Gaede KI, Fireman E, et al. Diagnoses of chronic beryllium disease within cohorts of sarcoidosis patients. Eur Respir J 2006;27:1190–5.

[27] Israel HL, Goldstein RA. Hepatic granulomatosis and sarcoidosis. Ann Intern Med 1973;79:669–78.

[28] Merrill PT, Kim J, Cox TA, et al. Uveitis in the southeastern United States. Curr Eye Res 1997;16: 865–74.

[29] Judson MA, Baughman RP, Teirstein AS, et al. Defining organ involvement in sarcoidosis: the ACCESS proposed instrument. ACCESS Research Group. A Case Control Etiologic Study of Sarcoidosis. Sarcoidosis Vasc Diffuse Lung Dis 1999;16:75–86.

[30] Siltzbach LE. The Kveim test in sarcoidosis. A study of 750 patients. JAMA 1961;178:476–82.

[31] Harris KM, McConnochie K, Adams H. The computed tomographic appearances in chronic berylliosis. Clin Radiol 1993;47:26–31.

[32] Fireman E, Haimsky E, Noiderfer M, et al. Misdiagnosis of sarcoidosis in patients with chronic beryllium disease. Sarcoidosis Vasc Diffuse Lung Dis 2003;20:144–8.

[33] Middleton DC, Lewin MD, Kowalski PJ, et al. The BeLPT: algorithms and implications. Am J Ind Med 2006;49:36–44.

[34] Rossman MD, Kern JA, Elias JA, et al. Proliferative response of bronchoalveolar lymphocytes to beryllium. A test for chronic beryllium disease. Ann Intern Med 1988;108:687–93.

[35] Judson MA. Gastrointesinal, hepatic, and splenic involvement with sarcoidosis. Semin Respir Crit Care Med 2002;23:529–41.

[36] Lewis PJ, Salama A. Uptake of fluorine-18-fluorodeoxyglucose in sarcoidosis. J Nucl Med 1994;35: 1647–9.

[37] Kaira K, Oriuchi N, Otani Y, et al. Diagnostic usefulness of fluorine-18-alpha-methyltyrosine positron emission tomography in combination with 18F-fluorodeoxyglucose in sarcoidosis patients. Chest 2007;131:1019–27.

[38] Manouvrier-Hanu S, Puech B, Piette F, et al. Blau syndrome of granulomatous arthritis, iritis, and skin rash: a new family and review of the literature. Am J Med Genet 1998;76:217–21.

[39] Kurokawa T, Kikuchi T, Ohta K, et al. Ocular manifestations in Blau syndrome associated with a CARD15/Nod2 mutation. Ophthalmology 2003; 110:2040–4.

[40] Brinker H. Granulomatous lesions of unknown significance: the GLUS syndrome. In: James DG, editor. Sarcoidosis and other granulomatous disorders. Philadelphia: W.B. Saunders; 1994. p. 69–86.

[41] Churg A, Carrington CB, Gupta R. Necrotizing sarcoid granulomatosis. Chest 1979;76:406–13.

[42] Dykhuizen RS, Smith CC, Kennedy MM, et al. Necrotizing sarcoid granulomatosis with extrapulmonary involvement. Eur Respir J 1997;10:245–7.

[43] Lazzarini LC, de Fatima do Amparo Teixeira M, Souza Rodrigues R, et al. Necrotizing sarcoid granulomatosis in a family of patients with sarcoidosis reinforces the association between both entities. Respiration 2007.

**ELSEVIER
SAUNDERS**

Clin Chest Med 29 (2008) 429–443

**CLINICS
IN CHEST
MEDICINE**

Cardiopulmonary Imaging in Sarcoidosis

Jason J. Akbar, MD*, Cris A. Meyer, MD, Ralph T. Shipley, MD,
Achala S. Vagal, MD

*Department of Radiology, University of Cincinnati Medical Center, 234 Goodman Street ML 0761,
Cincinnati, OH 45267-0761, USA*

Sarcoidosis was first described in 1877 and is a systemic granulomatous disorder with a wide range of radiologic and clinical manifestations. The first radiographic description of sarcoidosis occurred in 1915, 20 years after the discovery of the x ray [1]. Although the conventional chest radiograph remains the first imaging test of choice, the imaging options for the evaluation of sarcoidosis have significantly expanded. Clinically, sarcoidosis is a disease with protean clinical manifestations ranging from no symptoms to sudden death. Thus, radiologic tests often play a crucial role in the detection and diagnosis of this disorder. The armamentarium of advanced imaging options includes computed tomography (CT), standard high-resolution computed tomography (HRCT), and volumetric high-resolution computed tomography (VHRCT). Newer imaging technologies, such as gadolinium enhanced cardiac magnetic resonance (MR) imaging and positron emission tomography with computed tomography (PET/CT), proide physicians noninvasive methods to evaluate previously underrecognized areas of sarcoidosis involvement. Although sarcoidosis affects virtually every organ system, pulmonary involvement is most frequent. Previously underrecognized is the percentage of patients who have cardiac involvement, which has been implicated in up to 85% of sarcoidosis deaths in Japan [2]. In this article, we discuss current and future imaging technologies used in the diagnosis and follow-up of patients who have sarcoidosis, with a focus on cardiopulmonary involvement.

---

* Corresponding author.
E-mail address: akbarjj@uc.edu (J.J. Akbar).

Conventional chest radiograph in sarcoidosis

The conventional chest radiograph plays an important role in the diagnosis and prognosis of sarcoidosis. The minority (5%–10%) of patients who have sarcoidosis have a normal chest radiograph, with the vast majority of patients (75%–90%) demonstrating the typical symmetric mediastinal and hilar adenopathy. More than half of this majority are asymptomatic [3,4]. The finding of bilateral, symmetric hilar, and right paratracheal adenopathy is known by the eponym Garland's Triad (Fig. 1). Symmetric nodal involvement is important in distinguishing sarcoidosis from lymphoma, fungal disease, tuberculosis, and metastatic disease. On frontal chest radiograph, right paratracheal adenopathy manifests as thickening of the right paratracheal stripe with associated lobularity and increased density in this region. Other common sites of nodal involvement include the subcarina and aortopulmonary window [4,5]. Aortopulmonary window adenopathy can be recognized as a convex opacity between the aortic arch and pulmonary artery borders. Enlargement of the middle mediastinal nodes is unusual without concurrent hilar adenopathy [6]. Unilateral hilar adenopathy occurs in 1% to 3% of patients. Unilateral hilar adenopathy is the most frequent atypical manifestation of sarcoidosis in the older patient [7]. Although eggshell nodal calcifications can be seen in long standing sarcoidosis, it is not pathognomonic and can also be seen in histoplasmosis and silicosis [3].

In 25% to 50% of patients who have chest radiographic findings, pulmonary parenchymal disease is present. It is typically bilateral and symmetric with central and upper lobe

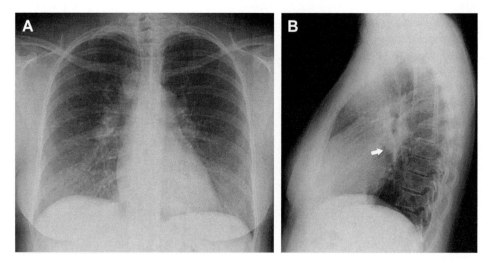

Fig. 1. (*A*) Stage I sarcoidosis PA radiograph demonstrating Garland's Triad, symmetric hilar, and right paratracheal adenopathy. (*B*) Lateral radiograph in the same patient with homogenous increased opacification of the hilar shadow with filling in of the infrahilar window (*arrow*), suggestive of hilar adenopathy.

predominance. Within the upper lobes, the posterior and apical segments are most severely affected, especially in the fibrotic stage [5,8,9]. Parenchymal involvement may be variable, with small nodules being most common in 30% to 60% of patients. These nodules range from 1 to 10 mm in size and predominate in the upper- and mid-lung zones. They may also be seen in combination with irregular linear opacities and architectural distortion indicating associated fibrosis (Fig. 2) [10]. Pleural effusion occurs in 1% to 4% of patients and is predominantly an incidental finding [11–13]. Pleural thickening or fibrothorax can be seen in association with pleural effusion. If the pleural thickening is apical or progressive, involvement with aspergillus should be suspected.

Primary cavitary sarcoidosis is rare. Central necrosis is due to confluence of granulomas and the cavities may be single, multiple, thick walled, thin walled, smooth, or irregular in contour. Cavitation is more common in necrotizing sarcoid angiitis in which the cavities abut the pleura. When cavities are present, aspergillosis with mycetoma formation can occur. The classic appearance of a mycetoma is a cavitary lesion with an intracavitary mass and an "air crescent" sign (Fig. 3A). Movement of the mass with positional maneuvers is essential to make this diagnosis (Fig. 3B,C). In one study of patients who had chronic sarcoidosis and abnormal cystic spaces, 53% of patients were found to have aspergillomas

[14]. Before the development of a fungus ball, new pleural thickening is often observed adjacent to the cystic space [15].

The classic chest radiograph staging system was defined by Scadding over 40 years ago and consists of stage 0 (normal chest radiograph), stage I (bilateral hilar adenopathy with or without paratracheal adenopathy), stage II (bilateral hilar lymphadenopathy with parenchymal disease)

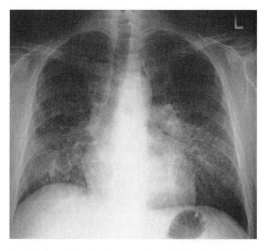

Fig. 2. Sarcoidosis with parenchymal fibrosis. PA chest radiograph reveals a pattern of small nodules with linear reticular opacities and parenchymal distortion in the midzones. Hilar enlargement is present, consistent with adenopathy.

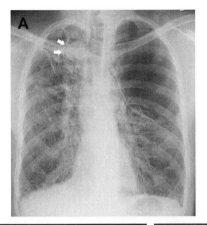

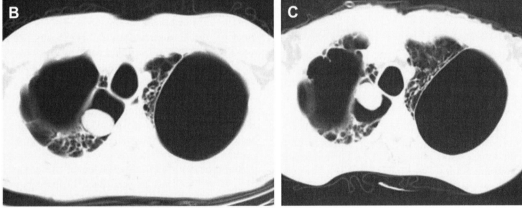

Fig. 3. (*A*) Extensive fibrocystic sarcoidosis and an aspergilloma in the right upper lobe (*arrows*). (*B* and *C*) Supine and prone CT of the chest demonstrates the freely mobile fungus ball in the right upper lobe. There is marked bullous disease in the apices.

(Fig. 4), stage III (parenchymal disease without bilateral hilar lymphadenopathy), and stage IV (parenchymal disease with pulmonary fibrosis) (Fig. 5). At presentation, 8% to 16% of patients are stage 0, 25% to 65% are stage I, 14% to 49% are stage II, approximately 10% are stage III, and approximately 5% are stage IV [3]. In patients who have stage I disease, spontaneous remission occurs in 55% to 90%. In stage I disease, chest radiographs often improve spontaneously or stabilize; significant morbidity or late sequelae in stage I disease is rare. The likelihood of remission declines with increasing stage. Forty percent to 70% of patients who have stage II disease, 10% to 20% of patients who have stage III disease, and 0% of patients who have stage IV disease remit spontaneously [9]. The likelihood of remission decreases after 2 years, regardless of initial stage and changes in stage are highly variable [3]. In patients who have stage II, III, or IV

disease (chronic parenchymal disease), complications are more frequent [9].

Abnormal pulmonary function tests are found in 20% of patients who have stage I disease and in 40% to 70% of patients who have stage II, III, and IV disease. Pulmonary function test findings do not correlate well with changes in the chest radiograph or radiographic stage [16]. Serial radiography is useful in monitoring for changes in stage and for complications of sarcoidosis, such as pneumothorax (prevalence of 2%–3% in patients who have sarcoidosis), bronchial stenosis, and aspergilloma (Fig. 6) [3,11,12].

For the one third of patients who do not spontaneously resolve, current therapeutic agents include corticosteroids and the newer anti–tumor necrosis factor–α antibodies such as infliximab. Infliximab inhibits the action of tumor necrosis factor–α, which is involved in the development of the noncaseating granulomas that are

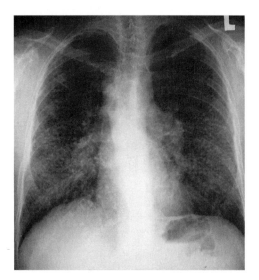

Fig. 4. Stage II sarcoidosis. The chest radiograph reveals right paratracheal and bilateral hilar adenopathy along with a diffuse bilateral fine nodular pattern in the lungs.

characteristic of sarcoidosis. In a randomized, double-blind, placebo-controlled, clinical study by Baughman and colleagues [17], conventional chest radiographs were taken at baseline, 6 weeks, and 24 weeks from patients being treated with infliximab. Of the 91 patients receiving infliximab, there was an approximately 26% decrease in the extent of reticulonodular infiltrates on

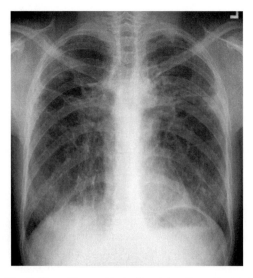

Fig. 5. Stage IV sarcoidosis. Frontal radiograph show lung architectural distortion with volume loss and bilateral hilar retraction.

conventional radiograph compared with placebo. Infliximab has been shown to induce rapid resolution of disease with relapse upon discontinuation [18]. Similarly, a significant reduction in size of mediastinal and hilar adenopathy on CT has been demonstrated with infliximab therapy [19]. Although infliximab may cause regression of sarcoidosis, there are several disease processes that can complicate therapy. These include reactivation of latent tuberculosis or histoplasmosis [20]. In addition, there is an increased incidence of lymphoma and pneumonia while on infliximab therapy [17].

Computed tomography imaging in sarcoidosis

The joint statement of the American Thoracic Society, the European Respiratory Society, and the World Association of Sarcoidosis and Other Granulomatous disorders states that the indications for chest CT scans are as follows: (1) atypical clinical and/or chest radiograph findings; (2) detection of complications of the lung disease, such as bronchiectasis, aspergilloma, pulmonary fibrosis, traction emphysema, or a superimposed infection or malignancy; and (3) a normal chest radiograph with clinical suspicion of the disease [16]. Chest CT can be performed in three basic formats: conventional chest CT, standard HRCT, and VHRCT. HRCT has the advantage of improved spatial resolution (490 μm), allowing for better definition of the distribution of disease relative to the anatomy of the secondary pulmonary lobule. Standard HRCT is a sampling technique that evaluates a 1-mm cross section of the thorax typically every 10 to 15 mm and as such evaluates only 10% of the lung parenchyma. This sampling technique has proven to be adequate in the evaluation of diffuse lung disease. With the advent of multidetector CT, VHRCT imaging has become feasible in a single breath hold with a collimation of 0.6 to 1.0 mm. VHRCT provides an isotropic data set, permitting the demonstration of anatomy in coronal and sagittal planes without loss of resolution (Fig. 7). Furthermore, imaging the entire chest in a volume makes comparison for interval change independent of sampling technique. Standard chest CT and volumetric HRCT have comparable radiation doses, whereas a conventional HRCT represents a 80% to 90% reduction in radiation dose based on the protocol used [21].

Conventional CT is superior to the conventional chest radiograph in the detailed assessment

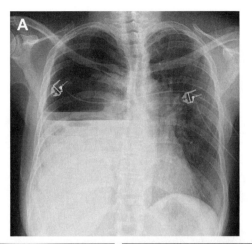

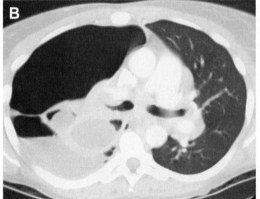

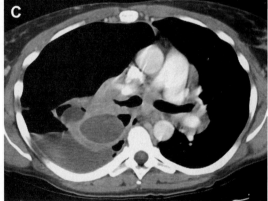

Fig. 6. A patient who has sarcoidosis presents with acute onset chest pain and shortness of breath. (*A*) PA chest radio-graph reveals a large hydropneumothorax and right lung collapse. (*B*) Contrast-enhanced CT in lung windows confirms the large hydropneumothorax and demonstrates two partially filled cavities in the collapsed right lung. (*C*) Contrast-enhanced CT in mediastinal windows reveals oval hypodense filling of these cavities, which was confirmed to be asper-gillomas at bronchoscopy.

of disease pattern and extent. It is also more sensitive in demonstrating nodules and adenopathy that may not be visible on chest radiograph. Conventional CT provides better definition of the parenchymal process relative to the bronchovascular bundle (Fig. 8). Subtle changes that may indicate complications such as cavitation or pleural thickening are more reliably detected. Typical conventional CT features include those found on conventional radiograph, such as thoracic lymphadenopathy, nodules, and ground glass opacities (Fig. 9). Lymphadenopathy in sarcoidosis is typically bilateral, nonnecrotic, and noncompressive (Fig. 10) [3]. Conventional CT examinations often demonstrate lymph nodes in the anterior or posterior mediastinum, previously thought to be unusual in sarcoidosis [22].

When parenchymal abnormalities are present at chest radiography, HRCT demonstrates small nodules in 90% to 100% of patients [10]. Although sarcoid granulomas are microscopic, nodules seen on CT typically measure 1 to 5 mm with an upper lobe predominance. The nodules are primarily found in a perilymphatic distribution. A perilymphatic distribution includes (1) the peribronchovascular regions, adjacent to the perihilar vessels and bronchi, (2) the subpleural interstitium including the fissures, (3) the interlobular septa, and (4) the centrilobular regions (Fig. 11) [23]. Identifying fine nodules along the major fissures is often key to recognition of a perilymphatic process. The distribution is variable among individual patients [24,25]. The small nodules may coalesce and form macroscopic nodules measuring 1 to 4 cm

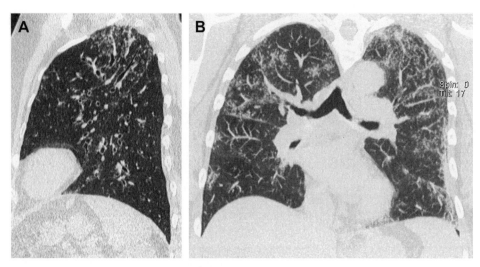

Fig. 7. Sagittal (*A*) and coronal (*B*) volumetric HRCT reformatted images demonstrating the perilymphatic distribution of nodules with an apical posterior predominance and cicatricial bronchiectasis.

in diameter and occur in up to 15% to 25% of patients. These larger nodules can appear consolidative with air bronchograms, also known as alveolar sarcoidosis, and rarely cavitate (Fig. 12) [25]. Confluent opacities show a predilection for the peripheral midzone and typically spare the costophrenic angles [26]. Histologic examination of the air bronchograms within these densely consolidated areas demonstrates bronchiolar dilation with surrounding fibrosis and microscopic honeycombing [27]. Patients who are older than 50 years of age at presentation have a higher prevalence of solitary and multiple mass-like opacities in the lung along with a high prevalence of atelectasis [7]. Recently, the term "sarcoid galaxy" was

coined by Nakatsu and colleagues [28] to describe a large nodule, usually with irregular margins, that is encircled by multiple tiny satellite nodules. In their study, 59 patients demonstrated this sarcoid galaxy sign, measuring 10 to 20 mm in diameter and with all but one being multiple (Fig. 13A,B). The galaxy sign is not unique to sarcoidosis and has also been described in mycobacterial infection [29].

More rarely, sarcoid granulomas distribute throughout the lung and within the secondary pulmonary lobule in a random distribution rather than the classic perilymphatic pattern. This miliary pattern of sarcoidosis manifests as innumerable tiny nodules and is defined by the absence of

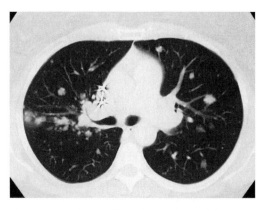

Fig. 8. Conventional CT chest at the level of the carina demonstrating larger nodules in a perilymphatic distribution.

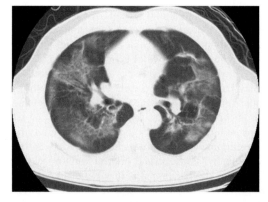

Fig. 9. CT chest reveals patchy ground glass haziness. Ground glass opacities are defined by the presence of increased parenchymal density without obscuration of underlying lung architecture.

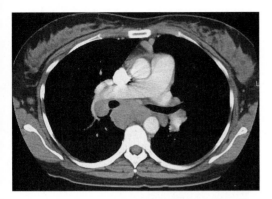

Fig. 10. Contrast-enhanced conventional CT shows enlarged bilateral hilar, subcarinal, and anterior mediastinal adenopathy.

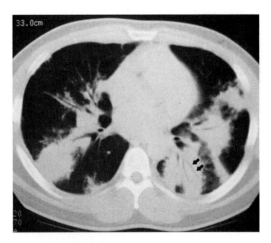

Fig. 12. Alveolar sarcoidosis with multifocal, bilateral areas of consolidation with air bronchograms (*arrows*). This atypical manifestation of sarcoidosis is seen in only 10% to 20% of patients.

a clear perilymphatic or centrilobular distribution (Fig. 14). Differential diagnosis for this pattern includes miliary tuberculosis, miliary fungal infection, and hematogenous metastatic disease.

On HRCT, there are a several disease processes in addition to sarcoidosis that manifest as perilymphatic nodules. These include pulmonary lymphangitic carcinomatosis (LC), coal worker's pneumoconiosis, silicosis, berylliosis, and lymphoproliferative disease. In LC, there is significant septal thickening along the secondary pulmonary lobule with fissural thickening and pleural effusions, not typical in sarcoidosis. The key to distinguishing LC from sarcoidosis is the

evaluation of lung architecture. LC preserves lung architecture, whereas sarcoidosis distorts lung architecture through fibrosis [30]. Silicosis, coal workers pneumoconiosis, and berylliosis can typically be differentiated from sarcoidosis by clinical history. In addition, the nodules in these entities are often more centrilobular in distribution with less associated linear fibrotic change until progressive massive fibrosis develops [5,25].

Although ground glass opacity, nodularity, and consolidation seen on HRCT tend to improve with time, fibrosis may progress or remain stable [25]. Early HRCT findings of fibrosis include posterior displacement of the main and upper lobe bronchi, which indicates volume loss in the posterior segments of the upper lobes (Fig. 15). As fibrosis progresses, irregular reticular opacities and irregular septal thickening develop [25]. Honeycombing may be seen, although it is found predominantly in patients who have severe fibrosis and central bronchial mass–like conglomeration, termed conglomerate or massive fibrosis [23]. Massive fibrosis is also seen in tuberculosis, talcosis, and silicosis [25].

HRCT has demonstrated bronchial abnormalities in up to 65% of patients, ranging from bronchial wall thickening to bronchial luminal abnormalities [25]. A study by Lenique and colleagues [31] found that when luminal abnormality was found on HRCT, follow-up bronchoscopy demonstrated mucosal thickening in 86% of patients, with a positive transbronchial biopsy in

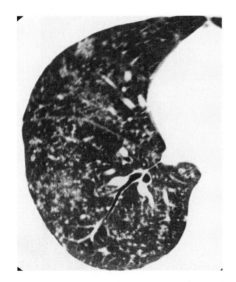

Fig. 11. HRCT of the right lung illustrating a classic perilymphatic distribution of nodules along vessels and pleural surfaces. In the appropriate clinical context, this pattern is virtually diagnostic of sarcoidosis.

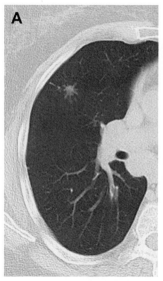
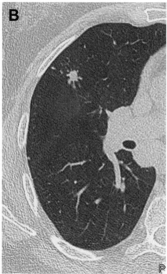

Fig. 13. (*A*) Conventional CT at 5 mm collimation reveals an apparent spiculated right upper lobe nodule with surrounding small nodules. (*B*) HRCT at 1 mm collimation demonstrates incorporated small nodules, the sarcoid galaxy sign.

93%. Bronchial wall thickening is more subjective at HRCT and can vary based upon window and level settings. In the same study, Lenique and colleagues [31] confirmed bronchial wall thickening in 59% of patients who had reported HRCT abnormality, whereas 43% of "normal" airways on HRCT were confirmed to be abnormal on bronchoscopy. The presence of air trapping with expiratory maneuvers at HRCT is common in patients who have sarcoidosis, with an incidence of 83.3% to 98% [3]. It can be recognized as patchy areas of low attenuation and may be a result of small airway obstruction secondary to intraluminal or peribronchiolar granulomas [3]. Hansell

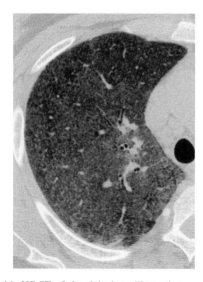

Fig. 14. HRCT of the right lung illustrating a miliary pattern of lung parenchymal involvement, an uncommon pattern of pulmonary sarcoidosis.

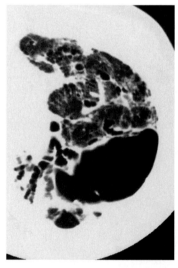

Fig. 15. HRCT of the left lung reveals extensive, irregular bronchovascular thickening with traction bronchiectasis. Note the architectural distortion indicated by posterior bronchial displacement.

and colleagues [32] demonstrated no correlation in the prevalence or extent of air trapping based on Scadding's stage. Conglomerate fibrotic masses are commonly seen in association with dilated bronchi, termed traction bronchiectasis.

Serial chest CTs typically do not correlate well with clinical or functional impairment. In a study of 27 patients by Muller and colleagues [33], conventional CT and radiographic assessment of disease extent had similar correlations to the severity of dyspnea. A newer study by Drent and colleagues [34] found that HRCT findings are more sensitive in depicting respiratory disability compared with conventional radiograph. Findings such as nodules, ground glass opacity, and interlobular septal thickening represent treatable or reversible disease, whereas fibrosis is generally irreversible. Normal radiologic studies do not rule out the diagnosis of pulmonary sarcoidosis because noncaseating granulomas have been reported in the setting of normal conventional radiographs, conventional CTs, and HRCTs.

Cardiac imaging in sarcoidosis

The clinical features of cardiac sarcoidosis are variable and include congestive heart failure, cor pulmonale, supraventricular and ventricular arrhythmias, conduction disturbances, ventricular aneurysms, pericardial effusion, and sudden death (Fig. 16A,B) [35]. Early diagnosis of cardiac sarcoidosis is crucial because up to 85% of deaths from sarcoidosis are a result of cardiac involvement [2]. Of patients who have sarcoidosis, only 5% develop symptoms from cardiac involvement, whereas 20% to 50% demonstrate noncaseating granulomatous infiltration of the myocardium at autopsy [36]. Other studies indicate myocardial involvement in 20% to 27% of patients who have sarcoidosis in the United States and up to 58% in Japan [2]. The pericardium may be involved by sarcoidosis causing inflammatory pericarditis. Cardiac MR imaging is a useful technique for evaluating patients who have recurrent pericardial effusion of unknown etiology [5].

The usefulness of gadolinium-enhanced cardiac MR imaging in the early detection of cardiac sarcoidosis has been studied and reported extensively [2,37–43]. No completed double-blind prospective study exists. Myocardial involvement on cardiac MR imaging manifests as increased signal on T2 and early gadolinium-enhanced imaging with thinning and segmental myocardial wall motion abnormalities [44]. The high T2 signal is thought to be due to edema associated with inflammation, and delayed enhancement with gadolinium is believed to be a result of myocardial degeneration in the regions of sarcoid involvement [36]. The pattern of myocardial enhancement is different than in ischemic heart disease; ischemic myocardial disease typically originates at the endocardium and progresses in an outward fashion to transmural involvement. In sarcoidosis, the increased signal is found in the mid-myocardium and epicardium and not in the endocardium (Fig. 17) [44]. Cardiac MR imaging may

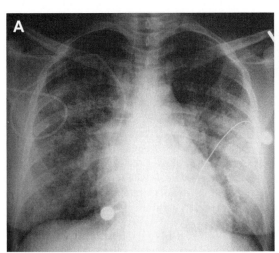
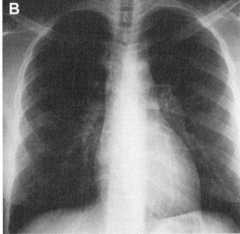

Fig. 16. (*A*) Chest radiograph at presentation in a biopsy proven case of cardiac sarcoidosis illustrating a cardiogenic pulmonary edema pattern of cardiomegaly and perihilar opacity. (*B*) Chest radiograph in the same patient after corticosteroid therapy documenting complete resolution of the pulmonary edema.

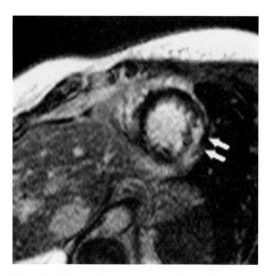

Fig. 17. Delayed-enhancement cardiac MR imaging demonstrating characteristic mid-myocardial enhancement in the lateral wall of the left ventricle (*arrows*).

also show a central portion with low signal on T1- and T2-weighted images (representing hyaline fibrosis) with a peripheral area of high signal on T2 (representing edema associated with granulomatous inflammation) [45]. Vignaux and colleagues [45] described three patterns in their series of 17 patients: (1) five patients had a pure nodular pattern with peripheral and central decreased intramyocardial signal intensity on T2 and postcontrast T1 images, (2) 10 patients had an inflammatory focal or patchy pattern with increased signal on postcontrast T1 images with or without myocardial thickening, and (3) two patients had a postinflammatory pattern with focal increased signal on T2 images (but no postcontrast enhancement) with or without myocardial thickening. Smedema and colleagues [46] used cardiac MR imaging to show that late gadolinium enhancement involving the basal and lateral segments is present in 73% of patients who have cardiac sarcoidosis. This study reported a sensitivity of 100%, a specificity 78%, a positive predictive value of 55%, a negative predictive value of 100%, and an overall accuracy of 83% in the detection of cardiac sarcoidosis. The predominant sites of myocardial involvement are, in decreasing frequency, the left ventricular free wall and papillary muscles, the basal aspect of the ventricular septum, the right ventricular free wall, and the atrial walls [44]. Advanced cardiac sarcoidosis demonstrates clinical and radiologic features that are similar to dilated

cardiomyopathy, predominantly heart failure. In addition, cine MR imaging has been shown to demonstrate myocardial akinesia in patients who have cardiac sarcoidosis [39]. A unique histologically proven case of cardiac sarcoidosis presenting as a broad-based mass in the basilar portion of the intraventricular septum protruding into the right ventricle has been reported [47].

Cardiac MR imaging is useful in evaluating response to therapy demonstrating normalization of abnormal myocardial delayed enhancement after corticosteroid administration [2,48–50]. It has been reported that there is good correlation between follow-up cardiac MR imaging findings and follow-up clinical findings while on therapy [51]. Cardiac MR imaging has also been used for targeting of endomyocardial biopsies [52].

Pulmonary hypertension (PH) is another recently recognized complication of sarcoidosis, especially in the advanced stages. Although not unique to sarcoidosis, the presence of PH remains a poor prognostic sign and can result in right ventricular enlargement and hypokinesis [53]. Radiologic signs of PH on CT include caliber alterations of the pulmonary arteries, mosaic perfusion, pulmonary edema/hemorrhage, and cardiac abnormalities. A main pulmonary artery larger than 2.9 cm in diameter or one that is larger than the ascending aorta is highly suggestive but not pathognomonic of PH (Fig. 18A) [25]. Recent studies have shown that in the setting of fibrosis, pulmonary arterial size is not as predictive of PH as previously thought. Evaluation of pulmonary artery size as a predictor of PH has been shown to be of limited value in sarcoidosis [54]. Decreased caliber of intrapulmonary arteries can be seen in patients who have PH as well. Pulmonary edema and hemorrhage and edema associated with PH appear as ground-glass opacity with interlobular septal thickening. Cardiac abnormalities seen with PH include dilation of the right-sided chambers and flattening of the ventricular septum (Fig. 18B,C) [25]. A cardiac MR imaging study by Roeleveld and colleagues [55] found that bowing of the intraventricular septum is present in patients who have PH and is proportional to systolic pulmonary arterial pressures. A ratio of the curvature of the left ventricular septal wall to free wall has also been demonstrated to be indicative of PH [56]. Even with the advances in radiologic imaging, cardiac catheterization remains the gold standard for the diagnosis of PH.

With the advent of cardiac multidetector CT, case reports of contrast-enhanced CT being used to

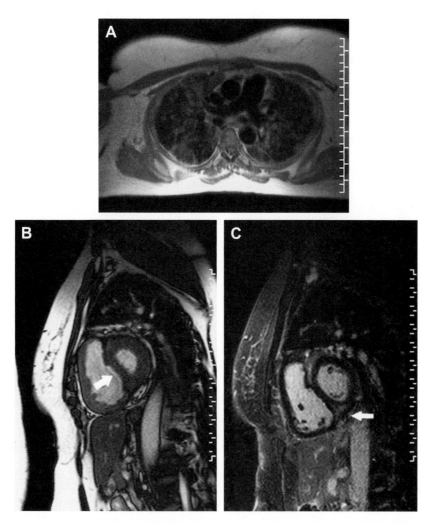

Fig. 18. MR imaging of a patient who has sarcoidosis and pulmonary hypertension. (*A*) Axial HASTE image at the level of the main pulmonary artery confirms enlargement and abnormal signal in the lung parenchyma. (*B*) A single frame from a bright blood cine sequence in end systole reveals flattening of the interventricular septum (*arrow*). (*C*) delayed enhancement cardiac MR imaging shows mid-myocardial scarring at RV insertion site and along the RV side of anterior septum (*arrow*). (*Courtesy of* Laura Heyneman, MD, Durham, NC.)

detect cardiac involvement in sarcoidosis are beginning to emerge. The use of CT in this setting permits simultaneous evaluation of the lung parenchyma and adenopathy in a single, cost–effective, and expedient scan [57]. The considerable additional radiation dose resulting from cardiac gating must be factored into the use of this emerging technology, and data in this application are sparse.

Positron emission tomography imaging in sarcoidosis

Another recent imaging technology that has been used in the diagnosis of patients who have

sarcoidosis is PET/CT. PET is a nuclear medicine study that uses positron-emitting radionuclides labeled to organic molecules to gain metabolic information. The most commonly used radionuclide in PET imaging is ^{18}F-fluorodeoxyglucose (^{18}F-FDG). ^{18}F-FDG is accumulated into malignant cells and sites of inflammation due to inherent enhanced glucose metabolism. After being transported into the cells, it is phosphorylated and becomes trapped, because it cannot be metabolized further. These areas demonstrate increased uptake on the scan relative to normal tissue (Fig. 19). ^{18}F-FDG provides nonspecific labeling of areas of metabolic activity and thus is of limited

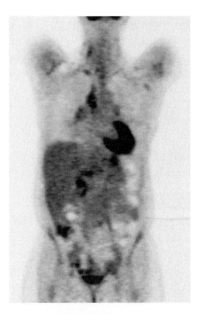

Fig. 19. Coronal PET image of a patient who has biopsy-proven sarcoidosis demonstrating uptake within right paratracheal and bilateral hilar lymph nodes.

value in distinguishing sarcoidosis from malignancy in the setting of large parenchymal nodules or lymphadenopathy [58,59]. Further complicating matters is the reported coexistence of malignancy in 1.2 to 2.5% of patients who have sarcoidosis, predominantly lung cancer, lymphoma, testicular cancer, and uterine cancer [60,61]. The association of malignancy with sarcoidosis remains incompletely delineated. The etiology of adenopathy requires a definitive answer, with sarcoidosis being a diagnosis of exclusion.

One proposed solution involves a novel radionuclide, ^{18}F-alpha-methyltyrosine (^{18}F-FMT). ^{18}F-FMT accumulates in malignant cells secondary to increased amino acid metabolism with increased active transport into the cells. This uptake is specific for malignancy and is not present in inflammation [60,62,63]. Kaira and colleagues [60] developed this radionuclide and reported high ^{18}F-FMT uptake in lung cancer and lymphoma without uptake in sarcoidosis. A two-phase PET scan with ^{18}F-FDG and ^{18}F-FMT should enable the differentiation of these common malignancies from sarcoidosis.

^{13}N-NH$_3$ is another commonly used PET radionuclide for the assessment of myocardial blood flow and coronary flow reserve [64]. Yamagishi and colleagues studied 17 patients using ^{13}N-NH$_3$ in combination with ^{18}F-FDG to diagnose

cardiac sarcoidosis. They found that ^{13}N-NH$_3$ defects were more commonly found in the basal anteroseptal wall of the left ventricle and that ^{18}F-FDG uptake was more commonly found in the basal and midanteroseptal-lateral wall of the left ventricle. After steroid therapy, the ^{18}F-FDG uptake was significantly diminished in size and intensity, with no change in the ^{13}N-NH$_3$ defects. This suggests that after treatment there is progression from active inflammatory granulomatous disease to healed scar. In addition, ^{18}F-FDG may be a sensitive marker of cardiac sarcoidosis activity because it has been successfully used to monitor response to corticosteroid therapy [62,65–67]. It has been reported that the pattern of cardiac uptake on ^{18}F-FDG PET in sarcoidosis is somewhat unique. Ishimaru and colleagues [68] studied 32 patients who had sarcoidosis and 30 control subjects who had ^{18}F-FDG PET, ^{99m}Tc-MIBI scintigraphy, and ^{67}Ga scintigraphy. The control subjects demonstrated no uptake or diffuse patterns. Patients who had sarcoidosis demonstrated no uptake (n = 16), diffuse (n = 7), focal (n = 8), or focal on diffuse (n = 2) patterns. The 32 patients who had sarcoidosis did not demonstrate abnormality on ^{67}Ga scintigraphy, and only four patients demonstrated abnormalities on ^{99m}Tc-MIBI scintigraphy. The authors propose that focal cardiac uptake is characteristic for sarcoidosis [68].

Other radioisotopes, such as Gallium-67 (^{67}Ga) and Technetium-99m-methoxyisobutlyisonitrile (^{99m}Tc-MIBI), have been used in the scintigraphic diagnosis of cardiac sarcoidosis. In a study of 22 patients, fasting ^{18}F-FDG PET was shown to be useful in detecting early cardiac sarcoidosis with higher sensitivity (100%) compared with ^{99m}Tc-MIBI SPECT (63.6%) or ^{67}Ga scintigraphy (36.3%) [69]. Other studies confirm these findings, demonstrating 100% sensitivity of ^{18}F-FDG PET for pulmonary sarcoidosis compared with 81% sensitivity for ^{67}Ga scintigraphy/SPECT and showing positive ^{18}F-FDG PET results in the face of negative ^{67}Ga scans [70,71].

^{18}F-FDG PET has been used to target video-assisted thorascopic surgery procedures with great success in obtaining diagnostic histologic samples [72]. These early reports demonstrate that PET imaging is evolving into a useful tool for the diagnosis and monitoring of sarcoidosis.

Summary

Sarcoidosis remains a challenging diagnosis with protean manifestations. Radiologic tests, such as chest radiography, CT, HRCT, cardiac MR imaging, and PET imaging, are often the key to making the diagnosis. Classic chest radiograph findings include bilateral symmetric hilar and mediastinal adenopathy with or without parenchymal distortion. CT findings typically include adenopathy, nodules distributed along the lymphatics, and ground glass opacities. On standard HRCT, the nodules and extent of parenchymal disease (ie, fibrosis) are better defined, in addition to a decreased radiation dose compared with conventional CT. It is important to note that sarcoidosis may be present even in the setting of normal conventional radiographs, conventional CTs, and HRCTs.

The diagnosis of cardiac sarcoidosis is critical because of its associated morbidity and mortality. Gadolinium-enhanced cardiac MR imaging is emerging as the new gold standard for diagnosis. Typical findings at MR imaging include delayed gadolinium enhancement and high T2 signal in the regions of cardiac involvement. Cardiac MR imaging may also be useful in diagnosing coexistent PH common to sarcoidosis. PET imaging has been used to document the extent of sarcoidosis and is being used in the detection of cardiac sarcoidosis. PET imaging may also be a reasonable alternative in patients who have sarcoidosis who have pacemakers or defibrillators for whom MR imaging is contraindicated. Dual-isotope PET imaging shows promise for delineating sarcoid from malignancy. Finally, PET and cardiac MR imaging have successfully been used to monitor response to therapy. Even with these promising results, large-scale prospective clinical trials for these techniques are needed.

Although sarcoidosis affects virtually every organ system, cardiopulmonary involvement is the most frequent and potentially devastating. The technologies reviewed in this article, including VHRCT, cardiac MR imaging, and PET, are the new noninvasive battery of imaging for diagnosing and monitoring treatment in this complex patient population.

References

[1] Martin L. Breathe easy: a guide to lung and respiratory diseases for patients and their families. Englewood Cliffs (NJ): Prentice-Hall; 1984. Available at: http://www.lakesidepress.com/pulmonary/books/breathe/Secto.htm. Accessed November 19, 2007.

[2] Shimada T, Shimada K, Sakane T, et al. Diagnosis of cardiac sarcoidosis and evaluation of the effects of steroid therapy by gadolinium-DTPA-enhanced magnetic resonance imaging. Am J Med 2001; 110(7):520–7.

[3] Nunes H, Brillet P, Valeyre D, et al. Imaging in sarcoidosis. Semin Respir Crit Care Med 2007;28(1): 102–20.

[4] Hansell D, Armstrong P, Lynch D. Imaging of diseases of the chest. 4th edition. Philadelphia: Elsevier Mosby; 2005. p. 631–52.

[5] Vagal A, Shipley R, Meyer C. Radiological manifestations of sarcoidosis. Clin Dermatol 2007;25(3): 312–25.

[6] Rockoff S, Rohatgi P. Unusual manifestations of thoracic sarcoidosis. AJR Am J Roentgenol 1985; 144:513–26.

[7] Conant E, Glickstein M, Mahar P, et al. Pulmonary sarcoidosis in the older patient: conventional radiographic features. Radiology 1988;169:315–9.

[8] Lynch J. Computed tomographic scanning in sarcoidosis. Semin Respir Crit Care Med 2003;24(4): 393–418.

[9] Muller N, Mawson J, Mathieson J, et al. Sarcoidosis: correlation of extent of disease at CT with clinical, functional, and radiographic findings. Radiology 1989;171:613–8.

[10] Fraser R, Muller N, Colman N, et al. Diagnosis of diseases of the chest. 4th edition. Philadelphia: W.B. Saunders; 1999. p. 1533–83.

[11] Soskel N, Sharma O. Pleural involvement in sarcoidosis: case presentation and detailed review of the literature. Semin Respir Med 1992;13:492–514.

[12] Sharma O, Gordonson J. Pleural effusion in sarcoidosis: a report of six cases. Thorax 1975;30: 95–101.

[13] Littner M, Schachter E, Putman C, et al. The clinical assessment of roentgenographically atypical pulmonary sarcoidosis. Am J Med 1977;62:361–8.

[14] Wollschlager C, Khan F. Aspergillomas complicating sarcoidosis: a prospective study in 100 patients. Chest 1984;86:585–8.

[15] Libshitz H, Atkinson G, Israel H. Pleural thickening as a manifestation of aspergillus superinfection. Am J Roentgenol Radium Ther Nucl Med 1974;120: 883–6.

[16] Statement on sarcoidosis. Joint Statement of the American Thoracic Society (ATS), the European Respiratory Society (ERS) and the World Association of Sarcoidosis and Other Granulomatous Disorders (WASOG) adopted by the ATS Board of Directors and by the ERS Executive Committee, February 1999. Am J Respir Crit Care Med 1999; 160(2):736–55.

[17] Baughman R, Drent M, Kavuru M, et al. Infliximab therapy in patients with chronic sarcoidosis and pulmonary involvement. Am J Respir Crit Care Med 2006;174(7):795–802 [Epub 2006 Jul 13].

[18] Atzeni F, Doria A, Carrabba M, et al. Potential target of infliximab in autoimmune and inflammatory diseases. Autoimmun Rev 2007;6(8):529–36 [Epub 2007 Apr 16].

[19] Uthman I, Touma Z, Khoury M. Cardiac sarcoidosis responding to monotherapy with infliximab. Clin Rheumatol 2007;26(11):2001–3 [Epub 2007 Mar 30].

[20] Doty J, Mazur J, Judson M. Treatment of sarcoidosis with infliximab. Chest 2005;127(3):1064–71.

[21] Mayo J, Aldrich J, Muller N. Fleischner Society. Radiation exposure at chest CT: a statement of the Fleischner Society. Radiology 2003;228(1):15–21.

[22] Sider L, Horton E. Hilar and mediastinal adenopathy in sarcoidosis as detected by computed tomography. J Thorac Imaging 1990;5(2):77–80.

[23] Lynch D, Webb W, Gamsu G, et al. Computed tomography in pulmonary sarcoidosis. J Comput Assist Tomogr 1989;13:405–10.

[24] Muller N, Kullnig P, Miller R. The CT findings of pulmonary sarcoidosis: analysis of 25 patients. AJR Am J Roentgenol 1989;152:1179–82.

[25] Webb R, Muller N, Naidich D. High-resolution CT of the lung. 3rd edition. Philadelphia: Lippincott, Williams & Wilkins; 2001. p. 286–301, 547–53.

[26] Battesti J, Saumon G, Valeyre D, et al. Pulmonary sarcoidosis with an alveolar radiographic pattern. Thorax 1982;37:448–52.

[27] Nishimura K, Itoh H, Kitaichi M, et al. Pulmonary sarcoidosis: correlation of CT and histopathologic findings. Radiology 1993;189:105–9.

[28] Nakatsu M, Hatabu H, Morikawa K, et al. Large coalescent parenchymal nodules in pulmonary sarcoidosis: "sarcoid galaxy"sign. AJR Am J Roentgenol 2002;178(6):1389–93.

[29] Heo J, Choi Y, Jeon S, et al. Pulmonary tuberculosis: another disease showing clusters of small nodules. AJR Am J Roentgenol 2005;184(2):639–42.

[30] Honda O, Johnkoh T, Ichikado K, et al. Comparison of high resolution CT findings of sarcoidosis, lymphoma and lymphangitic carcinoma: is there any difference of involved interstitium? J Comput Assist Tomogr 1999;23:374–9.

[31] Lenique F, Brauner M, Grenier P. CT assessment of bronchi in sarcoidosis: endoscopic and pathologic correlations. Radiology 1995;194(2):419–23.

[32] Hansell D, Milne D, Wilsher M, et al. Pulmonary sarcoidosis: morphologic associations of airflow obstruction at thin section CT. Radiology 1998;209: 697–704.

[33] Muller N, Mawson J, Mathieson J, et al. Correlation of CT with clinical, functional, and radiological findings. Radiology 1989;171.

[34] Drent M, De Vries J, Lenters M, et al. Sarcoidosis: assessment of disease severity using HRCT. Eur Radiol 2003;13(11):2462–71 [Epub 2003 Jun 17].

[35] Smedema J, Snoep G, van Kroonenburgh M, et al. Cardiac involvement in patients with pulmonary sarcoidosis assessed at two university medical centers in the netherlands. Chest 2005;128(1):30–5.

[36] Vignaux O. Cardiac sarcoidosis: spectrum of MRI features. AJR Am J Roentgenol 2005;184(1):249–54.

[37] Sato Y, Matsumoto N, Kunimasa T, et al. Multiple involvements of cardiac sarcoidosis in both left and right ventricles and papillary muscles detected by delayed-enhanced magnetic resonance imaging. Int J Cardiol 2007 Aug 7 [Epub ahead of print].

[38] Osman F, Foundon A, Leyva P, et al. Early diagnosis of cardiac sarcoidosis using magnetic resonance imaging. Int J Cardiol 2008;125(1):e4–5.

[39] Redheuil AB, Paziaud O, Mousseaux E. Ventricular tachycardia and cardiac sarcoidosis: correspondence between MRI and electrophysiology. Eur Heart J 2006;27(12):1430 [Epub 2005 Oct 24].

[40] Sanz J, Goyenechea M, Poon M. Cardiac sarcoidosis detected with magnetic resonance imaging. Eur Heart J 2006;27(14):1639 [Epub 2006 Jan 25].

[41] Chandra M, Silverman M, Oshinski J, et al. Diagnosis of cardiac sarcoidosis aided by MRI. Chest 1996; 110(2):562–5.

[42] Nemeth M, Muthupillai R, Wilson J, et al. Cardiac sarcoidosis detected by delayed-hyperenhancement magnetic resonance imaging. Tex Heart Inst J 2004;31(1):99–102.

[43] Serra J, Monte G, Mello E, et al. Images in cardiovascular medicine: cardiac sarcoidosis evaluated by delayed-enhanced magnetic resonance imaging. Circulation 2003;107(20):188–9.

[44] Doughan A, Williams B. Cardiac sarcoidosis. Heart 2006;92(2):282–8.

[45] Vignaux O, Dhote R, Duboc D, et al. Detection of myocardial involvement in patients with sarcoidosis applying T2-weighted, contrast-enhanced, and cine magnetic resonance imaging: initial results of a prospective study. J Comput Assist Tomogr 2002;26(5): 762–7.

[46] Smedema J, Snoep G, van Kroonenburgh M, et al. Evaluation of the accuracy of gadolinium-enhanced cardiovascular magnetic resonance in the diagnosis of cardiac sarcoidosis. J Am Coll Cardiol 2005; 45(10):1683–90.

[47] Slater G, Rodriguez E, Lima J, et al. A unique presentation of cardiac sarcoidosis. AJR Am J Roentgenol 2003;180(6):1738–9.

[48] Schulz-Menger J, Strohm O, Dietz R, et al. Visualization of cardiac involvement in patients with systemic sarcoidosis applying contrast-enhanced magnetic resonance imaging. MAGMA 2000;11(1–2):82–3.

[49] Doherty M, Kumar S, Nicholson A, et al. Cardiac sarcoidosis: the value of magnetic resonance imaging in diagnosis and assessment of response to treatment. Respir Med 1998;92(4):697–9.

[50] Stauder N, Bader B, Fenchel M, et al. Images in cardiovascular medicine: follow-up of cardiac sarcoidosis by magnetic resonance imaging. Circulation 2005;111(11):e158–60.

[51] Vignaux O, Dhote R, Duboc D, et al. Clinical significance of myocardial magnetic resonance abnormalities in patients with sarcoidosis: a 1-year follow-up study. Chest 2002;122(6):1895–901.

[52] Borchert B, Lawrenz T, Bartelsmeier M, et al. Utility of endomyocardial biopsy guided by delayed enhancement areas on magnetic resonance imaging in

the diagnosis of cardiac sarcoidosis. Clin Res Cardiol 2007;96(10):759–62 [Epub 2007 Aug 21].

[53] Shorr A, Helman D, Davies D, et al. Pulmonary hypertension in advanced sarcoidosis: epidemiology and clinical characteristics. Eur Respir J 2005;25(5):783–8.

[54] Baughman R, Engel P, Meyer C, et al. Pulmonary hypertension in sarcoidosis. Sarcoidosis Vasc Diffuse Lung Dis 2006;23(2):108–16.

[55] Roeleveld R, Marcus J, Faes T, et al. Interventricular septal configuration at MR imaging and pulmonary arterial pressure in pulmonary hypertension. Radiology 2005;234(3):710–7 [Epub 2005 Jan 5].

[56] Dellegrottaglie S, Sanz J, Poon M, et al. Pulmonary hypertension: accuracy of detection with left ventricular septal-to-free wall curvature ratio measured at cardiac MR. Radiology 2007;243(1):63–9.

[57] Kanao S, Tadamura E, Yamamuro M, et al. Demonstration of cardiac involvement of sarcoidosis by contrast-enhanced multislice computed tomography and delayed-enhanced magnetic resonance imaging. J Comput Assist Tomogr 2005;29(6):745–8.

[58] Taaleb K, Kaiser K, Wieler H. Elevated uptake of F-18 FDG in PET scans in nonmalignant disease. Clin Nucl Med 2000;25(11):939–40.

[59] Lewis P, Salama A. Uptake of fluorine-18-fluorodeoxyglucose in sarcoidosis. J Nucl Med 1994; 35(10):1647–9.

[60] Kaira K, Oriuchi N, Otani Y, et al. Diagnostic usefulness of fluorine-18-alpha-methyltyrosine positron emission tomography in combination with 18F-fluorodeoxyglucose in sarcoidosis patients. Chest 2007; 131(4):1019–27.

[61] Cohen P, Kurzrock R. Sarcoidosis and malignancy. Clin Dermatol 2007;25(3):326–33.

[62] Yamagishi H, Shirai N, Takagi M, et al. Identification of cardiac sarcoidosis with (13)N-NH(3)/ (18)F-FDG PET. J Nucl Med 2003;44(7):1030–6.

[63] Yamada Y, Uchida Y, Tatsumi K, et al. Fluorine-18-fluorodeoxyglucose and carbon-11-methionine

evaluation of lymphadenopathy in sarcoidosis. J Nucl Med 1998;39(7):1160–6.

[64] Khorsand A, Graf S, Eidherr H, et al. Gated cardiac 13N-NH3 PET for assessment of left ventricular volumes, mass, and ejection fraction: comparison with electrocardiography-gated 18F-FDG PET. J Nucl Med 2005;46(12):2009–13.

[65] Kaira K, Ishizuka T, Yanagitani N, et al. Value of FDG positron emission tomography in monitoring the effects of therapy in progressive pulmonary sarcoidosis. Clin Nucl Med 2007;32(2):114–6.

[66] Gyorik S, Ceriani L, Menafoglio A, et al. 18F-FDG PET scan as follow-up tool for sarcoidosis with symptomatic cardiac conduction disturbances requiring a pacemaker. Thorax 2007;62(6):560.

[67] Milman N, Mortensen J, Sloth C. Fluorodeoxyglucose PET scan in pulmonary sarcoidosis during treatment with inhaled and oral corticosteroids. Respiration 2003;70(4):408–13.

[68] Ishimaru S, Tsujino I, Takei T, et al. Focal uptake on 18F-fluoro-2-deoxyglucose positron emission tomography images indicates cardiac involvement of sarcoidosis. Eur Heart J 2005;26(15):1538–43 [Epub 2005 Apr 4].

[69] Okumura W, Iwasaki T, Toyama T, et al. Usefulness of fasting 18F-FDG PET in identification of cardiac sarcoidosis. J Nucl Med 2004;45(12):1989–98.

[70] Nishiyama Y, Yamamoto Y, Fukunaga K, et al. Comparative evaluation of 18F-FDG PET and 67Ga scintigraphy in patients with sarcoidosis. J Nucl Med 2006;47(10):1571–6.

[71] Xiu Y, Yu J, Cheng E, et al. Sarcoidosis demonstrated by FDG PET imaging with negative findings on gallium scintigraphy. Clin Nucl Med 2005;30(3):193–5.

[72] Luh S, Wu T, Wang Y, et al. Experiences and benefits of positron emitted tomography-computed tomography (PET-CT) combined with video-assisted thoracoscopic surgery (VATS) in the diagnosis of Stage 1 sarcoidosis. J Zhejiang Univ Sci B 2007;8(6):410–5.

**ELSEVIER
SAUNDERS**

Clin Chest Med 29 (2008) 445–458

CLINICS
IN CHEST
MEDICINE

Markers of Inflammation in Sarcoidosis: Blood, Urine, BAL, Sputum, and Exhaled Gas

E. Bargagli, MD, PhD, A. Mazzi, MD, Paola Rottoli, MD*

*Respiratory Diseases Section, Department of Clinical Medicine and Immunological Sciences, Siena University,
Le Scotte Hospital, Viale Bracci, 53100 Siena, Italy*

Sarcoidosis is a systemic granulomatous disease characterized by a T-helper-1 response with accumulation of $CD4^+$ lymphocytes and activated macrophages in the lungs and affected organs, resulting in granuloma formation [1]. The etiology of this disease is still unclear, although numerous hypotheses continue to be proposed [2]. An unidentified antigen induces an immune response mediated by alveolar macrophages and lymphocytes [3] that release a wide spectrum of mediators, such as cytokines, chemokines, oxygen radicals, and other mediators, which are involved in the pathogenesis of sarcoidosis [4,5]. This multisystem disorder has an unpredictable clinical course: acute and chronic progressive variants are distinguished. Approximately 15% to 25% of cases are chronic progressive and may lead to lung fibrosis [6,7]. The unpredictable clinical course of sarcoidosis has prompted research into biomarkers that could help predict outcome. The need for diagnostic and prognostic markers is a very topical subject for all chest physicians involved with sarcoidosis patients.

Serum angiotensin-converting enzyme (ACE) is the first widely used marker of sarcoidosis, but its concentrations in serum and bronchoalveolar lavage (BAL) seem to have poor predictive value [8–10]. Because ACE may be elevated in various lung diseases it has low specificity as a marker and is associated with genetic polymorphisms that modify its expression in different populations [8,9]. Other markers of inflammation in sarcoidosis include lysozyme, cytokines, chemokines, and

various molecules produced by activated macrophages or lymphocytes [10–13]. These mediators, which could be involved in the pathogenesis of the disease, have been analyzed in different human body fluids and tissues. Most of these studies have been performed in serum and BAL, although some also consider expired breath condensate (a noninvasive method of obtaining samples directly from the respiratory system) and other biologic fluids. Sarcoidosis has been the disease most widely studied through BAL since the advent of this procedure [14]. Analysis of cell pattern and cytokine profile of sarcoidosis by the Th1/Th2 model in BAL has contributed to the definition of its pathogenesis and identified some reliable markers with potential clinical applications [12,15,16]. Sarcoidosis is a good model for analyzing immune response by virtue of its complex pathogenesis, which involves many different cells and mediators. This is why the literature abounds in papers proposing new markers for clinical use (prevalently for activity evaluation). Sufficient specificity, sensitivity, and reproducibility, however, have been demonstrated for very few of them.

This article examines the principal literature on the different markers of inflammation in sarcoidosis analyzed in serum, BAL, expired breath, and urine. It also looks at oxidative stress mediators and various potential markers of the disease, most in the course of study.

Angiotensin-converting enzyme

Serum ACE activity has been used as a diagnostic and prognostic marker of sarcoidosis

* Corresponding author.
E-mail address: rottoli@unisi.it (P. Rottoli)

0272-5231/08/$ - see front matter © 2008 Elsevier Inc. All rights reserved.
doi:10.1016/j.ccm.2008.03.004

chestmed.theclinics.com

since Lieberman [17] revealed its elevation in patients with active disease in 1975. ACE is an acid glycoprotein (molecular weight 140,000 d) that converts angiotensin I into angiotensin II by cleaving the dipeptide histidine and leucine C-terminal of angiotensin I [17]. It is secreted by monocytes and macrophages and in sarcoidosis by pulmonary endothelial cells that release ACE into blood vessels where it exerts its functions. ACE is produced by different tissues and its serum concentrations may reflect monocyte-macrophage system activity. ACE activity is elevated in lungs of sarcoidosis patients, secondary to the macrophage alveolitis [18] and enhanced expression of epithelial cells. Epithelial cells are involved in granuloma formation and are an important source of ACE and other enzymes, such as lysozyme and elastase. Serum ACE activity is not influenced by human gender, although children and young adults may have higher ACE levels than older people. Different studies have documented significantly elevated concentrations of ACE in serum and other biologic fluids of sarcoidosis patients with respect to controls. Some of these papers also report a correlation between serum ACE concentrations and radiologic stages of sarcoidosis [17]. In 1981, the Ninth International Conference of Sarcoidosis approved the concept that serum concentrations of ACE can be a useful diagnostic and prognostic tool; however, normal levels do not exclude sarcoidosis and false-positives are quite frequent. Indeed, serum concentrations of ACE may also be elevated in granulomatous diseases, such as pulmonary silicosis [19], miliary tuberculosis [20], berylliosis [21], and leprosy [22]. Gaucher's disease [23], diabetes mellitus [24], hyperthyroidism [25], and liver cirrhosis [26] are other diseases in which serum concentrations of ACE are generally enhanced.

ACE activity in serum is currently considered a marker of granuloma formation with limited sensitivity (50%–60% positivity at clinical onset) and specificity. It must be analyzed together with other markers of sarcoidosis and needs to be correlated with clinical phenotypes and radiologic findings to be used for diagnosis and follow-up [27,28]. Because its concentration generally decreases with therapy or remission, it can be useful for follow-up of patients with elevated levels at onset.

ACE concentrations in specific biologic fluids are also influenced by genetic polymorphism. An insertion (I)/deletion (D) polymorphism in the ACE gene is associated with variations in serum levels of ACE [29]. Documented in several populations, the polymorphism is caused by a 287-bp fragment inserted in intron 16 [30]. Absence of the inserted fragment is caused by a deletion. Homozygous carriers of the deletion (DD) or insertion (II) express the highest and lowest ACE levels, respectively, whereas heterozygous ID individuals express intermediate ACE levels [31]. ACE activity may be underestimated in patients homozygous for insertion (II) and overestimated in DD patients. The introduction of genotype-specific reference intervals for ACE activity (II, DD, ID) prevents this underestimation or overestimation.

I/D allele frequencies may also differ between ethnic groups. Indeed, in whites the D and I allele distributions are the same [31], whereas in the Japanese population the I is more frequent than the D allele. Because this relatively simple genetic profile can indicate a more precise reference interval, ACE I/D genotyping may improve assessment of disease activity, both at diagnosis and during follow-up of treated and untreated patients [31,32].

ACE can also be measured in BAL of sarcoidosis patients where it is generally found to be elevated (particularly in active disease). ACE activity in BAL is generally considered a good marker of sarcoidosis severity with higher prognostic value than ACE in serum [33]. ACE concentrations have been assayed in other biologic fluids, including cerebrospinal fluid and urine, and in different tissues, leading to the proposal that their elevation may signal the presence of sarcoidosis in patients with extrapulmonary localizations [34].

ACE concentrations in serum are generally analyzed by a colorimetric method as described by Lieberman and colleagues [21]. The same method with some modifications can be used to detect ACE levels in BAL and other biologic fluids [35].

Lysozyme

Lysozyme, produced by the monocyte-macrophage system, is another enzyme that can be considered a potential marker of sarcoidosis severity. Enhanced activity of phagocytes in sarcoidosis may determine an increase in lysozyme in serum of these patients. This enzyme was first discovered in 1922 by Fleming who reported that it had antibacterial activity through cleavage of β1-4 glycoside bonds in cell walls of certain bacteria. Lysozyme is normally present in the granules of monocytes, macrophages, and polymorphonuclear leukocytes, whence it may be released into biologic fluids, such as saliva, tears, and airway secretions [36,37]. In sarcoidosis, lysozyme is mainly produced by macrophages and epithelioid cells involved in granuloma formation and is generally not expressed by old granuloma cells. Because it is filtered by renal glomeruli, absorbed, and finally metabolized in the proximal tubular epithelium, an increase in serum concentrations of lysozyme may also be a consequence of renal dysfunction. Serum levels of lysozyme are generally independent of gender and smoking habits [38]. Elevated serum levels have been reported in serum of sarcoidosis patients (about 30% of patients at clinical onset) and also in other lung diseases, including pulmonary tuberculosis, silicosis, asbestosis, and berylliosis [39–41]. Its use as a clinical marker of sarcoidosis is recommended to monitor the course and severity of disease rather than for diagnosis [42]. Research has demonstrated that serum concentrations of lysozyme may be positively correlated with serum levels of ACE, number of organs involved, and radiologic stages of sarcoidosis, although specificity and sensitivity are lower than for other markers [42].

Chitotriosidase

Chitotriosidase is a member of family 18 of glycosylhydrolases (or chitinases), enzymes involved in the degradation of chitin (an abundant polymer of *N*-acetylglucosamine) and chitin-like substrate [43]. The enzyme is expressed by activated macrophages and elevated activity has been observed in serum of patients with atherosclerosis, β-thalassemia, acute *Plasmodium falciparum* malaria, and visceral leishmaniasis, and in cerebrospinal fluid of patients with multiple sclerosis [44–46]. Chitotriosidase is considered a selective marker of macrophage activation [47] and the principal biochemical marker of Gaucher's disease [48]. The authors' research group found significantly higher levels of chitotriosidase in serum of patients with sarcoidosis than in controls (more than 90% of patients had increased chitotriosidase levels) [49], with a particularly evident difference between patients with active and inactive sarcoidosis. Chitotriosidase concentrations were also positively correlated with serum concentrations of ACE, soluble interleukin-2 receptor (sIL-2R), and radiographic stages (Fig. 1) [50].

Expression of chitotriosidase at alveolar level and its possible involvement in the pathogenesis

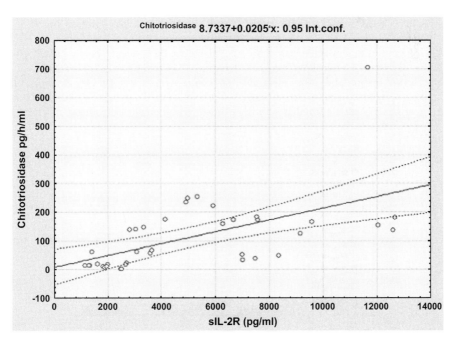

Fig. 1. Correlation between chitotriosidase levels in serum and sIL2R in sarcoidosis. (*From* Bargagli E, Bianchi N, Margollicci M, et al. Chitotriosidase and soluble IL-2 receptor: comparison of two markers of sarcoidosis severity. Scand J Clin Lab Invest 2008, in press; with permission.)

of sarcoidosis were analyzed in a recent study that compared chitotriosidase levels in progressive and stable sarcoidosis patients [35]. Significantly higher chitotriosidase activity was demonstrated in BAL of sarcoidosis patients than in controls, and in progressive than in stable disease [35]. Chitotriosidase activity in BAL was correlated with sarcoidosis radiologic stages, serum levels of ACE, and fibrotic lung involvement quantified by a CT-based quantitative visual score. Comparison of chitotriosidase and ACE in BAL revealed that the chitinase had higher sensitivity (more than 85% of sarcoidosis patients had increased chitotriosidase) and prognostic value, being the only marker correlated with the quantitative score [35].

The sensitivity of chitotriosidase as a marker of sarcoidosis has been analyzed by detecting it in serum of patients with granulomatous lung diseases, such as pulmonary tuberculosis, and different interstitial lung diseases, including pulmonary fibrosis associated with systemic sclerosis and idiopathic pulmonary fibrosis [51,52]. Chitotriosidase was not significantly elevated in serum of patients with other interstitial or granulomatous lung diseases but was only significantly higher in serum of sarcoidosis patients with respect to controls (Fig. 2) [52].

Brunner and colleagues [53] recently analyzed serum chitotriosidase levels in a group of juvenile sarcoidosis patients, finding significantly higher chitotriosidase concentrations in active sarcoidosis than inactive disease. These authors assessed chitotriosidase levels before and after medical treatment, finding a significant reduction during oral steroid therapy. They concluded that serum chitotriosidase can also be proposed as a marker of juvenile sarcoidosis [53].

Although the role of chitotriosidase in the pathogenesis and progression of sarcoidosis is not yet clearly understood, this chitinase secreted by activated macrophages may reasonably induce overexpression of profibrotic type-2 cytokines and play a relevant role in the pathogenesis of sarcoidosis [52,53]. It can be recommended as a clinical marker of sarcoidosis severity and to monitor follow-up; its use for diagnostic purposes has never been evaluated. Chitotriosidase activity can be determined in serum and BAL by a fluorimetric test [49].

Cytokines and chemokines

Many cytokines and chemokines have been analyzed in serum and BAL of sarcoidosis patients [3,54]; some of these mediators, together with immunocompetent cells, are involved in the inflammatory processes occurring in this disease and may have a potential clinical application (Box 1, Fig. 3) [1,12]. They have been studied singly and in panels to evaluate Th1/Th2 profile. BAL seems to have the potential to provide useful diagnostic parameters; however, no single biochemical marker sufficiently sensitive for diagnosis of sarcoidosis has yet been found in the fluid component. A cell pattern typical of lymphocytic alveolitis (lymphocyte count greater than 15%) and a T cell $CD4^+/CD8^+$ ratio over 3.5 has been recognized as an aid for diagnosis of sarcoidosis, however, in the absence of biopsy in patients without tuberculosis or fungal infections and with

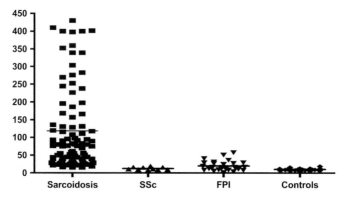

Fig. 2. Chitotriosidase concentrations in serum of sarcoidosis patients, idiopathic pulmonary fibrosis, and pulmonary fibrosis associated with systemic sclerosis patients and in healthy controls. (*From* Bargagli E, Margollicci MA, Luddi A, et al. Chitotriosidase in BAL of patients with diffuse lung diseases. Respir Med 2007;101:2176–81; with permission.)

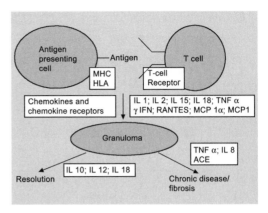

Fig. 3. Immune responses that induce granuloma formation in sarcoidosis. ACE, angiotensin-converting
enzyme; IFN, interferon; IL, interleukin; MCP, monocyte chemoattractant protein; MHC, major histocompatibility complex; TNF, tumor necrosis factor. (*From
Baughman RP, Lower EE, du Bois RM. Sarcoidosis.
Lancet 2003;361:1111–8; with permission.*)

a compatible clinical and radiologic picture
[1,6,8,14]. The CD4/CD8 ratio is only elevated
in about 50% of cases, and it may be enhanced
under different clinical conditions [13]. The role
of the CD4/CD8 ratio of T lymphocytes in the diagnostic work-up of sarcoidosis has been the subject of much debate [1,3,13,14,55,56].

Among the cytokines released by Th1 lymphocytes, IL-2 induces T-cell proliferation and activation after interaction with its receptor [51,57].
sIL-2R is a T-cell surface receptor. Its concentrations are elevated in serum and BAL of sarcoidosis patients because of the increased number and
enhanced activation of T lymphocytes characteristic of this disease [10,11,58]. It is a widely used serologic marker of sarcoidosis, easily detectable in
serum and BAL. It has been recently shown that
this receptor has a prognostic value, being

associated with peculiar disease phenotypes [59].
sIL-2R concentrations correlated with BAL T-
cell numbers and activity (ie, sIL-2R levels are significantly higher in patients with active sarcoidosis
than in patients with inactive disease); its use as
marker of activity is recommended [58,59]. Comparing other serologic inflammatory markers (eg,
C-reactive proteins and serum amyloid A) with
markers of T-cell activation (sIL-2R) and granuloma formation (ACE), Drent and coworkers
[10] concluded that only sIL-2R could be predictive of sarcoidosis severity (Fig. 4).

Another marker of T-cell activation that has
been related to sarcoidosis activity is neopterin,
a metabolite of guanosine triphosphate, released
in vitro by macrophages activated by interferon-γ.
Its concentrations in serum [60] and urine [61]
have been found higher in patients with sarcoidosis than in controls, and in patients with active
than in those with inactive sarcoidosis [62]. Serum
neopterin concentrations were found to have similar predictive value to sIL-2R in a cohort of
newly diagnosed pulmonary sarcoidosis patients
[11]. A recent study of 225 sarcoidosis patients
showed elevated concentrations of sIL-2R and
neopterin in BAL cell cultures of patients with
acute disease and also in those with nonacute disease requiring long-term therapies. These two
markers were studied by a multivariate statistical
analysis that showed correlations with clinical parameters [59].

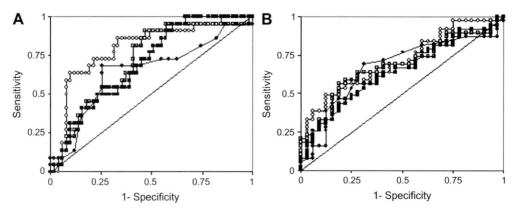

Fig. 4. ROC curves for the inflammatory markers to determine respiratory functional impairment (RFI) in untreated (*A*) and treated (*B*) patients. ●, ACE; sIL2R; SAA; hs-CRP. The diagonal line indicates an AUC of 0.5 (no discrimination between the two states). RFI was defined as present if DLCO was less than 80%, FEV_1 was less than 80%, or FVC was less than 80% of the predicted value and as absent if DLCO was 80%, FEV_1 was 80%, or FVC was 80% of the predicted value. For group I (all untreated patients; *A*), the AUCs (95% confidence intervals [CI]) were 0.799 (0.686–0.913) for sIL2R; 0.650 (0.504–0.795) for ACE; 0.708 (0.583–0.832) for hs-CRP; and 0.701 (0.580–0.821) for SAA. For group II (all treated patients; *B*), the AUCs (95% CI) were 0.711 (0.592–0.829) for sIL2R; 0.671 (0.541–0.801) for ACE; 0.681 (0.556–0.806) for hs-CRP; and 0.645 (0.518–0.773) for SAA. (*From* Rothkrantz-Kos S, van Dieijen-Visser MP, Mulder PGH, et al. Potential usefulness of inflammatory markers to monitor respiratory functional impairment in sarcoidosis. Clin Chem 2003;49:1510–7; with permission.)

Tumor necrosis factor (TNF)-α is a relevant cytokine with a major role in the development and maintenance of granuloma [62]. Alveolar macrophages are the main source of TNF-α in the lungs, although also producing it are activated T-cells and pulmonary epithelial cells [63–70]. Fehrenbach and colleagues [64] demonstrated an association between high levels of TNF-α in BAL cells and granuloma precursors (clusters of alveolar macrophages). They sustained the fundamental role of alveolar macrophages and TNF-α in the initial phase of sarcoidosis. TNF-α concentrations did not seem to be influenced by TNF-α polymorphism in sarcoidosis patients [71]. A recent meta-analysis showed that TNF-α genotype, but not ACE genotype, may be associated with increased risk of sarcoidosis [72]. The receptors of this cytokine have several immunologic functions. TNF receptors (TNFRs) include TNFR-1 (CD120a) or TNFR-2 (CD120b). CD120a determines the apoptotic activity of TNF-α, whereas CD120b induces cytokine activation and cell stimulation by NFkB. Expression of these receptors and concentrations of TNF-α are higher in alveolar macrophages from sarcoidosis patients than in those from controls [73,74]. Increased levels of TNFRs have been reported in serum and BAL of sarcoidosis patients [75].

TNF-β is another cytokine of the TNF family. It is mainly produced by activated T

cells and interacts with the same receptors as TNF-α. The first study that reported a link between a cytokine gene polymorphism and sarcoidosis prognosis was performed on TNF-β. It was concluded that the TNFB*1 allele was a marker of long clinical course in sarcoidosis patients [76].

Transforming growth factor-β is an important profibrotic growth factor involved in lung fibrosis development [77]. It induces synthesis of extracellular matrix molecules, such as fibronectin and type I collagen [78], and inhibits cytokine release by activated macrophages [79] and lymphocytes [80]. Epithelioid histiocytes of sarcoid granuloma contain abundant transforming growth factor-β [81] and some authors reported increased transforming growth factor-β levels in cultures of BAL cells from sarcoidosis patients in spontaneous remission [82]. Kruit and colleagues [83] recently suggested that transforming growth factor-β3 genetic polymorphism could be related to the development of pulmonary fibrosis in sarcoidosis patients. Clinical application of this marker cannot yet be recommended.

Interferon-γ is the main cytokine of Th1 immune response and has a pivotal role in the pathogenesis of sarcoidosis [1,84–86]. It is produced in great quantity by BAL Th1 activated cells of sarcoidosis patients. It induces activation of alveolar macrophages and expression of chemokines, such as CXCL10, and participates in granuloma formation. A deficit in IL-12 and the interferon-γ/interferon-γR system has been associated with altered granuloma development [87]. It is usually assayed with other cytokines, rather than alone, to characterize the Th1 pattern in sarcoidosis and its prevalence over Th2 [84,86]. It could be useful for therapeutic purposes in a panel of cytokines to identify patients with Th1/Th2 imbalance.

IL-8 (CXCL8) is produced by mononuclear cells and has a role in attracting leukocytes, neutrophils, and mononuclear phagocytes to inflamed tissue. IL-8 is usually increased in BAL of patients with chronic sarcoidosis and its concentrations are close to those of idiopathic pulmonary fibrosis (IPF) patients [88]. IL-8 levels in BAL may have a prognostic value in sarcoidosis patients [88].

The IL-12 and IL-18 cytokine families are also Th1 cytokines [89–91]. Antigen-presenting cells are the main source of IL-12 in vivo [91]. Cytokines of the IL-12 family are also produced by lymphocytes, macrophages, and natural killers [89], whereas IL-18 is expressed as an inactive precursor molecule, mainly by macrophages and dendritic cells at sites of chronic Th1-mediated inflammatory diseases [89]. The cytokines of the IL-12 and IL-18 families are potent inducers of Th1 differentiation by stimulation of interferon-γ production and enhancement of T cells and NK cytotoxicity [89]. Moreover, IL-12 induces differentiation of naive T cells into Th1 cells [90]. Several studies report an increase in IL-12 and IL-18 levels in tissues, BAL, and serum of patients with sarcoidosis, showing an involvement of these cytokines in the disease pathogenesis [89–91]. There are no data in the literature of their correlation with lung function tests or radiologic stage, so clinical application as single cytokines seems unlikely.

IL-10 is mainly released by CD8 lymphocytes involved in down-regulation of activated T-helper lymphocytes and macrophages [79]. No concordant data are available on its increased expression in sarcoidosis patients [82] and no positive association has been demonstrated between IL-10 gene functional polymorphism and susceptibility to sarcoidosis [92].

Macrophage colony–stimulating factor and granulocyte-macrophage colony–stimulating factor induce proliferation and differentiation of alveolar macrophages and are released by activated T cells. Although increased levels of these factors have been reported in BAL cells of sarcoidosis patients [93], they cannot be considered clinically significant inflammatory markers of the disease.

Among cell growth factors, YKL-40 is a molecule recently proposed as a potential biomarker of sarcoidosis activity. Its serum levels have been found higher in sarcoidosis patients than controls and correlated with sACE levels and lung function parameters [94].

A variety of chemokines, such as CCL5 (RANTES), CCL9 (MIG), and CCL10 (IP-10), are expressed more abundantly in biologic fluids of sarcoidosis patients and are responsible for the attraction of CD4-lymphocytes at sites of disease [3,54]. CCL18 (or PARC) is a Th2 chemokine produced by alternatively activated alveolar macrophages [95]. There is evidence that CCL18 levels are elevated in BAL and BAL-derived cell cultures from patients with interstitial lung diseases including IPF, sarcoidosis, and hypersensitivity pneumonitis. Prasse and colleagues [96] documented significantly higher BAL levels of CCL18 in idiopathic pulmonary fibrosis patients than healthy controls and in stage IV sarcoidosis patients than those with stage I to II disease. CCL18 is a promising chemokine involved in the fibrotic remodeling typical of diffuse lung diseases. It could be useful for early identification of patients at risk for progressive pulmonary fibrosis [96].

Another chemokine with prognostic significance analyzed in BAL of interstitial lung disease patients is monocyte chemoattractant protein-1. It has been found elevated in serum and BAL of sarcoidosis patients, the increase being more evident in patients with persistent recurrent sarcoidosis. monocyte chemoattractant protein-1 and metalloproteinase-9 induce activation of the receptor DDR1, another molecule associated with susceptibility to sarcoidosis [97].

Markers of oxidative stress

Oxidative stress is the result of an imbalance between oxidant and antioxidant molecules and may cause cell damage. Inflammatory cells, such as neutrophils and macrophages, release reactive oxygen species, such as superoxide anions, hydrogen peroxide, and hydroxyl radicals, which act as oxidants during inflammatory processes, damaging neighboring cells [98]. Reactive oxygen species affect different cell components, such as cell membrane lipids, DNA, and proteins [98]. Oxidative stress can be quantified in biologic materials by measuring concentrations of reactive oxygen species themselves (eg, H_2O_2) or products of oxidative stress [99]. It has been shown that alveolar macrophages, isolated from sarcoidosis patients and cultured in vitro, produce more superoxide anions than those from normal subjects [100]. Moreover, the products of lipid peroxidation have been found elevated in expired breath condensate and BAL of sarcoidosis patients, particularly those with active disease. F_2 isoprostanes are stable prostaglandin-F_2–like compounds derived from nonenzymic oxidation of cell membrane arachidonic acid [101]. 8-Isoprostane is the most frequent F_2 isoprostane in humans and its concentration is significantly elevated in expired breath condensate of patients with different lung diseases (chronic obstructive pulmonary disease, acute respiratory distress syndrome, and so forth) including sarcoidosis. 8-Isoprostane concentrations are also elevated in BAL and can be a useful marker of inflammation and oxidative damage in this disease; however, clinical correlations have not yet been shown [102].

The most widely studied oxidative stress–induced modification of proteins is the formation of carbonyl groups on lysine, proline, arginine, and threonine residues. Oxidative damage to polypeptide chains is quantified by the number of carbonyls [103]. Carbonylated proteins have been analyzed in BAL of sarcoidosis patients by different methods [104]. Quantitative detection showed significantly higher concentrations in BAL of patients than controls because of respiratory burst activation of alveolar phagocytes present in this disease. BAL protein targets of oxidation had also been identified in sarcoidosis patients by a proteomic approach using two-dimensional electrophoresis and immunoblotting with specific antibodies for carbonyl groups [104].

A decrease of redox state has been documented in the erythrocytes of female sarcoidosis patients as another consequence of the occurrence of oxidative stress [105]. Furthermore, the transcription factor NF-kB, of which it is known that it is activated by radical damage, is increased in alveolar macrophages and mononuclear blood cells of active sarcoidosis patients compared with those of healthy controls [106].

Analysis of oxidative stress markers in BAL of sarcoidosis patients by proteomics promises insights into the composition of alveolar microenvironment relevant for the immunopathogenesis of sarcoidosis. Reactive oxygen species and products of oxidative stress in BAL and expired breath cannot yet be considered prognostic markers.

More research is needed into their potential clinical applications, particularly for new therapeutic approaches.

Other markers of sarcoidosis

Immunologic studies on serum, tissue, and BAL have highlighted a polyclonal hypergammaglobulinemia (with a predominance of IgG) in sarcoidosis patients [33,57,107] and formation of circulating immune-complexes [107]. Their clinical value, however, is poorly defined.

Other markers of inflammation have been analyzed in different human biologic fluids by different methods. For example, endothelin-1, a vasoactive bronchoconstrictive peptide involved in lung fibroproliferative processes, has been analyzed in serum, BAL, urine, and lung tissue of sarcoidosis patients [108,109]. Its concentrations were found higher in biologic samples of sarcoidosis patients, especially those with radiologically documented lung involvement, than in samples of controls [110]. Recently Terashita and colleagues [110] observed elevated endothelin-1 levels in 25% of a population of sarcoidosis patients. Endothelin-1 concentrations were found correlated with the number of BAL macrophages. It was postulated that the peptide is involved in the development of pulmonary fibrosis and hypertension, although further studies are required to evaluate its potential as a target for new treatments.

D dimer is a product of the fibrinolytic system. In 1988, Hasday and colleagues [111] implicated coagulation and fibrinolytic systems in the pathogenesis of sarcoidosis, noting enhanced expression of certain procoagulant factors in BAL fluid of sarcoidosis patients. It was later found that protein C activity was depressed in BAL [112] and that circulating D dimer levels were frequently altered in serum and BAL of sarcoidosis patients. D dimer levels were correlated with the radiologic stages of the disease and were proposed as markers of sarcoidosis severity [113]. More recently, Perez and colleagues [114] underlined the potential of D dimer levels in BAL as a prognostic indicator, especially in African Americans. It is not yet clear whether D dimer alteration is a result of general stimulation of different inflammatory cascades or a more specific pathophysiologic process.

Proteins, such as thioredoxin and thioredoxin reductase [115], alpha-defensin [116], serum amyloid A, and C-reactive protein, have been proposed as inflammatory markers in sarcoidosis. C-reactive protein and amyloid A are acute-phase proteins released by the liver under IL-1 and IL-6 stimulation. Drent and colleagues [117] reported higher levels of C-reactive protein in serum of sarcoidosis patients than serum of controls. Serum amyloid A is an acute-phase reactant, produced in response to cytokines synthesized by activated macrophages, and is related to high-density lipoprotein cholesterol. Serum amyloid A levels are much higher in sarcoidosis patients with active inflammatory disease than in those with inactive disease [10,118].

β_2-Microglobulin, a marker of lymphocyte activation, was studied for clinical application, especially in the 1980s. β_2-Microglobulin is a low-molecular-weight protein, reflecting lymphocyte activity, produced by all cells except mature red cells. High concentrations of β_2-microglobulin have been described in various inflammatory, immunologic, and neoplastic diseases. Various authors have noted that about 25% of sarcoidosis patients have elevated serum concentrations of β_2-microglobulin. Selroos and Klockars [119] measured serum concentrations of ACE and β_2-microglobulin in patients with sarcoidosis in different clinical stages and in healthy subjects. β_2-Microglobulin levels were correlated with granuloma formation in initial phases, whereas ACE values reflected later phases. These results suggested that simultaneous determinations of serum ACE and β_2-microglobulin may be useful for describing disease activity [119]. β_2-Microglobulin concentrations have also been assayed in cerebrospinal fluid where they were found elevated in 68% of neurosarcoidosis patients but not in patients without neurologic involvement [120]. With its low specificity and sensitivity, however, this marker is of little value in clinical practice.

Impaired calcium metabolism is a classical clinical feature of sarcoidosis. Hypercalcemia (prevalence 5%–10%) and hypercalciuria (prevalence 40%–62%) are the most frequent disorders [6]. The pathogenesis of abnormal calcium metabolism in sarcoidosis is not fully understood, but hyperabsorption of calcium seems to depend on serum concentrations of the active form of vitamin D, $1\alpha,25(OH)2D3$, which is overproduced by sarcoid granuloma [121]. High serum concentration of $1\alpha,25(OH)2D3$ down-regulates parathyroid hormone release. Alterations in parathyroid hormone–related proteins have also been demonstrated. Hypercalcemia and hypercalciuria are simple indices of disease activity; however, they have limited prevalence and prognostic value [121,122].

Proteomic approach

A more recent approach to the analysis of sarcoidosis markers is the application of proteomics. Proteome analysis enables one simultaneously to analyze all proteins present in a biologic sample and to define protein profiles characteristic of a disease [86,123]. This approach is independent of any a priori hypothesis about specific proteins, implying high potential for new discoveries [86,104,124–132]. Many techniques with different advantages and disadvantages are actually available for proteomic approach and some of them have been applied to the study of sarcoidosis [129]. The groups of Wattiez and colleagues, Lindahl and colleagues, Grunewald and colleagues, and the authors were among the first to work in this field contributing to the identification of BAL proteins with the aim to create a database and to characterize disease-specific protein patterns [124–126,130].

According to the authors' experience, the most interesting findings on proteomic analysis of interstitial lung disease were in BAL, where huge amounts of plasma and locally produced proteins were found [86,104,124]. A total of 85 proteins were identified by two-dimensional electrophoresis and mass spectrometry, 38 for the first time in BAL [124]. These proteins had different origins (plasma derived, locally secreted, or products of cell damage and proteolytic activity) and functions (eg, antiprotease, anti-inflammatory or proinflammatory, antioxidant, coagulation-related, and so forth), and different protein profiles characteristic of each interstitial lung disease were identified [86]. Two-dimensional electrophoretic studies on BAL demonstrated that some acute-phase proteins (eg, ceruloplasmin, haptoglobin β, α_1-antichymotrypsin) were more abundant in sarcoidosis than in idiopathic pulmonary fibrosis patients [86,124].

Applying narrow-range pH gradients a new group of proteins in BAL of sarcoidosis patients was identified [126]. Comparison of BAL protein composition with serum showed three proteins simultaneously increased in serum and BAL of the same patients: immunoglobulin kappa light chain, β_2-microglobulin, and β_2-microglobulin 1 [131]. In 2007 the same authors applied difference gel electrophoresis proteomics to the analysis of BAL protein profiles in patients with high risk of developing chronic sarcoidosis (HLA-DRB1*15 positive) compared with chronic beryllium disease and controls [127]. A total of 37 protein spots were differently expressed in sarcoidosis patients versus controls and 14 of these proteins were identified [127]. Another recent approach to the study of protein composition is the use of SELDI-TOF mass spectrometry, which facilitates the discovery of disease-related protein patterns. It has been used to identify different protein profiles in BAL linked to a particular sarcoidosis clinical course [132]. Some protein peaks were specifically associated with the radiologic stages of sarcoidosis, although the proteins corresponding to these peaks were not yet identified, with the exception of albumin, α_1-antitrypsin, and protocadherin-2 precursor [132]. Very recently, SELDI-TOF mass spectrometry technique has been used to identify new serologic markers of sarcoidosis, such as the $\alpha2$ chain of haptoglobin [128].

The use of proteome analysis to study BAL and serum of sarcoidosis patients allowed the identification of several proteins differently expressed compared with controls or other interstitial lung diseases; some of them may represent markers of the disease. They need to be validated further by other easier methods applied to a greater number of samples and by adequate statistical analysis [86,104,124].

Summary

Sarcoidosis is characterized by intense inflammation at the different sites of localization fullstop. According to a recent classification, has also been included among autoinflammatory diseases [133]. Many different mediators, such as cytokines, chemokines, and other proteins with various functions, participate in its complex pathogenesis and some have been proposed as markers of inflammation. These generally increase during the active phase of the disease and they are considered markers of activity, although the concept of activity has not yet been clearly defined in sarcoidosis. The clinical course of sarcoidosis varies in different patients. The disease may resolve spontaneously or progress leading to lung fibrosis [6]. Because no tests at diagnosis can predict the outcome for a patient, prognosis is difficult.

This review of inflammatory biomarkers used for monitoring sarcoidosis shows that most have been studied in BAL fluid, because lungs are the most frequently involved organ [134]. Identification of biomarkers in serum or expired breath condensate [101,102] would be preferable, because they are less invasive than BAL to obtain.

After many years of research, no single marker sufficiently sensitive and specific for diagnosis of sarcoidosis has yet been found. Only the T lymphocyte CD4/CD8 ratio in BAL has been recognized as an aid for diagnosis of sarcoidosis [6,134], although it has some limits. With regard to prognosis, the best evidence of clinical correlations is for sIL-2R and chitotriosidase, which seem more promising than ACE [10,35]. Other mediators, such as TNF-α and CCL18, could help to identify patients at risk for fibrosis or progressive disease [64,96]. Sophisticated methods applied to the study of BAL and serum are providing new markers useful for further characterizing the immunoinflammatory mechanisms of this disease; however, greater correlation with clinical parameters is needed and proper validation in large cohorts of patients [13].

It must be clarified which and how many inflammatory markers are needed to characterize the patient clinical pattern. It is important to determine which are early markers of progression toward chronic disease and lung fibrosis, disease relapse, and response to therapy. It is necessary to assess their cost-benefit ratio in relation to the clinical information they provide. These relevant aspects need to be discussed by a panel of experts and a common project drawn up to coordinate future research in this field. Groups of markers have to be selected, and they may also be useful for better defining the clinical phenotypes of sarcoidosis [59].

Acknowledgments

The authors thank C. Madioni, C. Olivieri, and F, Mezzasalma for their contribution.

References

[1] Baughman RP, Lower EE, du Bois RM. Sarcoidosis. Lancet 2003;361:1111–8.

[2] Moller DR. Potential etiologic agents in sarcoidosis. Proc Am Thorac Soc 2007;4:465–8.

[3] Drent M, Costabel U. Sarcoidosis. European Respiratory Monograph 2005;10(32):13.

[4] Dai H, Guzman J, Chen B, et al. Production of soluble TNF receptor and TNF alpha by alveolar macrophages in sarcoidosis and extrinsic allergic alveolitis. Chest 2005;127:251–6.

[5] Ziegenhagen MW, Rothe ME, Zissel G, et al. Exaggerated TNF alpha release of alveolar macrophages in corticosteroid resistant sarcoidosis. Sarcoidosis Vasc Diffuse Lung Dis 2002;19:185–90.

[6] Iannuzzi MC, Rybicki BA, Teirstein AS. Sarcoidosis. N Engl J Med 2007;357:2153–65.

[7] Aladesanmi OA. Sarcoidosis: an update for the primary care physicians. MedGenMed 2004;6:7.

[8] Sharma OP, Smith I, Maguire G, et al. Clinical value of ACE genotyping in diagnosis of sarcoidosis. Lancet 1997;349:1602–3.

[9] Stokes GS, Monaghan JC, Schrader AP, et al. Influence of ACE genotype on interpretation of diagnostic tests for serum ACE activity. Aust N Z J Med 1999;29:315–8.

[10] Rothkrantz-Kos S, van Dieijen-Visser MP, Mulder PGH, et al. Potential usefulness of inflammatory markers to monitor respiratory functional impairment in sarcoidosis. Clin Chem 2003;49:1510–7.

[11] Ziegenhagen MW, Rothe ME, Schlaak M, et al. BAL and serological parameters reflecting the severity of sarcoidosis. Eur Respir J 2003;21:407–13.

[12] Rottoli P, Bargagli E. Is bronchoalveolar lavage obsolete in the diagnosis of interstitial lung disease? Curr Opin Pulm Med 2003;9:418–25.

[13] Kantrow SP, Meyer KC, Kidd P, et al. The CD4/CD8 ratio in BAL fluid is highly variable. Eur Respir J 1997;10:2716–21.

[14] Hunninghake GW, Crystal RG. Pulmonary sarcoidosis: a disorder mediated by excess helper T lymphocyte activity at sites of disease activity. N Engl J Med 1981;305:429–34.

[15] Haslam PL, Baughman RP. Guidelines for measurement of acellular components and standardization of BAL. Eur Respir J 1999;9:25–7.

[16] Baughman RP, Drent M. Role of BAL in interstitial lung diseases. Clin Chest Med 2001;22:331–41.

[17] Lieberman J. Elevation of serum angiotensin-converting enzyme (ACE) level in sarcoidosis. Am J Med 1975;59:365–72.

[18] Studdy PR, Lapworth R, Bird R. Angiotensin-converting enzyme and its clinical significant: a review. J Clin Pathol 1983;36:938–47.

[19] Gronhagen-Riska C, Kuppa K, Fyhrquist F, et al. Angiotensin-converting enzyme and lysozyme in silicosis and asbestosis. Scand J Respir Dis 1978;59:228–31.

[20] Brice EA, Friedlander W, Bateman ED, et al. Serum angiotensin-converting enzyme activity, concentration, and specific activity in granulomatous interstitial lung disease, tuberculosis, and COPD. Chest 1995;107(3):706–10.

[21] Lieberman J, Nosal A, Schleissner LA, et al. Update on SACE assays for diagnosis and evaluation of sarcoidosis. Baltimore (MD): University Park Press; 1974.

[22] Lieberman J, Rea TH. Serum angiotensin-converting enzyme in leprosy and coccidioidomycosis. Ann Intern Med 1977;87:422–5.

[23] Casal JA, Lacerda L, Perez LF, et al. Relationships between serum markers of monocyte/macrophage activation in type 1 Gaucher's disease. Clin Chem Lab Med 2002;40:52–5.

[24] Kennon B, Konnell JM. ACE gene polymorphism and diabetic complications: is there a connection? BioDrugs 2000;14:73–81.

[25] Smallridge RC, Rogers J, Verma PS. Serum angiotensin-converting enzyme: alterations in hyperthyroidism, hypothyroidism and subacute thyroiditis. JAMA 1983;250:2489–93.

[26] Matsuki K, Sakata T. Angiotensin-converting enzyme in diseases of the liver. Am J Med 1982;73:549–51.

[27] Lieberman J, Schleissner LA, Nosal A, et al. Clinical correlations of serum angiotensin-converting enzyme in sarcoidosis: a longitudinal study of serum ACE, 67 gallium scans, chest roentgenograms and pulmonary functions. Chest 1983;84:522–8.

[28] Schurmann M. Angiotensin converting enzyme gene polymorphism in patients with pulmonary sarcoidosis: impact on disease severity. Am J Pharmacogenomics 2003;3:233–43.

[29] Cambien F, Alhenc-Gelas F, Herbeth B, et al. Familial resemblance of plasma ACE level: the Nancy study. Am J Hum Genet 1998;43:774–80.

[30] Rigat B, Hubert C, Alhenc-Gelas F, et al. An insertion/deletion polymorphism in the angiotensin I converting enzyme gene accounting for half the variance of serum enzyme levels. J Clin Invest 1990;86:1343–6.

[31] Kruit A, Grutters JC, Gerritsen WBM, et al. ACE I/D-corrected Z-scores to identify normal and elevated ACE activity in sarcoidosis. Respir Med 2007;101:510–5.

[32] Alia P, Mana J, Capdevila O, et al. Association between ACE gene I/D polymorphism and clinical presentation and prognosis of sarcoidosis. Scand J Clin Lab Invest 2005;65:691–7.

[33] Costabel U, Tescheler H. Biochemical changes in sarcoidosis. Clin Chest Med 1997;18:827–42.

[34] Baudin B. Angiotensin I-converting enzyme (ACE) for sarcoidosis diagnosis. Pathol Biol 2005;53:183–8 [in French].

[35] Bargagli E, Margollicci M, Perrone M, et al. Chitotriosidase levels in BAL of patients with sarcoidosis. Sarcoidosis Vasc Diffuse Lung Dis 2007;24:59–64.

[36] Hankiewicz J, Swierczek E. Lysozyme in human body fluids. Clin Chim Acta 1974;57(3):205–9.

[37] Prior C, Barbee RA, Evans PM, et al. Lavage versus serum measurements of lysozyme, angiotensin-converting enzyme and inflammatory markers in pulmonary sarcoidosis. Eur Respir J 1990;3:1146–54.

[38] Selroos OB. Biochemical marker in sarcoidosis. Crit Rev Clin Lab Sci 1986;24:185–216.

[39] Gronhagen-Riska C. Angiotensin-converting enzyme: activity and correlation with serum lysozime in sarcoidosis, other chest or lymph node disease

and healthy persons. Scand J Respir Dis 1979;60: 83–93.

[40] Khan K, Perillie PE, Finch SC. Serum lysozyme in pulmonary tuberculosis. Am J Med Sci 1973;265: 297–302.

[41] Turton CWG, Grundy E, Firth G, et al. Value of measuring serum angiotensin-converting enzyme and serum lysozyme in the management of sarcoidosis. Thorax 1979;34:57–62.

[42] Tomita H, Sato S, Matsuda R, et al. Serum lysozyme levels and clinical features of sarcoidosis. Lung 1999;177:161–7.

[43] Boot RG, Bussink AP, Verhoek M, et al. Marked differences in tissue-specific expression of chitinases in mouse and man. J Histochem Cytochem 2005; 53:1283–92.

[44] Wajner A, Michelin K, Burin MG, et al. Biochemical characterisation of chitotriosidase enzyme: comparison between normal individuals and patients with Gaucher and with Niemann-Pick diseases. Clin Biochem 2004;37:893–7.

[45] Michelakakis H, Dimitriou E, Labadaridis I. The expanding spectrum of disorders with elevated plasma chitotriosidase activity: an update. J Inherit Metab Dis 2004;27:705–6.

[46] Artieda M, Cennaro A, Ganan A, et al. Serum chitotriosidase in subjects with atherosclerosis disease. Arterioscler Thromb Vasc Biol 2003;23:1645–52.

[47] Vellodi A, Foo Y, Cole TJ. Evaluation of three biochemical markers in the monitoring of Gaucher disease. J Inherit Metab Dis 2005;28:585–92.

[48] Brinkman J, Wijburg FA, Hollak CE, et al. Plasma chitotriosidase and CCL18: early biochemical surrogate markers in type B Niemann-Pick disease. J Inherit Metab Dis 2005;28:13–20.

[49] Grosso S, Margollicci MA, Bargagli E, et al. Serum levels of chitotriosidase as a marker of disease activity and clinical stage in sarcoidosis. Scand J Clin Lab Invest 2004;64:57–62.

[50] Bargagli E, Bianchi N, Margollicci M, et al. Chitotriosidase and soluble IL-2 receptor: comparison of two markers of sarcoidosis severity. Scand J Clin Lab Invest, in press.

[51] Bargagli E, Margollicci M, Nikiforakis N, et al. Chitotriosidase activity in serum of patients with sarcoidosis and pulmonary tuberculosis. Respiration 2007;74:548–52.

[52] Bargagli E, Margollicci MA, Luddi A, et al. Chitotriosidase in BAL of patients with diffuse lung diseases. Respir Med 2007;101:2176–81.

[53] Brunner J, Scholl-Burgi S, Zimmerhackl LB. Chitotriosidase as a marker of disease activity in sarcoidosis. Rheumatol Int 2007;27:1171–2.

[54] Gurrieri G, Bortoli M, Brunetta E, et al. Cytokines, chemokines and other biomolecular markers in sarcoidosis. Sarcoidosis Vasc Diffuse Lung Dis 2005; 22:S9–14.

[55] Antoniou K, Tsiligianni I, Kyriakou D, et al. Perforin down-regulation and adhesion molecules

activation in pulmonary sarcoidosis. Chest 2006; 129:1592–8.

[56] Kurumagawa T, Seki S, Kobayashi H, et al. Characterization of bronchoalveolar lavage T cell subsets in sarcoidosis on the basis of CD57, CD4 and CD8. Clin Exp Immunol 2003;133(3):438–47.

[57] Semenzato G, Bortoli M, Agostini C. Applied clinical immunology in sarcoidosis. Curr Opin Pulm Med 2002;8(5):441–4.

[58] Grutters JC, Fellrath JM, Mulder L, et al. Serum soluble IL2 receptor measurement in patients with sarcoidosis. Chest 2003;124:186–95.

[59] Prasse A, Katic C, Germann M. Phenotyping sarcoidosis from a pulmonary perspective. Am J Respir Crit Care Med 2008;177(3):330–6.

[60] Eklund A, Blaschke E. Elevated serum neopterin levels in sarcoidosis. Lung 1986;164(6):325–32.

[61] Lacronique J, Auzeby A, Valeyre D, et al. Urinary neopterin in pulmonary sarcoidosis: relationship to clinical and biologic assessment of the disease. Am Rev Respir Dis 1989;139(6):1474–8.

[62] Muller-Quernheim J. Serum markers for the staging of disease activity of sarcoidosis and other interstitial lung diseases of unknown etiology. Sarcoidosis Vasc Diffuse Lung Dis 1998;15:22–37.

[63] Müller-Quernheim J. Sarcoidosis: immunopathogenetic concepts and their clinical application. Eur Respir J 1998;12:716–38.

[64] Fehrenbach H, Zissel G, Goldmann T, et al. Alveolar macrophages are the main source for tumour necrosis factor-α in patients with sarcoidosis. Eur Respir J 2003;21:421–8.

[65] Prasse A, Georges CG, Biller H, et al. Th1 cytokine pattern in sarcoidosis is expressed by bronchoalveolar CD4+ and CD8+ T cells. Clin Exp Immunol 2000;122:241–8.

[66] Mollers M, Aries SP, Dromann D, et al. Intracellular cytokine repertoire in different T cell subsets from patients with sarcoidosis. Thorax 2001;56: 487–93.

[67] Wahlström J, Katchar K, Wigzell H, et al. Analysis of intracellular cytokines in CD4(+) and CD8(+) lung and blood T cells in sarcoidosis. Am J Respir Crit Care Med 2001;163:115–21.

[68] Marques LJ, Zheng L, Poulakis N, et al. Pentoxifylline inhibits TNF alpha production from human alveolar macrophages. Am J Respir Crit Care Med 1999;159:508–11.

[69] Zissel G, Ernst M, Rabe K, et al. Human alveolar epithelial cells type II are capable of regulating T-cell activity. J Investig Med 2000;48:66–75.

[70] Piguet PF, Ribaux C, Karpuz V, et al. Expression and localization of tumor necrosis factor-alpha and its mRNA in idiopathic pulmonary fibrosis. Am J Pathol 1993;143:651–5.

[71] Somoskovi A, Zissel G, Seitzer U, et al. Polymorphism at position -308 in the promoter region of the TNF-α and in the first intron of the TNF-β genes and spontaneous and lipopolysaccharide-induced

TNF-α release in sarcoidosis. Cytokine 1999;11: 882–7.

[72] Medica I, Kastrin A, Maver A, et al. Role of genetic polymorphisms in ACE and TNF-alpha gene in sarcoidosis: a meta-analysis. J Hum Genet 2007; 52(10):836–47.

[73] Dai H, Guzman J, Chen B, et al. Increased expression of apoptosis signalling receptors by alveolar macrophages in sarcoidosis. Eur Respir J 1999;13:1451–4.

[74] Kieszko R, Krawczyk P, Chocholska S, et al. Tumor necrosis factor receptors (TNFRs) on T lymphocytes and soluble TNFRs in different clinical courses of sarcoidosis. Respir Med 2007;101: 645–54.

[75] Hino T, Nakamura H, Shibata Y, et al. Elevated levels of type II solubile tumor necrosis factor receptors in the bronchoalveolar lavage fluids of patients with sarcoidosis. Lung 1997;175:187–93.

[76] Yamaguchi E, Itoh A, Hizawa N, et al. The gene polymorphism of tumor necrosis factor-ß, but not that of tumor necrosis factor-α, is associated with the prognosis of sarcoidosis. Chest 2001;119:753–61.

[77] Border WA, Noble NA. Transforming growth factor β in tissue fibrosis. N Engl J Med 1994;10:1286–92.

[78] Moses HL, Yang EY, Pietenpol JA. TGF β stimulation and inhibition of cell proliferation: new mechanistic insights. Cell 1990;63:245–7.

[79] Zissel G, Schlaak J, Schlaak M, et al. Regulation of cytokine release by alveolar macrophages treated with interleukin-4, interleukin-10, or trasforming growth factor beta. Eur Cytokine Netw 1996;7: 59–66.

[80] Yamamoto H, Hirayama M, Genyea C, et al. TGF β mediates natural suppressor activity of IL-2 activated lymphocytosec. J Immunol 1994;149: 197–204.

[81] Limper AH, Colby TV, Sanders MS, et al. Immunohistochemical localization of TGF β1 in the non necrotizing granulomas of pulmonary sarcoidosis. Am J Respir Crit Care Med 1994;149:197–204.

[82] Zissel G, Homolka J, Schlaak J, et al. Anti-inflammatory cytokine release by alveolar macrophages in pulmonary sarcoidosis. Am J Respir Crit Care Med 1996;154:713–9.

[83] Kruit A, Grutters JC, Ruven HJ, et al. Transforming growth factor-ß gene polymorphisms in sarcoidosis patients with and without fibrosis. Chest 2006;129:1584–91.

[84] Bäumer I, Zissel G, Schlaak M, et al. Th1/Th2 cell distribution in pulmonary sarcoidosis. Am J Respir Cell Mol Biol 1997;16:171–7.

[85] Moller DR. Pulmonary fibrosis of sarcoidosis: new approaches, old ideas. Am J Respir Cell Mol Biol 2003;29(Suppl 3):S37–41.

[86] Rottoli P, Magi B, Perari MG, et al. Cytokine profile and proteome analysis in BAL of patients with sarcoidosis pulmonary fibrosis associated with systemic sclerosis and idiopathic pulmonary fibrosis. Proteomics 2005;5:1423–30.

[87] Wysoczanska B, Bogunia-Kubik K, Suchnicki K, et al. Combined association between IFN-gamma 3,3 homozygosis and DRB1%66D03 in Lofgren's syndrome patients. Immunol Lett 2004;91:127–31.

[88] Baughman RP, Keeton D, Lower EE. Relationship between IL-8 and neutrophils in the BALF of sarcoidosis. Sarcoidosis Vasc Diffuse Lung Dis 1994; 11:S217–20.

[89] Shigehara K, Shijubo N, Ohmichi M, et al. IL-12 and IL-18 are increased and stimulate IFN-γ production in sarcoid lungs. J Immunol 2001;166:642–9.

[90] Shigehara K, Shijubo N, Ohmichi M, et al. Increased circulating interleukin-12 (IL-12) p40 in pulmonary sarcoidosis. Clin Exp Immunol 2003; 132:152–7.

[91] Sinigaglia F. IL-12 in lung diseases. Sarcoidosis Vasc Diffuse Lung Dis 2000;17:122–4.

[92] Murakozy G, Gaede KI, Zissel G, et al. Analysis of gene polymorphisms in interleukin-10 and transforming growth factor-ß1 in sarcoidosis. Sarcoidosis Vasc Diffuse Lung Dis 2001;18:165–9.

[93] Kreipe H, Radzun HJ, Heidorn K, et al. Proliferation, macrophage colony-stimulating factor-receptor expression of alveolar macrophage in active sarcoidosis. Lab Invest 1990;62:697–703.

[94] Johansen JS, Milman N, Hansen M, et al. Increased serum YKL-40 in patients with pulmonary sarcoidosis: a potential marker of disease activity? Respir Med 2005;99(4):396–402.

[95] Mrazek F, Sekerova V, Drabek J, et al. Expression of the chemokine PARC in BAL of patients with sarcoidosis. Immunol Lett 2002;84:17–22.

[96] Prasse A, Pechkovsky DV, Toews GB, et al. A vicious circle of alveolar macrophages and fibroblast perpetuates pulmonary fibrosis via CCL18. Am J Respir Crit Care Med 2006;173:781–92.

[97] Matsuyama W, Mitsuyama H, Watanabe M, et al. Involvement of discoidin domain receptor 1 in the deterioration of pulmonary sarcoidosis. Am J Respir Crit Care Med 2005;33:565–73.

[98] Rahman I, Biswas SK, Kode A. Oxidant and antioxidant balance in the airways and airway diseases. Eur J Pharmacol 2006;533:222–39.

[99] Das KK, Buchner V. Effect of nickel exposure on peripheral tissues: role of oxidative stress in toxicity and possible protection by ascorbic acid. Rev Environ Health 2007;22:157–73.

[100] Baughman RP, Lower EE, Pierson G, et al. Spontaneous hydrogen peroxide release from alveolar macrophages of patients with active sarcoidosis: comparison with cigarette smokers. J Lab Clin Med 1998;111:399–404.

[101] Psathakis K, Papatheodorou G, Plataki M, et al. 8-Isoprostane, a marker of oxidative stress, is increased in the expired breath condensate of patients with pulmonary sarcoidosis. Chest 2004;125: 1005–11.

[102] Piotrowski WJ, Antczak A, Marczak J, et al. Eicosanoids in exhaled breath condensate and BAL fluid

of patients with sarcoidosis. Chest 2007;132(2): 589–96.

[103] Dalle-Donne I, Scaloni A, Giustarini D, et al. Proteins as biomarkers of oxidative/nitrosative stress in diseases: the contribution of redox proteomics. Mass Spectrom Rev 2005;24:55–99.

[104] Rottoli P, Magi B, Cianti R, et al. Carbonylated proteins in BAL of patients with sarcoidosis, pulmonary fibrosis associated with systemic sclerosis and idiopathic pulmonary fibrosis. Proteomics 2005;5:2612–8.

[105] Rothkrantz-Kos S, Drent M, Vuil H, et al. Decreased redox state in red blood cells from patients with sarcoidosis. Sarcoidosis Vasc Diffuse Lung Dis 2002;19:114–20.

[106] Drent M, van den Berg R, Haenen GR, et al. NF-KappaB activation in sarcoidosis. Sarcoidosis Vasc Diffuse Lung Dis 2001;18:50–6.

[107] Daniele RP, Dauber JH, Rossman MD. Immunological abnormalities in sarcoidosis. Ann Intern Med 1980;92:406–16.

[108] Sofia M, Mormile M, Faraone S, et al. Endothelin-1 escretion in urine in active pulmonary sarcoidosis and in other interstitial lung diseases. Sarcoidosis 1995;12:118–23.

[109] Reichenberger F, Schauer J, Kellner K, et al. Different expression of endothelin in the BAL in patients with pulmonary diseases. Lung 2001;179:163–74.

[110] Terashita K, Kato S, Sata M, et al. Increased endothelin-1 levels of BAL fluid in patients with pulmonary sarcoidosis. Respirology 2006;11(2):145–51.

[111] Hasday JD, Backwich PR, Lynch JP, et al. Procoagulant and plasminogen activator activities of bronchoalveolar lavage fluid in patients with pulmonary sarcoidosis. Exp Lung Res 1988;14:261–78.

[112] Kobayashi H, Gabazza EC, Taguch O, et al. Protein C anticoagulant system in patients with interstitial lung disease. Am J Respir Crit Care Med 1998;157:1850–4.

[113] Shorr AF, Hnatiuk OW. Circulating D dimer in patients with sarcoidosis. Chest 2000;117:1012–6.

[114] Perez RL, Kimani AP, King TE Jr, et al. Emory Interstitial Lung Disease Center. Bronchoalveolar lavage fluid D dimer levels are higher and more prevalent in black patients with pulmonary sarcoidosis. Respiration 2007;74(3):297–303.

[115] Tiitto L, Kaarteenaho-Wiik R, Sormunen R, et al. Expression of the thioredoxin system in interstitial lung disease. J Pathol 2003;201(3):363–70.

[116] Ashitani J, Matsumoto N, Nakazato M. Elevated alpha-defensin levels in plasma of patients with pulmonary sarcoidosis. Respirology 2007;12(3):339–45.

[117] Drent M, Wirnsberger RM, de Vries J, et al. Association of fatigue with an acute phase response in sarcoidosis. Eur Respir J 1999;13:718–22.

[118] Salazar A, Pinto X, Manà J. Serum amyloid A and high-density lipoprotein cholesterol: serum markers of inflammation in sarcoidosis and other systemic disorders. Eur J Clin Invest 2001;31: 1070–7.

[119] Selroos O, Klockars M. Relation between clinical stage of sarcoidosis and serum values of angiotensin converting enzyme and beta2-microglobulin. Sarcoidosis Vasc Diffuse Lung Dis 1987;4: 13–7.

[120] Oksanen V. New cerebrospinal fluid, neurophysiological and neuroradiological examinations in the diagnosis and follow up of neurosarcoidosis. Sarcoidosis Vasc Diffuse Lung Dis 1987;4:105–10.

[121] Barnard J, Newman LS. Sarcoidosis: immunology, rheumatic diseases, and therapeutics. Curr Opin Rheumatol 2001;13:84–91.

[122] Rottoli P, Gonnelli S, Solitro S, et al. Alterations in calcium metabolism and bone mineral density in relation to the activity of sarcoidosis. Sarcoidosis 1993;10:161–2.

[123] Kauffmann F, Post Genome Respiratory Epidemiology Group. Post-genome respiratory epidemiology: a multidisciplinary challenge. Eur Respir J 2004;24(3):471–80.

[124] Magi B, Bini L, Perari MG, et al. BAL fluid protein composition in patients with sarcoidosis and IPF: a 2DE study. Electrophoresis 2002;23:3434–44.

[125] Wattiez R, Falmagne P. Proteomics of bronchoalveolar lavage fluid. J Chromatogr B Analyt Technol Biomed Life Sci 2005;815(1–2):169–78.

[126] Sabounchi-Schütt F, Astrom J, Eklund A, et al. Detection and identification of human BAL proteins using narrow-range immobilized pH gradient DryStryp and the paper bridge sample application method. Electrophoresis 2001;22:1851–60.

[127] Silva E, Bourin S, Sabounchi-Shutt F, et al. A quantitative proteomic analysis of soluble BAL fluid proteins from patients with sarcoidosis and chronic beryllium disease. Sarcoidosis Vasc Diffuse Lung Dis 2007;24:24–32.

[128] Bons JA, Drent M, Bowman FG, et al. Potential biomarkers for diagnosis of sarcoidosis using proteomics in serum. Respir Med 2007;101:1687–95.

[129] Magi B, Bargagli E, Bini L, et al. The proteomic analysis of BAL in lung diseases. Proteomics 2006;6(23):6354–69.

[130] Lindahl M, Ekstrom T, Sorensen J, et al. Two dimensional protein patterns of BAL fluid from non-smokers, smokers, and subjects exposed to asbestos. Thorax 1996;51:1028–35.

[131] Sabounchi-Schutt F, Astrom J, Hellman U, et al. Changes in BAL fluid proteins in sarcoidosis: a proteomics approach. Eur Respir J 2003;21:414–20.

[132] Kriegova E, Melle C, Kolek V, et al. Protein profiles of bronchoalveolar lavage fluid from patients with pulmonary sarcoidosis. Am J Respir Crit Care Med 2006;173(10):1145–54.

[133] Kanazawa N, Furukawa F. Autoinflammatory syndromes with a dermatological perspective. J Dermatol 2007;34(9):601–18.

[134] Meyer KC. Bronchoalveolar lavage as a diagnostic tool. Semin Respir Crit Care Med 2007;28(5): 546–60.

ELSEVIER
SAUNDERS

Clin Chest Med 29 (2008) 459–473

CLINICS
IN CHEST
MEDICINE

Pulmonary Sarcoidosis

Violeta Mihailovic-Vucinic, MD, PhD[a,b,c,*], Dragana Jovanovic, MD, PhD[a,c]

[a]Medical School, University of Belgrade, Dr Subotica 8, 11000 Belgrade, Serbia
[b]Yugoslav Association of Sarcoidosis, Visegradska 26/20, 11 000 Belgrade, Serbia
[c]Vth Clinical Department, Institute of Pulmonary Diseases, University Clinical Center, Visegradska 26/20, 11 000 Belgrade, Serbia

Sarcoidosis is an inflammatory granulomatous disease that is characterized by diverse organ system manifestations, a variable clinical course, and a predilection for affecting relatively young adults worldwide [1]. Abnormalities on chest radiographs are detected in 85% to 95% of patients with sarcoidosis [1–5]. Approximately 20% to 50% of patients who have sarcoidosis present with respiratory symptoms, including dyspnea, cough, chest pain, and tightness of the chest [4]. The clinical course and manifestations of pulmonary sarcoidosis are protean: spontaneous remission occurs in approximately two thirds of patients; up to 30% of patients have chronic course of the lung disease, resulting in progressive, (sometimes life-threatening) loss of lung function. Morbidity that correlates to sarcoidosis occurs in 1% to 4% of patients [6–8].

An epidemiologic study by British scientists identified 1019 cases of sarcoidosis between 1991 and 2003. Mortality rates at 3 and 5 years for sarcoidosis patients were 5% and 7%, respectively, compared with 2% and 4%, respectively, among age- and gender-matched controls without sarcoidosis. Causes of death were not reported [4,9,10].

Clinical symptoms of pulmonary sarcoidosis

The clinical manifestations of sarcoidosis are heterogeneous and overlap with many infectious and noninfectious granulomatous disorders. Although the lung is involved in more than 90% of patients, multisystemic involvement is characteristic of the disease, and virtually any organ can be affected [1–4]. In some patients, extrapulmonary manifestations are the presenting and predominant features. Recognition of extrapulmonary features of sarcoidosis is critical to ensure prompt diagnosis and appropriate treatment. Approximately one third of patients initially complain of nonspecific symptoms of fever, anorexia, fatigue, malaise, and weight loss, and approximately 20% to 50% of patients who have sarcoidosis present with respiratory symptoms, such as dyspnea, cough, chest pain, and tightness of the chest [11].

Constitutional symptoms

Fever

Sarcoidosis is an important cause of "fever of unknown origin" [11,12], although fever is more common in tuberculosis, fungal infection, and some other granulomatous infections. Fever may occur in the early course of sarcoidosis, but fever that lasts longer than 6 weeks occurs in less than 5% of patients who have sarcoidosis [11–16]. The fever of an early stage of sarcoidosis spontaneously remits within a few weeks in most patients [10]. Fever can be combined with polyarthritis, erythema nodosum, and bilateral hilar lymphadenopathy (Löfgren's syndrome) (Fig. 1).

* Corresponding author. Vth Clinical Department, Institute of Pulmonary Diseases, University Clinical Center, Visegradska 26/20, 11 000 Belgrade, Serbia.
E-mail address: violeta.vucinic@kcs.ac.yu (V. Mihailovic-Vucinic).

0272-5231/08/$ - see front matter © 2008 Elsevier Inc. All rights reserved.
doi:10.1016/j.ccm.2008.03.002

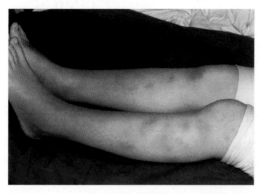

Fig. 1. Erythema nodosum, the hallmark of acute sarcoidosis, fever, and polyarthralgia are usual at the onset. The skin lesions show a play of colors from the onset to the end. The period ranges from 1 to 20 weeks. Recurrences of erythema nodosum are seen in 10% of patients usually within 3 months [17].

Fatigue

Fatigue occurs in many diseases. Fatigue is also common in patients who have sarcoidosis, although the exact incidence of fatigue in sarcoidosis is not known [1]. Patients use the term "fatigue" to describe malaise associated with infections. It may also indicate muscle weakness and tiredness and limited exercise tolerance. Patients who have acute sarcoidosis and patients who have with chronic lung fibrosis suffer from fatigue. Many patients who have sarcoidosis have a "flu-like" syndrome, which may last for weeks or months. Fatigue may be mild or severe, or it can be so overwhelming that patients are not able to participate in any activity either at home or at work [10,13].

Clinical appearance of sarcoidosis

Clinical manifestations of sarcoidosis show various symptoms and signs depending on the organ involved. Commonly, sarcoidosis is the disease with an acute onset. In some patients, sarcoidosis is a chronic disease with an atypical, unusual onset, which clinically may represent a broad spectrum of any other infectious or noninfectious disease. Possible clinical manifestations of sarcoidosis are shown in Box 1.

Chest radiographic features in sarcoidosis

Chest radiographs in patients who have sarcoidosis have been classified into four stages [1]:

- Stage 0 (clear chest radiograph)

- Stage I (bilateral hilar lymphadenopathy [BHL])
- Stage II (bilateral hilar adenopathy and parenchymal infiltration)
- Stage III (parenchymal infiltrations)
- Stage IV (irreversible fibrosis)

Box 2 summarizes common clinical symptoms and common differential diagnosis of radiographic sarcoidosis stages I, II, and III [17–19].

Stage 0: clear chest radiograph

In some patients, this stage can be a relatively late phase of sarcoidosis, whereas in others, it may be the earliest phase of the disease. Up to 10% of patients at the time of initial presentation or during the course of the disease have normal results on chest radiographs. In some of these patients, lung biopsy procedures would probably reveal granulomatous inflammation [3,15,16,20,21].

Box 1. Clinical manifestations of sarcoidosis

Acute sarcoidosis (with symptoms and signs persistent for less than 2 years)
- The disease has an abrupt onset and tends to clear spontaneously
- Patients are usually asymptomatic
- Chest radiographs show bilateral hilar lymphadenopathy or diffuse parenchymal infiltrations
- The chest radiograph clears within a year in more than 60% of patients
- Treatment with steroids is seldom needed [1–7,10]

Chronic sarcoidosis (with symptoms for more than 2 years)
- The disease has a subtle onset and progressive variable course
- Chest radiographs show extensive parenchymal infiltrates without fibrosis
- Lupus pernio, skin plaques, chronic uveitis, glaucoma, and persistent parotitis are frequent findings
- Hypercalcemia and hypercalciuria may lead to nephrocalcinosis and renal failure
- Therapy with corticosteroids only relieves symptoms [1–6,11]

Box 2. Common clinical symptoms and common differential diagnosis of radiographic sarcoidosis stages I, II, and III

Common clinical manifestations of pulmonary sarcoidosis
Stage I
    BHL, fever, polyarthralgias, erythema nodosum
Stage II
    Fever, weight loss, cough, and dyspnea asymptomatic in some patients
Stage III
    Common clinical symptoms: dry cough, dyspnea
    Rare clinical symptoms: productive cough (caused by bronchopulmonary infection), haemoptysis in some patients
Stage IV
    Clinical features vary broadly, but most patients complain of dyspnea, cough, and expectoration
    Complications such as pneumothorax, cor pulmonale, and aspergillosis are present

Common differential diagnosis
Lymphoma
Pneumoconiosis
Bronchogenic carcinoma
Lymph node metastasis
Beryllium lung disease
Silicosis
Tuberculosis
Lymphangitic carcinoma
Coccidioidomycosis
Brucellosis
Idiophatic pulmonary fibrosis (IPF)
Pneumoconiosis
Scleroderma
Rheumatoid lung
Lupus erythematosus: lung involvement
Extrinsic alveolitis
Lymphangitic carcinomatosis
Tuberculosis (upper lobe localization)
Eosinophilic granuloma
Hemosiderosis
Drug reaction

Stage I: bilateral hilar lymphadenopathy

This stage occurs in more than 50% of all patients who have sarcoidosis. The stage is characterized by an enlargement of bronchopulmonary, tracheobronchial, and paratracheal lymph nodes (Fig. 2). A translucent space between the enlarged lymph nodes and the cardiovascular margin (clearer on the right side) is often noted. BHL may be associated with either right paratracheal (25%) or bilateral paratracheal lymphadenopathy [3,8,9,11]. Enlargement of left paratracheal, para-aortic, and subcarinal lymph node groups may be detected by CT scans [3,18,21] but are not usually evident on plain chest radiographs [3]. Subcarinal adenopathy may lead to distortion of the main carina, which is appreciated during bronchoscopy (Fig. 3).

Prognosis of pulmonary sarcoidosis stage I. In 60% to 80% of patients with only BHL, complete remission of the radiographic finding occurs within 2 years; the lymph nodes rarely enlarge again. Approximately 10% of patients follow a persistent course (ie, patients with chronic skin lesions and bone cysts).The remaining 10% to 15% of patients with stage I disease may remain stationary or advance only slowly to stage II [3,17]. Box 2 shows common clinical symptoms of lung sarcoidosis and common differential diagnosis of lung sarcoidosis at stages I, II, and III [17–19].

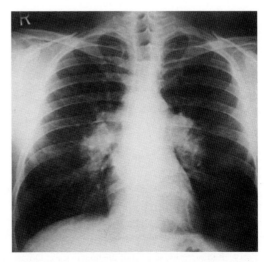

Fig. 2. Radiographic stage I of lung sarcoidosis with BHL.

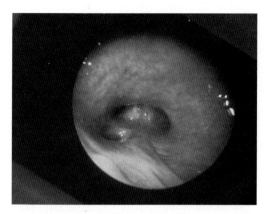

Fig. 3. Bronchoscopic view of carina distended by extramural lymph node compression. Small granulomas of the bronchial mucosa are also visible.

Stage II: bilateral hilar adenopathy and parenchymal infiltrations

This stage occurs in 25% to 50% of patients who have sarcoidosis [3,5,6,11]. The parenchymal infiltration is bilateral, but the pattern of the infiltrates varies: parenchymal infiltrates may be patchy or diffuse and preferentially involve the upper and mid-lung zones [22]. Fig. 4 shows an example of stage II disease. In approximately 70% of patients who have stage II, the symptoms eventually resolve. Symptoms in the remaining 30% of patients are stationary or progress into stage III.

Pulmonary sarcoidosis stage III

This stage involves parenchymal infiltration without hilar adenopathy. Approximately 15% of patients who have sarcoidosis present with this stage of the disease. Radiographic findings may present in several ways: (1) reticulonodular, (2) acinar or alveolar, (3) segmental or lobar infiltrate with fluffy margins, or (d) with air bronchograms. The reticulonodular form is the most common parenchymal abnormality, with a mixture of linear densities and small nodules 3 to 5 mm in diameter. The infiltration is almost always bilateral, although unilateral or localized involvement of the lung parenchyma may occur. There is a tendency of sparing apices or extreme bases (Fig. 5).

Pulmonary sarcoidosis stage IV

This stage involves irreversible fibrosis/bullae formation. The overall prevalence is approximately 20% of all patients who have sarcoidosis. Lung lesions include irreversible fibrosis with hilar retraction (Fig. 6), bullae formation, and emphysema. With pulmonary fibrosis as in stage IV, loss of volume, hilar retraction, and coarse linear bands may be observed on chest radiographs. With advanced fibrocystic sarcoidosis, large bullae (Fig. 7), cystic radiolucencies, distortion [23,24], mycetomas [25,26], or bronchiectasis may be observed [27,28].

Clinical features of stage IV vary broadly, but most patients complain of dyspnea, cough, and expectoration. Respiratory failure caused by loss of lung volume occurs in almost all patients in stage IV of this lung disease. Complications such as pneumothorax, cor pulmonale, or aspergillosis are present in patients with stage IV sarcoidosis [17].

Uncommon radiographic presentations of lung sarcoidosis include pleural effusion, pneumothorax, nodular sarcoidosis, cavitary sarcoidosis,

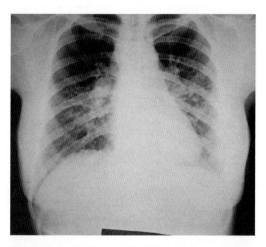

Fig. 4. Radiographic stage II of the lung disease. Diffuse micronodular lesions on both sides. Hilar lymph nodes are also enlarged in this stage.

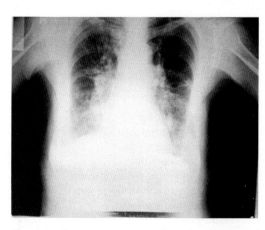

Fig. 5. Radiographic stage III. Parenchymal infiltrates producing the "ground glass" formation.

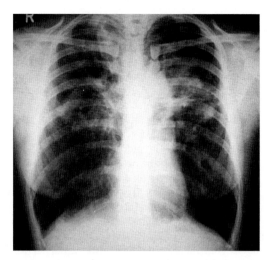

Fig. 6. Radiographic stage IV of lung sarcoidosis. Hilar retraction with rough linear bands.

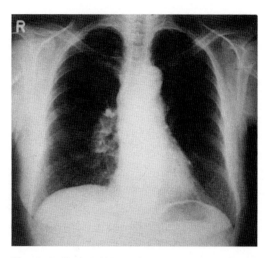

Fig. 8. Unilateral hilar enlargement: an uncommon manifestation of sarcoidosis.

peripheral infiltration with eosinophilia, calcifications (including egg shell calcifications of the lymph nodes), and unilateral hilar adenopathy. Unilateral hilar adenopathy (Fig. 8) can be a diagnostic dilemma in patients who are suspected of having sarcoidosis. When found, the enlargement of hilar lymph nodes usually occurs on the right side. Unilateral adenopathy is more frequently found in primary tuberculosis, lymphoma, coccidioidomycosis, and histoplasmosis. It also can be mimicked by a lesion of the apical segment of lower lobe and pulmonary valve stenosis. Other uncommon causes of unilateral adenopathy (or its appearance) besides sarcoidosis are amyloidosis, aneurysm of a pulmonary artery, pulmonary

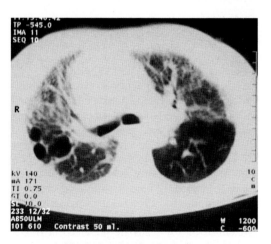

Fig. 7. Large bullae formation.

embolism, and poststenotic pulmonary artery dilatation. Rarely is the finding of unilateral hilar adenopathy caused by brucellosis or infectious mononucleosis [17].

Sarcoidosis of the airways: endobronchial sarcoidosis

The bronchial mucosa is often involved in sarcoidosis. In one study, 40% of patients with stage I and approximately 70% of patients with stages II and III had noncaseating granulomas in bronchial biopsy specimens [3]. Endobronchial sarcoidosis is commonly found as nodular elevation on the bronchial mucosa, with the nodules 2 to 3 mm in diameter. Uncommonly, there are gross mucosal abnormalities [19]. Rarely, granulomatous involvement may produce narrowing of bronchi with resulting atelectasis and pulmonary infections distal to the obstruction (Fig. 9) [17,19]. Endobronchial involvement is usually asymptomatic, although some patients complain of cough, wheezing, and even hemoptysis [17].

Influence of clinical findings on prognosis of pulmonary sarcoidosis

Clinical manifestations of sarcoidosis may have some prognostic value. Löfgren's syndrome (manifested as BHL, erythema nodosum polyarthritis, and fever) in acute onset of sarcoidosis has excellent prognosis [6,29,30]. Patients have high

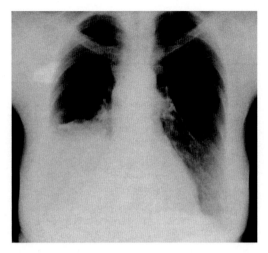

Fig. 9. Sarcoidosis granulomatous involvement may produce narrowing of bronchi.

rates of spontaneous remission. Clinical manifestations associated with poor prognosis include age at onset older than 40 years [29,31], hypercalcemia [29], extrapulmonary involvement (ie, chronic eye, bone, or sarcoidosis of the upper respiratory tract lesions) [29], and parenchymal infiltrates on chest radiographs.

Influence of chest radiographic findings on prognosis

Although the chest radiographic staging system was developed approximately 50 years ago, currently it still has a certain prognostic value [4,9]. Scandinavian authors emphasized the predominance of stages I and II with good prognosis among patients who have sarcoidosis in that part of the world [4]. The prognosis is best with radiographic stage I in patients who have sarcoidosis all over the world. In a study by Scadding [9], patients who had sarcoidosis were followed for 5 years. At the end of this follow-up period, 31 of 32 patients (97%) with stage I were asymptomatic; only 58% of stage II and 25% of stage III patients were asymptomatic at the end of the 5-year follow-up period.

Almost 20 years later, investigators from the same part of the world followed up 818 patients with sarcoidosis [29]. The highest rate of radiographic remission occurred in patients who had stage I sarcoidosis (59%) compared with stage II (39%) and stage III (38%). Treated and untreated patients were included in study. Japanese investigators found radiographic resolution within

3 years in 68% of patients who had sarcoidosis [30]. Mana and colleagues [31] from Spain analyzed 193 patients who had sarcoidosis and found nearly the same percent of chest radiograph resolution (78%) but within 2 years. In the same study, parenchymal infiltrates that persisted for years predicted a chronic form of the disease. In A Case Control Epidemiologic Study of Sarcoidosis, a study performed in the United States, 215 patients who had sarcoidosis were followed up for 2 years. Most of the observed patients showed no significant changes on chest radiographic findings, lung function, or dyspnea scale during the 2-year follow-up period [6].

Prognosis of sarcoidosis is definitely related to ethnic and geographic factors, although referral biases contribute to the prognostic variety. Positive outcome is evident in patients with stage I sarcoidosis, although even these patients might experience a progression into stage II or III. On the contrary, some patients with initial stage III sarcoidosis experienced radiographic remission within a prolonged period of 5-year follow-up [32–36]. Spontaneous remission is an important part of the prognosis. Authors from the United States who analyzed 337 patients who had sarcoidosis found a rate of spontaneous remission of 36% [37]. Only 8% of patients with spontaneous remission experienced relapse of sarcoidosis later, whereas 74% of patients with corticosteroid therapy experienced late relapse of their disease.

The prognosis of sarcoidosis is undeniably worse among African Americans [5,6,29,37], in whom the clinical and radiographic course of the disease is associated with chronic progressive pulmonary disease, worse long-term prognosis, and extrapulmonary involvement.

CT scans

A routine CT chest scan is not necessary in managing sarcoidosis [38]. Thoracic CT scans may be helpful in patients who have sarcoidosis and atypical chest radiographic findings or atypical clinical manifestations of the disease or in patients with normal chest radiographic findings but clinical suspicion for sarcoidosis [1,22]. A thoracic CT scan is indicated to detect specific complications of sarcoidosis, such as bronchiectasis, aspergilloma, pulmonary fibrosis with honeycombing, and superimposed infection or malignancy. Specific complications with characteristic findings of sarcoidosis on CT scans are presented in Box 3. Individual patients may have multiple CT findings

Box 3. Indications for CT scans and characteristic findings
Thoracic CT scan is indicated to detect specific complications of sarcoidosis • Bronchiectasis • Aspergilloma • Pulmonary fibrosis • Superimposed infection or malignancy *Characteristic findings of sarcoidosis on CT scans include* • Mediastinal or hilar adenopathy • Nodular opacities • Micronodules along bronchovascular bundles • Pleural or subpleural nodules • Septal and nonseptal lines • Consolidations • Ground-glass opacities [1,22]

evolving over time [1,22]. High-resolution CT is indicated to outline parenchymal, mediastinal, and hilar structures, emphasize details in the lung parenchyma, and distinguish inflammation from fibrosis [4,39].

Lung function impairments in sarcoidosis

"With no other disease did pulmonary physiologists have so much fun as with sarcoidosis. More is yet to come, because so much remains unexplained" [19,40–43]. This observation was written 20 years ago to introduce the topic on functional impairments in sarcoidosis at the Meeting of Sarcoidosis in Milan, Italy in 1988. Considering lung function in sarcoidosis, this introduction remains appropriate two decades later.

Respiratory tract involvement occurs at some time during the course of the disease of almost all patients who have sarcoidosis. The disease is an interstitial lung disorder that involves alveoli, blood vessels, and bronchioles and produces clinical findings of dry cough, restricted lung volumes, and gas exchange abnormalities. The airways are also susceptible to granulomatous involvement. Limitation of airflow is one of the expected pulmonary physiologic abnormalities [44–46].

The results of lung function investigations have been compared with clinical findings, radiologic appearances, and pathologic changes. Sarcoid granulomas occur in interstitial tissue in almost all patients who have sarcoidosis regardless of radiographic stage of the disease. Granuloma formations are clustered in the small lymphatic vessels, alveolar walls, perivascular and peribronchial areas, and subpleural areas of the lung [46,47], thus producing consecutive impairments of the lung function.

In chronic sarcoidosis, long-standing granulomatous formations make dense fibrotic tissue with distorted bronchioles, the areas of bronchiectases, and surrounding emphysematous areas. In the number of patients with chronic progressive disease, the final result is an extensive pulmonary fibrosis [47]. These structural changes determine the variety of physiologic abnormalities. Some clinicians concentrate on early treatment to prevent the definite structural changes of the lung. Early treatment may include inhaled corticosteroids [48].

Overall, lung function impairments are present in approximately 20% of patients who have sarcoidosis with radiographic stage I and 40% to 80% of patients with parenchymal infiltrations (stages II, III, and IV) [3,29,49–51].

Sarcoidosis is an interstitial lung disease. It leads to a restrictive pattern of lung function changes (with reduced lung volumes vital capacity and total lung capacity), usually in patients with severe, parenchymal involvement (lung disease stage III and IV) [49–57]. Diffusing capacity for carbon monoxide is the most sensitive pulmonary function test for interstitial lung disease [58]. Diffusing capacity for carbon monoxide is reduced in 15% to 50% of patients who have sarcoidosis [49,59].

Airflow obstruction with reduced forced expiratory volume in 1 second and expiratory flow rates occurs in 30% to 50% of patients who have sarcoidosis [50,54,58,60]. Airflow obstruction occurs in a high rate even in acute sarcoidosis stage I [61,62]. This airway disease also can manifest as increased bronchial hyperreactivity, which has been reported in increased frequency on some studies of patients who have sarcoidosis [61,62]. For example, in a study of Serbian authors, the bronchial hyperreactivity was found in 58% of patients who have sarcoidosis [62].

Respiratory muscle functional impairments may contribute to the subjective feeling of dyspnea or actual exercise limitation in patients who have sarcoidosis. Dyspnea does not always correlate with lung function parameters (ie, lung volumes or diffusing capacity for carbon monoxide). Baydur and coworkers [63] studied respiratory muscle function by mouth inspiratory pressure and expiratory muscle pressure and found a significant linear correlation between the decreased respiratory muscle function and increased dyspnea. The mouth inspiratory pressure is also related to lung volume; dyspnea is multifactorial in patients who have sarcoidosis [4].

Lung function impairments and prognosis of sarcoidosis

Criteria of assessing the response to therapy or the actual improvement of the lung function parameters have not been validated. Most authors define the increase of forced vital capacity of more than 10% to 15% and diffusing capacity for carbon monoxide of more than 20% as significant [4,64,65]. Several studies on lung function impairments in sarcoidosis showed the importance of lung function testing in following the course and assessing the response to the treatment. In these studies, the average improvement in lung function was often less than 10%. It is clear that the prognosis is worse in patients with serious lung function impairments at the onset of the disease [54,57,58,60–65].

Diagnosis of pulmonary sarcoidosis

The diagnosis of pulmonary sarcoidosis is based on (1) recognizing the possible clinical manifestations of sarcoidosis, (2) recognizing the chest radiographic abnormalities, and (3) finding the histologic evidence of noncaseating granuloma. Finding the histologic evidence of non-caseating granuloma, the hallmark of sarcoidosis, requires lung biopsy procedures in patients with suspected pulmonary sarcoidosis. The initial procedure is flexible fiberoptic bronchoscopy with transbronchial lung biopsy. Sensitivity of this diagnostic procedure ranges from 60% to 90% [59,66]. Some investigations confirmed that the combination of transbronchial needle aspiration biopsies and transbronchial needle biopsies have higher rates of positive findings than either procedure alone [67].

CT-guided transthoracic fine needle aspiration may be useful for diagnosing malignant or benign lesions of mediastinal or subcarinal lymph nodes [4,68]. Endoscopic ultrasound endobronchial ultrasound-guided fine needle aspiration has been used to diagnose mediastinal lymph node enlargement in patients with malignancy [69], but investigations are limited in patients who have pulmonary

sarcoidosis. Mediastinoscopy to obtain samples of the mediastinal lymph nodes is often performed when bronchoscopy is nondiagnostic or there is concern about underlying malignancy or lymphoma. Open lung biopsy as a surgical procedure is not always required to diagnose sarcoidosis, but when the other diagnostic procedures do not contribute to the definite diagnosis, surgical biopsy can be done.

Pleural sarcoidosis

Pleural involvement is an uncommon manifestation of sarcoidosis. It may manifest as a pleural effusion, pneumothorax, pleural thickening and nodules, hydropneumothorax, trapped lung, hemothorax, or chylothorax [4,70–76]. Clinically significant pleural manifestations (eg, pneumothorax, pleural effusions or chylothorax) occur in 2% to 4% of patients who have sarcoidosis [4,70,72,77–81]. With the introduction of CT scan, especially high-resolution CT, awareness of pleural manifestations of sarcoidosis has increased, allowing detection of more subtle cases of pleural involvement. Pleural manifestations of sarcoidosis may arise at initial presentation or at a later stage in the development of known sarcoidosis. The development of pleural sarcoidosis does not seem to have any clear prognostic value. Often the diagnosis is based on clinical finding without histologic proof, because when the disease is present elsewhere, most pleural sarcoidosis does not require a biopsy to treat the patient properly. A summary of a total of 145 biopsy-proven cases of pleural involvement with sarcoidosis was reported in 2000 [72].

Pleural effusions

Pleural effusions complicate sarcoidosis in less than 3% of patients; when present, they are usually asymptomatic [4,72]. The incidence of pleural effusion with sarcoidosis ranges from 0 to 5% [71,72,78] but has been reported to be as high as 7.5% [81]. An analysis of the published references up to 1985 that included reports of pleural involvement with sarcoidosis [14,77,78,81–94] showed that out of a total of 3146 cases of sarcoidosis, 76 had pleural effusions (2.4%) [82]. In another report, however, only three pleural effusions were detected among 2775 patients who had pulmonary sarcoidosis [95].

Because sarcoid-related pleural effusions are rare, it should not be assumed that a pleural effusion that occurs in a patient who has sarcoidosis is sarcoid related; other causes should be considered [70]. A definitive diagnosis of a sarcoid pleural effusion relies on a biopsy that demonstrates noncaseating granuloma, with the exclusion of alternate granulomatous diseases.

In a recent prospective study, thoracic ultrasonograms were performed in 181 consecutive outpatients who had sarcoidosis [70]. Pleural effusions were detected in five patients (2.8%), but only three were attributed to sarcoidosis (1.1%); two were a manifestation of congestive heart failure.

The mechanism of pleural effusion formation in patients with sarcoidosis is presumably similar to that of other infiltrative diseases. Involvement of the pleura may lead to increased capillary permeability. Superior vena cava obstruction [75], endobronchial sarcoidosis leading to bronchial stenosis and lobar atelectasis [76], trapped lung [96,97], and lymphatic disruption with the development of chylothorax have been reported as a cause of sarcoid-related pleural effusions [75].

Sarcoidosis-related pleural effusions occur slightly more commonly in the right lung (45%) than in the left lung (33%) [72]. The reason for right-sided predominance is unclear and not related to organ involvement. Bilateral effusions have been reported in 22% of cases [72]. The onset of pleural effusion ranges from being coincidental with the first diagnosis of sarcoidosis [98] to occurring several years after the diagnosis was made. In most cases, the effusions were incidental findings [70,72,73,77,78,98–101]. Patients with sarcoid pleural effusion usually have extensive parenchymal disease (radiographic stage II or stage III) and frequently have extrathoracic sarcoidosis [78,81,87,102]. In series of pleural sarcoidosis with biopsy of visceral and parietal pleural surfaces performed, most cases were radiographic stage II and III sarcoidosis [103]. It seems that with progression of parenchymal disease, the prevalence of pleural effusions decreases, whereas pleural thickening and pneumothorax increase [72]. Sarcoid-related pleural effusions can occur in all Scadding radiographic stages. There are no specific radiologic features of pleural effusions that occur in sarcoidosis to suggest the cause, except for the presence of associated parenchymal disease or intrathoracic lymphadenopathy.

Although generally small to medium, occasionally effusions can be massive [73,77,78,87, 99–102,104], sometimes bilateral [76,77,81,87,97, 101–103,105], and rarely loculated [106].

Sarcoid-related pleural effusions have been described as exudates or transudates. Most series have not reported the criteria used to classify these pleural effusions [72–78,81,87,96,97,99–103,107–112]. Higgins and colleagues [70] summarized the pleural fluid characteristics of all sarcoid-related pleural effusions reported in the literature. When either the protein or lactate dehydrogenase (LDH) criterion is used, most sarcoid-related pleural effusions are exudative. The appearance of the pleural fluid is most commonly serous. Occasionally it is serosanguinous [87,96,100,103]; bloody pleural effusion is an extremely rare finding [73]. The nucleated cell count is typically low at 1100 cells/μL or less. Lymphocytosis occurs in two thirds of cases [4,70,72,77,78], with predominance of CD_4 lymphocytes [4,72,113,114]. Few cases of pleural fluid eosinophilia have been reported [115–117].

The typical finding in sarcoid pleural effusions is a paucicellular, lymphocyte-predominant exudate with a pleural fluid/serum protein ratio more consistently in the exudative range than the pleural fluid LDH criterion. Dyssynchrony between the pleural fluid protein and LDH ratios suggests that the pathogenesis of sarcoid-related pleural effusions is most consistent with increased capillary permeability with minimal pleural space inflammation. A definitive diagnosis of sarcoid pleural effusion relies on a pleural biopsy sample that demonstrates noncaseating granulomas, with the exclusion of granulomatous diseases of known origin. Sarcoid pleural effusions may resolve spontaneously or require corticosteroids for resolution. Most of these effusions resolve spontaneously. The time of spontaneous resolution is variable, but most resolve in 1 to 3 months [70,77,78,81,99,109,110]. There are reports of resolution at 2 weeks with steroid therapy [73,101] and as long as 6 months with or without steroid administration [76,78]. If the effusion is symptomatic and recurrent, steroid therapy is recommended for symptomatic relief and hastening the resolution of the effusion. Incomplete resolution of these effusions has been reported with eventual progression to chronic pleural thickening [81] or a trapped lung [96,97]. Decortication was successful in relieving dyspnea in a patient who had lung entrapment from sarcoidosis [4,72,96,109].

Pneumothorax

Pneumothorax occurs in 2% to 4% of patients who have sarcoidosis (Fig. 10) [4,118,119]. The

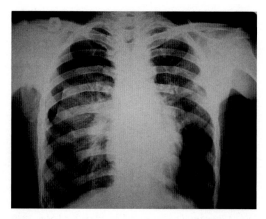

Fig. 10. Pneumothorax as a complication of pulmonary sarcoidosis.

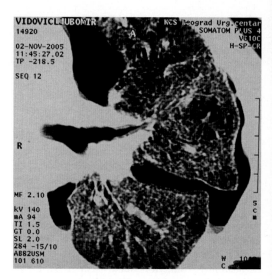

Fig. 11. Loculated pneumothorax in patient with fibrocystic sarcoidosis.

necrosis of subpleural granuloma or the rupture of bullae or both seem to be the mechanism of this rare manifestation of sarcoidosis [71,82]. Since the first description by Freiman in 1948, numerous reports have described the association between pneumothorax and sarcoidosis [14,84,85,92,93,118–125]. Pneumothorax may be the presenting manifestation of pulmonary sarcoidosis [126] but more often is a complication of already diagnosed sarcoidosis [82,85,93,119,126–128], may be recurrent, and involves both sides on different occasions [128].

In a series of 180 patients who had sarcoidosis, 5 (2.7%) patients with pneumothorax were noted [118]. Another series reported two cases of pneumothorax out of 52 patients who had sarcoidosis (3.7%) [119], and Froudarakis and colleagues [126] noted 5 patients (2.5%) who had sarcoidosis. The large series of 2775 sarcoidosis cases contained only 2 patients who had pneumothorax [95].

Pneumothorax was reported in 32% of all pleural cases of sarcoidosis [72]. Most cases occurred in association with diffuse pulmonary parenchymal disease, particularly fibrocystic disease [82,93,118]. Although pneumothorax is more commonly observed in the late evolution of sarcoidosis (Fig. 11), it can occur in the early stages [126,127]. Few authors have reported the occurrence of pneumothorax at the early stage of the disease [126,127,129,130]. Bilateral spontaneous pneumothorax also was reported in patients who had sarcoidosis [129,131]. According to literature data, no preference as to side of pneumothorax was shown [93,118,119,126].

Other pleural manifestations can be present in association with pneumothorax, such as hemothorax [129] and pleural effusion [130]. The superimposition of pneumothorax on an already compromised ventilatory function can be fatal [121]. Thoracostomy tube therapy seems effective despite the restrictive nature of the lung diseases [72]. There are several reported cases of chylothorax caused by sarcoidosis [71,74,132–136]. This type of effusion tends to be large and sometimes recurrent [134].

Pleural thickening and nodules

Pleural thickening is much more common in sarcoidosis than has been emphasized in the literature [4,71,72,81,82,88,106,111]. It has been found often at thoracotomy [106] and autopsy. It is rarely extensive enough to produce clinical or physiologic consequences [105]. Pleural thickening is usually not associated with clinical symptoms [4,72,82]. Pleural thickening and abnormalities of the subpleural region have been recognized increasingly in sarcoidosis by use of high-resolution CT scanning [105]. Use of CT in pulmonary sarcoidosis demonstrates a high incidence of minor pleural abnormalities (Fig. 12) [39,71,72,82]. Two studies using high-resolution CT cited pleural thickening in 9% [39] and 11% [137] of patients who had sarcoidosis, respectively. The incidence is higher in patients who have chronic fibrocystic sarcoidosis. A study of 61

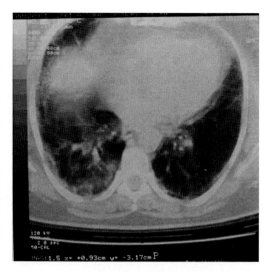

Fig. 12. Pleural thickening as demonstrated by CT scan.

patients who had chronic sarcoidosis (>2 years' duration) cited pleural involvement on chest CT in 25 (41%), which included 20 cases of pleural thickening and five effusions [138].

Pleural thickening or fibrothorax is usually seen after or in association with pleural effusion and most frequently in association with extensive parenchymal fibrocystic disease [4,71,72]. It is predominantly confined to the lower hemithoraces but is infrequently apical [71,72], when it sometimes precedes the development of *Aspergillus* superinfection [139].

Subpleural or pleural nodules [4,71,72,105,140] may be observed by high-resolution CT in 22% to 76% of sarcoidosis cases [105,141], but they rarely cause symptoms. They are often described as masses [72,105] and correspond to nodules seen on parietal and visceral surfaces at thoracotomy [140] and autopsy, which may be associated with pleural thickening [72,142]. A solid, pleural mass is rarely seen in sarcoidosis [104].

Summary

Sarcoidosis, an enigmatic multisystemic disease, has many different faces. Every patient has his or her own story, and every sarcoidologist has a unique but complex approach to maintaining the disease. Although multisystemic involvement is characteristic of the disease and virtually any organ can be affected, lungs are involved in more than 90% of patients who have sarcoidosis. Radiographic features and lung function impairments are supportive in managing how serious the disease is in an individual patient but are not the parameters for definite prognosis. Pleural involvement is a rare but serious presentation of this perplexing disease.

References

[1] Joint Statement of the American Thoracic Society (ATS), the European Respiratory Society (ERS) and the World Association of Sarcoidosis and Other Granulomatous Disorders (WASOG) adopted by the ATS Board of Directors and by the ERS Executive Committee. Statement on sarcoidosis. February 1999. Am J Respir Crit Care Med 1999; 160:736–55.

[2] Newman LS, Rose CS, Maier LA. Sarcoidosis. N Engl J Med 1997;336:1224–34.

[3] Lynch JP III, Kazerooni EA, Gay SE. Pulmonary sarcoidosis. Clin Chest Med 1997;18:755–85.

[4] Lynch JP III, Ma YL, Koss MN, et al. Pulmonary sarcoidosis. Semin Respir Crit Care Med 2007; 28(1):53–74.

[5] Baughman RP, Teirstein AS, Judson MA, et al. Clinical characteristics of patients in a case control study of sarcoidosis. Am J Respir Crit Care Med 2001;164(10 Pt 1):1885–9.

[6] Judson MA, Baughman RP, Thompson BW, et al. Two year prognosis of sarcoidosis: the ACCESS experience. Sarcoidosis Vasc Diffuse Lung Dis 2003;20:204–11.

[7] Gribbin J, Hubbard RB, Le Jeune I, et al. The incidence and mortality of idiopathic pulmonary fibrosis and sarcoidosis in the UK. Thorax 2006;61: 980–5.

[8] Reich JM. Mortality of intrathoracic sarcoidosis in referral vs population-based settings: influence of stage, ethnicity, and corticosteroid therapy. Chest 2002;121:32–9.

[9] Scadding JG. Prognosis of intrathoracic sarcoidosis in England: a review of 136 cases after five years' observation. BMJ 1961;2:1165–72.

[10] Hillerdal G, Nou E, Osterman K, et al. Sarcoidosis: epidemiology and prognosis: a 15-year European study. Am Rev Respir Dis 1984;130:29–32.

[11] Sharma O. Sarcoidosis: clinical management. London: Butterworth & Co (Publishers), Ltd.; 1984.

[12] Katz S. Clinical presentation and natural history of sarcoidosis. In: Fanburg BL, editor. Sarcoidosis and other granulomatous diseases of the lung. New York: Marcel Dekker; 1983. p. 3–36.

[13] Petersdorf R, Beeson P. Fever of obscure origin: report of 100 cases. Medicine 1961;40:1.

[14] Mayock R, Bertrand P, Morrison C, et al. Manifestations of sarcoidosis: analysis of 145 patients, with review of nine series selected from the literature. Am J Med 1963;35:67–89.

[15] Silzbach L, James D, Neville E. Course and prognosis of sarcoidosis around the world. Am J Med 1974;57:847–52.

[16] Thomas P, Hunninghake G. Current concepts of the pathogenesis of sarcoidosis. Am Rev Respir Dis 1987;135:747–60.

[17] Vucinic Mihailovic V, Sharma OP. Atlas of sarcoidosis. London: Springer; 2005.

[18] Bergin CJ, Bell DY, Coblentz CL, et al. Sarcoidosis: correlation of pulmonary parenchymal pattern at CT with results of pulmonary function tests. Radiology 1989;171:619–24.

[19] Teirstein A, Siltzbach L. Sarcoidosis of the upper lung fields simulating pulmonary tuberculosis. Chest 1973;64:303–8.

[20] Peuringer R, Schwartz D, Dayton C, et al. The relationship between alveolar macrophage, TNF, IL-1 and PGE2 release, alveolitis and disease severity in sarcoidosis. Chest 1993;103:832–8.

[21] Winterbauer R, Belic M, Moores K. A clinical interpretation of bilateral hilar adenopathy. Ann Intern Med 1973;78:65–71.

[22] Lynch JP III. Computed tomographic scanning in sarcoidosis. Semin Respir Crit Care Med 2003;24: 393–418.

[23] Packe GE, Ayres JG, Citron KM, et al. Large lung bullae in sarcoidosis. Thorax 1986;41:792–7.

[24] Zar HJ, Cole RP. Bullous emphysema occurring in pulmonary sarcoidosis. Respiration 1995;62:290–3.

[25] Biem J, Hoffstein V. Aggressive cavitary pulmonary sarcoidosis. Am Rev Respir Dis 1991;143: 428–30.

[26] Israel HL, Lenchner GS, Atkinson GW. Sarcoidosis and aspergilloma: the role of surgery. Chest 1982;82:430–2.

[27] Tomlinson JR, Sahn SA. Aspergilloma in sarcoid and tuberculosis. Chest 1987;92:505–8.

[28] Lewis MM, Mortelliti MP, Yeager H Jr, et al. Clinical bronchiectasis complicating pulmonary sarcoidosis: case series of seven patients. Sarcoidosis Vasc Diffuse Lung Dis 2002;19:154–9.

[29] Neville E, Walker A, James DG. Prognostic factors predicting the outcome of sarcoidosis: an analysis of 818 patients. Q J Med 1983;52(208): 525–33.

[30] Nagai S, Shigematsu M, Hamada K, et al. Clinical courses and prognoses of pulmonary sarcoidosis. Curr Opin Pulm Med 1999;5:293–8.

[31] Mana J, Salazar A, Manresa F. Clinical factors predicting persistence of activity in sarcoidosis: a multivariate analysis of 193 cases. Respiration 1994;61: 219–25.

[32] Mana J, Gomez-Vaquero C, Montero A, et al. Lofgren's syndrome revisited: a study of 186 patients. Am J Med 1999;107:240–5.

[33] Gibson GJ, Prescott RJ, Muers MF, et al. British Thoracic Society Sarcoidosis study: effects of long term corticosteroid treatment. Thorax 1996;51: 238–47.

[34] Hunninghake GW, Gilbert S, Pueringer R, et al. Outcome of the treatment for sarcoidosis. Am J Respir Crit Care Med 1994;149(4 Pt 1):893–8.

[35] Chappell AG, Cheung WY, Hutchings HA. Sarcoidosis: a long-term follow-up study. Sarcoidosis Vasc Diffuse Lung Dis 2000;17:167–73.

[36] Pietinalho A, Ohmichi M, Lofroos AB, et al. The prognosis of pulmonary sarcoidosis in Finland and Hokkaido, Japan: a comparative five-year study of biopsy-proven cases. Sarcoidosis Vasc Diffuse Lung Dis 2000;17:158–66.

[37] Gottlieb JE, Israel HL, Steiner RM, et al. Outcome in sarcoidosis: the relationship of relapse to corticosteroid therapy. Chest 1997;111:623–31.

[38] Mana J, Teirstein AS, Mendelson DS, et al. Excessive thoracic computed tomographic scanning in sarcoidosis. Thorax 1995;50:1264–6.

[39] Brauner M, Grenier P, Mompoint D, et al. Pulmonary sarcoidosis: evaluation with high-resolution CT. Radiology 1989;172:467–71.

[40] Huang C, Heurich A, Rosen Y, et al. Pulmonary sarcoidosis: roentgenographic, functional and pathologic correlations. Respiration 1979;37: 467–71.

[41] Olsson T, Bjornstad-Petterson H, Stjernberg N. Bronchostenosis due to sarcoidosis: a cause of atelectasis and airway obstruction simulating pulmonary neoplasm and chronic obstructive pulmonary disease. Chest 1979;75:337.

[42] Sharma O. Pulmonary sarcoidosis: radiographic features. In: James DO, editor. Sarcoidosis and other granulomatous disorders. New York: Marcel Dekker; 1994. p. 213–45.

[43] Sharma OP. Functional impairment in sarcoidosis: state of the art. Sarcoidosis and other granulomatous disorders. Proceedings of the XI Congress on Sarcoidosis and other Granulomatous Disorders. Milan, September 6-11, 1987. Amsterdam: EXCEPTA MEDICA; 1988. p. 341–51.

[44] Harrison BDW, Shaylor JM, Stokes TC, et al. Airflow limitation in sarcoidosis: a study of pulmonary function in 107 newly diagnosed patients. Respir Med 1991;85:59–64.

[45] Crystal RG, Gadek JE, Ferrans VJ, et al. Interstitial lung disease: current concepts of pathogenesis, staging and therapy. Am J Med 1981;70:542–68.

[46] Fraser RG, Pare JAP. Diagnosis of diseases of the chest. Philadelphia: W.B. Saunders Co; 1979. p. 1659–89.

[47] Marshal R, Smellie H, Baylish JH, et al. Pulmonary function in sarcoidosis. Thorax 1988;13:48–58.

[48] Pietinalho A, Tukiainen P, Haahtela T, et al, Finnish Pulmonary Sarcoidosis Study Group. Early treatment of stage II sarcoidosis improves 5-year pulmonary function. Chest 2002;121:24–31.

[49] Alhamad EH, Lynch JP III, Martinez FJ. Pulmonary function tests in interstitial lung disease: what role do they have? Clin Chest Med 2001;22: 715–50, ix.

[50] Sharma OP, Johnson R. Airway obstruction in sarcoidosis: a study of 123 nonsmoking black American patients with sarcoidosis. Chest 1988;94:343–6.

[51] Sharma OP. Pulmonary sarcoidosis and corticosteroids. Am Rev Respir Dis 1993;147(6 Pt 1): 1598–600.

[52] Kaneko K, Sharma OP. Airway obstruction in pulmonary sarcoidosis. Bull Eur Physiopathol Respir 1977;13:231–40.

[53] Levinson RS, Metzger LF, Stanley NN, et al. Airway function in sarcoidosis. Am J Med 1977;62: 51–9.

[54] Harrison B, Shaylor J, Stokes T, et al. Airflow limitation in sarcoidosis: a study of pulmonary function in 107 patients with newly diagnosed disease. Respir Med 1991;85:59–64.

[55] Laverne F, Clerici B, Saoun D, et al. Airway obstruction in bronchial sarcoidosis: outcome with treatment. Chest 1999;116:1194–9.

[56] Benatar SR, Clark TJH. Pulmonary function in a case of endobronchial sarcoidosis. Am Rev Respir Dis 1974;110:490–6.

[57] Miller A, Teirstein AS, Jackler I, et al. Airway function in chronic pulmonary sarcoidosis with fibrosis. Am Rev Respir Dis 1974;109:179–89.

[58] Subramanian I, Flaherty K, Martinez F. Pulmonary function testing in sarcoidosis. In: Baughman RP, editor. Sarcoidosis, vol. 210. New York: Taylor and Francis Group; 2006. p. 415–33.

[59] Gilman MJ, Wang KP. Transbronchial lung biopsy in sarcoidosis: an approach to determine the optimal number of biopsies. Am Rev Respir Dis 1980;122:721–4.

[60] McCann BG, Harrison BD. Bronchiolar narrowing and occlusion in sarcoidosis: correlation of pathology with physiology. Respir Med 1991;85: 65–7.

[61] Ohrn MB, Skold CM, van Hage-Hamsten M, et al. Sarcoidosis patients have bronchial hyperreactivity and signs of mast cell activation in their bronchoalveolar lavage. Respiration 1995;62:136–42.

[62] Mihailovic-Vucinic V, Zugic V, Videnovic-Ivanov J. New observations on pulmonary function changes in sarcoidosis. Curr Opin Pulm Med 2003;9:436–41.

[63] Baydur A, Alsalek M, Louie SG, et al. Respiratory muscle strength, lung function, and dyspnea in patients with sarcoidosis. Chest 2001;120:102–8.

[64] Winterbauer RH, Hutchinson JF. Use of pulmonary function tests in the management of sarcoidosis. Chest 1980;78:640–7.

[65] Goldstein DS, Williams MH. Rate of improvement of pulmonary function in sarcoidosis during treatment with corticosteroids. Thorax 1986;41:473–4.

[66] Poe RH, Israel RH, Utell MJ, et al. Probability of a positive transbronchial lung biopsy result in sarcoidosis. Arch Intern Med 1979;139:761–3.

[67] Trisolini R, Lazzari Agli L, Cancellieri A, et al. Transbronchial needle aspiration improves the diagnostic yield of bronchoscopy in sarcoidosis. Sarcoidosis Vasc Diffuse Lung Dis 2004;21:147–51.

[68] Zwischenberger JB, Savage C, Alpard SK, et al. Mediastinal transthoracic needle and core lymph node biopsy: should it replace mediastinoscopy? Chest 2002;121:1165–70.

[69] Larsen SS, Krasnik M, Vilmann P, et al. Endoscopic ultrasound guided biopsy of mediastinal lesions has a major impact on patient management. Thorax 2002;57:98–103.

[70] Higgins JT, Doelken P, Sahn SA, et al. Pleural effusions in a series of 181 outpatients with sarcoidosis. Chest 2006;129:1599–604.

[71] Battesti JP, Azoulay E. Formes atypique de sarcoidose. Ann Med Interne 2001;152(1):51–7 [in French].

[72] Soskel NT, Sharma OP. Pleural involvement in sarcoidosis. Curr Opin Pulm Med 2000;6:455–68.

[73] De Vuyst P, DeTroyer A, Vernault JC. Bloody pleural effusion in a patient with sarcoidosis. Chest 1979;76:607–9.

[74] Aberg H, Bah M, Waters AW. Sarcoidosis complicated by chylothorax. Minn Med 1966;57:1065–70.

[75] Gordonson J, Trachtenberg S, Sargent EN. Superior vena cava obstruction due to sarcoidosis. Chest 1973;63:292–3.

[76] Poe RH. Middle-lobe atelectasis due to sarcoidosis with pleural effusion. N Y State J Med 1978;78: 2095–7.

[77] Nicholls AJ, Friend JA, Legge JS. Sarcoid pleural effusion: three cases and review of the literature. Thorax 1980;35:277–81.

[78] Sharma OP, Gordonson J. Pleural effusion in sarcoidosis: a report of six cases. Thorax 1975;30: 95–101.

[79] Soskel N, Sharma OP. Pleural involvement in sarcoidosis: case presentation and detailed review of the literature. Semin Respir Med 1992;13:492–514.

[80] Warshawsky ME, Shanies HM, Rozo A. Sarcoidosis involving the thyroid and pleura. Sarcoidosis Vasc Diffuse Lung Dis 1997;14:165–8.

[81] Wilen SB, Rabinowitz JG, Ulreich S, et al. Pleural involvement in sarcoidosis. Am J Med 1974;57: 200–9.

[82] Rockoff SD, Rohatgi PK. Unusual manifestations of thoracic sarcoidosis. AJR Am J Roentgenol 1985;144:513–28.

[83] Garland LH. Pulmonary sarcoidosis: the early roentgen findings. Radiology 1947;48:333–54.

[84] Kirks DR, McCormick VD, Greenspan RH. Pulmonary sarcoidosis: roentgenologic analysis of 150 patients. Am J Roentgenol Radium Ther Nucl Med 1973;117:777–86.

[85] Freundlich IM, Libshitz HI, Glassman LM, et al. Sarcoidosis: typical and atypical thoracic manifestations and complications. Clin Radiol 1970;21: 376–83.

[86] Ellis K, Renthal G. Pulmonary sarcoidosis: roentgenographic observations on course of disease.

Am J Roentgenol Radium Ther Nucl Med 1962;88: 1070–83.

[87] Chusid EL, Siltzbach LE. Sarcoidosis of the pleura. Ann Intern Med 1974;81:190–4.

[88] Rabinowitz JG, Ulreich S, Soriano C. The usual unusual manifestations of sarcoidosis and the "hilar haze": a new diagnostic aid. Am J Roentgenol Radium Ther Nucl Med 1974;120:821–31.

[89] Israel HL, Sones M. Sarcoidosis. Arch Intern Med 1958;102:766–76.

[90] Kampfer A. Uber extrapulmonale organ manifestationen des Morbus-Boeck). Prax Pneumol 1964; 4:204–17 [in German].

[91] McCort JJ, Wood RH, Hamilton JB, et al. Sarcoidosis: a clinical and roentgenologic study of 28 proved cases. Arch Intern Med 1947;80: 293–321.

[92] Longcope WT, Freiman DG. A study of sarcoidosis based on a combined investigation of 160 cases including 30 autopsies from the Johns Hopkins Hospital and Massachusetts General Hospital. Medicine 1952;31:32.

[93] Scadding JG. Sarcoidosis. London: Eyre and Spotisswoode; 1967. p. 136–8.

[94] Lebacq E. La sarcoidose de Besnier-Boeck-Schaumann. Paris: Librairie Maloine SA; 1964. p. 186–7 [in French].

[95] Kostina ZI, Ivanovskii VB, Voloshko IV, et al. Diagnosis and treatment of pleural lesions in sarcoidosis of the respiratory organs). Probl Tuberk 1992; 78:21–3 [in Russian].

[96] Heidecker JT, Judson MA. Pleural effusion caused by a trapped lung. South Med J 2003;96:510–1.

[97] Claiborne RA, Kerby GR. Pleural sarcoidosis with massive pleural effusion and lung entrapment. Kans Med 1990;91:103–5.

[98] Gardiner IT, Uff JS. Acute pleurisy in sarcoidosis. Thorax 1978;33:124–7.

[99] Selroos O. Exudative pleurisy and sarcoidosis. Br J Dis Chest 1966;60:191–6.

[100] Berte SJ, Pfotenhauer MA. Massive pleural effusion in sarcoidosis. Am Rev Respir Dis 1962;86: 261–4.

[101] Johnson NM, Martin N, McNicol MW. Sarcoidosis presenting with pleurisy and bilateral pleural effusions. Postgrad Med J 1980;56:266–7.

[102] Beekman JF, Zimmert SM, Chun BK, et al. Spectrum of pleural involvement in sarcoidosis. Arch Intern Med 1976;136:323–30.

[103] Salazar A, Mana J, Corbella X, et al. Sarcoid pleural effusion: a report of two cases. Sarcoidosis 1994; 11:135–7.

[104] Tice F, Sweany H. A fatal case of Besnier-Boeck-Schaumann's disease with autopsy findings. Ann Intern Med 1941;15:597–609.

[105] Loughney E, Higgins BG. Pleural sarcoidosis: a rare presentation. Thorax 1997;52:200–1.

[106] Everett E, Overholt E. Sarcoidosis and pleural effusion. Mil Med 1968;133:731–3.

[107] Kovnat PJ, Donohoe RF. Sarcoidosis involving the pleura. Ann Intern Med 1965;62:120–4.

[108] Tommasini A, Vittorio GD, Facchinetti F, et al. Pleural effusions in sarcoidosis: a case report. Sarcoidosis 1994;11:138–40.

[109] Cohen M, Sahn SA. Resolution of pleural effusions. Chest 2001;119:1547–62.

[110] Durand DV, Dellinger A, Guerin C, et al. Pleural sarcoidosis: one case presenting with an eosinophilic effusion. Thorax 1984;39:468–9.

[111] Nelson DG, Loudon RG. Sarcoidosis with pleural involvement. Am Rev Respir Dis 1973;108:647–51.

[112] Ilan Y, Yehuda AB, Breuer R. Pleural effusion: the presenting radiological manifestation of sarcoidosis. Isr J Med Sci 1994;30:535–6.

[113] Flammang d'Ortho MP, Cadranel J, Milleron BJ, et al. Pleural, alveolar and blood T-lymphocyte subsets in pleuropulmonary sarcoidosis. Chest 1990;98:782–3.

[114] Groman GS, Castele RJ, Altose MD, et al. Lymphocyte subpopulations in sarcoid pleural effusion. Ann Intern Med 1984;100:75–7.

[115] Chao DC, Hassenpflug M, Sharma OP. Multiple lung masses, pneumothorax, and psychiatric symptoms in a 29-year-old African-American woman. Chest 1995;108:871–3.

[116] Vander Werf TS, Vennik PHW. Rare presentation or lead time bias in pleural sarcoidosis? Thorax 1997;52:782–3.

[117] Tudela P, Haro M, Marti S, et al. Eosinphilic pleuritis as the presenting form of sarcoidosis. Med Clin (Barc) 1992;99:75–7.

[118] Sharma OP. Sarcoidosis: unusual pulmonary manifestations. Postgrad Med J 1977;61:67–73.

[119] Riley EA. Boeck's sarcoid: a review based upon a clinical study of 52 cases. Am Rev Tuberc 1950; 62:231–85.

[120] Harden KA, Barkthakur A. "Cavitary" lesions in sarcoidosis. Dis Chest 1958;35:607–14.

[121] Gendel BR, Luton EF. Sarcoidosis complicated by spontaneous pneumothorax. Am Pract Dig Treat 1951;2:339–40.

[122] Aussakoff AH. Massive pulmonary hemorrhage due to sarcoidosis: report of two cases. Dis Chest 1954;26:217–23.

[123] Felson B. Uncommon roentgen patterns of pulmonary sarcoidosis. Dis Chest 1958;34:357–67.

[124] Selroos O. The frequency, clinical picture and prognosis of pulmonary sarcoidosis in Finland. Acta Med Scand Suppl 1969;503:1–73.

[125] Thygesen K, Viskum K. Manifestations and cause of disease in intrathoracic sarcoidosis. Scand J Respir Dis 1972;53:174–80.

[126] Froudarakis ME, Bouros D, Voloudaki A, et al. Pneumothorax as a first manifestation of sarcoidosis. Chest 1997;112:278–80.

[127] Fein A, Gupta A, Goodman P. Spontaneous pneumothorax as a presenting pulmonary manifestation of early sarcoidosis. Chest 1980;77:455–6.

[128] Ross RJM, Empey DW. Bilateral spontaneous pneumothorax in sarcoidosis. Postgrad Med J 1983;59:106–7.

[129] Gomm SA. An unusual presentation of sarcoidosis: spontaneous haemopneumothorax. Postgrad Med J 1984;60:621–3.

[130] Ravichander P. Hydropneumothorax in sarcoidosis. Respir Med 1989;83:251–3.

[131] Akelsson IG, Eklund A, Skold CM, et al. Bilateral spontaneous pneumothorax and sarcoidosis. Sarcoidosis 1990;7:136–8.

[132] Carlier ML, Roux JP, Perez T, et al. Chylothorax and sarcoidosis. Rev Mal Respir 1997;14:315–7.

[133] Parker JM, Torrington KG, Phillips YY. Sarcoidosis complicated by chylothorax. South Med J 1994;87:860–2.

[134] Lengyel RJ, Shanley DJ. Recurrent chylothorax associated with sarcoidosis. Hawaii Med J 1995;54:817–8.

[135] Cappell MS, Friedman D, Mikhail N. Chyloperitoneum associated with chronic severe sarcoidosis. Am J Gastroenterol 1993;88:99–101.

[136] Jarman PR, Whyte MK, Sabroe I, et al. Sarcoidosis presenting with chylothorax. Thorax 1995;50:1324–5.

[137] Ohmichi M, Hiraga Y, Hirasawa M. Pulmonary involvements of sarcoidosis). Nihon Kyobu Shikkan Gakkai Zasshi 1990;28:48–55 [in Japanese].

[138] Szwarcberg JB, Glajchen N, Teirstein AS. Pleural involvement in chronic sarcoidosis detected by thoracic CT scanning. Sarcoidosis Vasc Diffuse Lung Dis 2005;22:58–62.

[139] Libshitz HI, Atkinson GW, Israel HL. Pleural thickening as a manifestation of *Aspergillus* superinfection. Am J Roentgenol Radium Ther Nucl Med 1974;120:883–6.

[140] Remy-Jardin M, Beuscart R, Sault MC, et al. Subpleural micronodules in diffuse infiltrative lung diseases: evaluation with thin-section CT scans. Radiology 1990;177:133–9.

[141] Bergstrom CE, Eklund A. Sarcoidosis with pleural involvement mimicking a coin lesion. Sarcoidosis 1990;7:78–9.

[142] Miller BH, Rosado-de-Christenson ML, McAdams HP, et al. Thoracic sarcoidosis: radiologic-pathologic correlation. Radiographics 1995;15:421–37.

**ELSEVIER
SAUNDERS**

Clin Chest Med 29 (2008) 475–492

**CLINICS
IN CHEST
MEDICINE**

Neurosarcoidosis

Elyse E. Lower, MD[a],*, Kenneth L. Weiss, MD[b]

[a]*Interstitial Lung Disease and Sarcoidosis Center, University of Cincinnati Medical Center,
3235 Eden Avenue, Cincinnati, OH 45267, USA*
[b]*University of Cincinnati Medical Center, 3235 Eden Avenue, Cincinnati, OH 45267, USA*

Although neurosarcoidosis is a less common manifestation of sarcoidosis, its symptoms can be devastating and occasionally life-threatening. The diagnosis of neurosarcoidosis can be challenging because the disease can present with a myriad of symptoms and diverse roentgenographic findings [1–5]. Although neurologic complications of sarcoidosis are reported in 5% to 10% of patients who have known sarcoidosis [6–8], a prospective series identified neurologic complications in 32 of 123 (26%) patients who had sarcoidosis [9]. In addition, the prospective epidemiologic study of 736 newly diagnosed patients who had sarcoidosis in the United States (ACCESS) identified 34 (4.6%) who had definite or probable neurosarcoidosis [10]. Autopsy studies confirm more neurologic involvement than antemortem reports. Neurosarcoidosis can provide a diagnostic dilemma, particularly for patients who do not carry a known diagnosis of sarcoidosis [2]. This entity is a diagnostic consideration for any patient who has known sarcoidosis who presents with symptoms related to the central or peripheral nervous systems. It is also a diagnostic consideration for patients who do not have confirmed sarcoidosis but who have neurologic symptoms suggestive of neurosarcoidosis. Most patients who have neurosarcoidosis have findings suggestive of multisystem disease, particularly lung and cardiac involvement. Approximately half of patients who have neurosarcoidosis experience neurologic symptoms at the time of the initial sarcoidosis diagnosis [3,11,12].

Neurologic manifestations

Because the granulomas of sarcoidosis can affect virtually any part of the central or peripheral nervous system, patients may present to a variety of health care professionals, including primary care specialists, ophthalmologists, neurologists, otolaryngologists, endocrinologists, infectious disease experts, oncologists, or pulmonologists. Cranial neuropathies are identified in 50% to 75% of patients who have neurosarcoidosis, with facial palsy reported in 25% to 50% [2,13–16]. Diplopia, impaired visual acuity, pain, and facial palsy are frequent initial complaints. One series identified optic nerve involvement as the most frequent cranial nerve involved [17]. Meningeal disease, including aseptic meningitis and mass lesions, is seen in 10% to 20% of patients [18,19], and hydrocephalus is identified in 10% [2,20]. Patients who have meningeal disease typically present with symptoms of meningitis, including headache and neck stiffness. Approximately 50% of patients who have neurosarcoidosis experience parenchymal brain disease, which can involve endocrinopathies (10%–15%) [21], mass lesions (5%–10%) [22,23], encephalopathy (5%–10%) [24], psychiatric symptoms (19%), and seizures (5%–10%) [3,8]. Psychosis has been the presenting feature of neurosarcoidosis with diffuse meningeal and hypothalamic disease [25–28]. Seizures may be the presenting symptom of patients who have neurosarcoidosis. In the past, seizures were considered a poor prognostic indicator associated with higher mortality perhaps due to the association of seizures with hydrocephalus or mass lesions [8]. More recent series do not confirm this association, suggesting that contemporary cytotoxic therapies may improve prognosis [16,29].

Because the base of the brain is frequently abnormal in neurosarcoidosis, patients may present with evidence of pituitary or hypothalamic dysfunction (Fig. 1) [21,30]. Presenting

* Corresponding author.
E-mail address: elower@ohcmail.com (E.E. Lower).

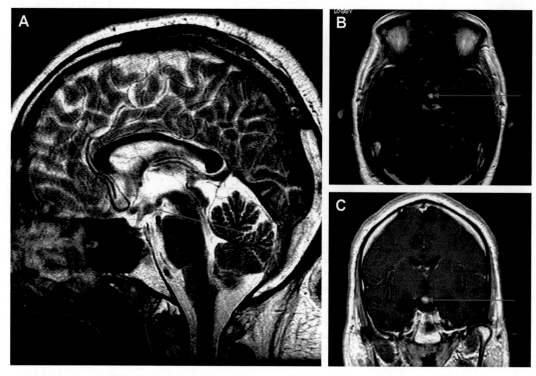

Fig. 1. (*A*) Midline sagittal T2-weighted image. (*B*) Axial postcontrast T1-weighted image and abnormal thick enhancing leptomeninges coating the anterior brainstem and within the cerebellar sulci. (*C*) Coronal postcontrast T1-weighted image. Red arrow points to enlarged contrast enhancing tubercinerium of the hypothalamus.

endocrinologic symptoms can include galactorrhea or altered menses, libido, or potency [31]. Altered sleep, body temperature, and appetite may be reported. Excessive thirst may be a symptom of diabetes insipidus [32], altered calcium levels, or diabetes mellitus. Hypothalamic hypothyroidism may develop, creating increased fatigue and changes in weight, hair, and skin [33,34].

Previous data suggest that spinal cord involvement occurs in less than 5% of patients who have sarcoidosis and in less than 10% of patients who have neurosarcoidosis [3,35–37]. Newer studies using magnetic resonance (MR) imaging criteria suggest that spinal cord involvement may be more prevalent than previously reported. Spinal cord involvement may be the initial presentation of sarcoidosis. In a study by Bradley and colleagues [38], only 4 of 17 patients who had spinal cord sarcoidosis were previously diagnosed with sarcoidosis before spinal cord involvement. Patients who have spinal cord sarcoidosis frequently present with insidious, progressive, but nonspecific paresthesias and weakness that can progress to paraplegia [39]. Many patients may experience progressive debilitating symptoms for months

before diagnosis. In a recent report, 5 of 17 patients developed paraplegia before a confirmed diagnosis [38]. Compared with spinal cord compression associated with malignancy, patients who have spinal cord sarcoidosis are less likely to experience back pain [38]. Studies suggest that the granulomas of sarcoidosis may have an affinity for the cervical level with extension over multiple cord segments [40–42]. Most clinically apparent spinal sarcoid lesions are intramedullary [43,44], with rare cases reported of intradural extramedullary [45] or cauda equina lesions [46–50]. Schaller and colleagues [51] suggest that intradural extramedullary disease may represent early stage spinal sarcoidosis. Unlike intramedullary disease, extramedullary sarcoid lesions can be surgically excised with favorable results.

Audiovestibular dysfunction is a rare neurologic complication of sarcoidosis. Hearing loss is usually sensorineural, bilateral, and asymmetric. Vestibular impairment is frequently encountered and usually associated with abnormal vestibular testing. A review of 48 case reports concluded that the manifestations are the result of vestibulocochlear nerve neuropathy [52].

Approximately 15% of patients experience a variety of peripheral neuropathy manifestations, including axonal, sensory, motor, mononeuropathy, mononeuropathy multiplex, demyelinating, and Gullain-Barre syndrome [4,53]. The pathologic process may be focal or multifocal, with virtually all levels and classes of nerve fibers being involved [54,55]. Of equal frequency is myopathy (15%), which can present as nodules, polymyositis, or atrophy [56]. Symptomatic improvement is usually noted with corticosteroids [54]. The prognosis is usually better for patients who have peripheral symptoms of paresthesias, muscle weakness, and stocking-glove numbness compared with patients who have central nervous system (CNS) symptoms.

The diverse manifestations and percentage of individual neurosarcoidosis involvement are summarized in Table 1. The range of presentations may be due to differences in ethnic background, methods of detection, or interest of the reporting physicians.

The diagnostic dilemma of neurosarcoidosis

Because of the diverse clinical presentations, patients are often classified as having definite, probable, or possible neurosarcoidosis based on the confirmed diagnosis of multisystem sarcoidosis, the pattern of neurologic disease, and the

response to treatment. Two groups have proposed criteria for neurosarcoidosis based on the probability of neurologic involvement [17,57]. Table 2 compares the two proposals in terms of definite, probable, and possible neurosarcoidosis diagnosis. In Judson and colleagues' [57] proposal, all patients are required to have biopsy confirmation of sarcoidosis in the nervous system or elsewhere. Consequently, patients who have known sarcoidosis with features supportive of neurosarcoidosis are considered "definite." Zajicek and colleagues [17] assigned a "definite" neurosarcoidosis category to patients who had biopsy confirmation of neurologic involvement. This approach has been supported by others [58]. From a practical perspective, the presence of "definite" or "probable" disease categorization has been used as an indication for therapy [59].

Confirming the diagnosis of neurosarcoidosis depends on whether the symptoms develop in a patient who has known sarcoidosis or in a patient who does not have known sarcoidosis. Patients who have confirmed sarcoidosis who develop symptoms or findings suggestive of neurologic sarcoidosis should be evaluated for exclusion of other disease entities, such as cerebrovascular disease, complications of metabolic diseases such as diabetes, and malignancies. Infections can be a consequence of sarcoidosis, treatment for the sarcoidosis [60], or other conditions. Fig. 2 reveals the MR image of a patient followed at our clinic for pulmonary and cutaneous sarcoidosis. This patient had discontinued systemic therapy for more than 5 years when she presented with ataxia, and the MR imaging revealed a cerebellar lesion (Fig. 2). Because of the atypical presentation after many years off therapy, a biopsy was performed, which revealed toxoplasmosis. The patient was confirmed to be infected with HIV.

Clinicians can be challenged to diagnose neurosarcoidosis in patients who have suggestive neurologic findings but have no confirmed diagnosis of sarcoidosis. An extensive differential diagnosis includes primary neurologic diseases, such as multiple sclerosis (MS) [61], lymphoma, craniopharyngioma, primary CNS neoplasia, primary CNS infections including neurosyphillis, HIV, or toxoplasmosis, brucellosis, Whipple's disease, and autoimmune diseases (including systemic lupus erythematosis, Sjogren syndrome, Behcet's disease, Vogt-Koyanagi-Harada disease, lymphocytic hypophysitis, pachymeningitis, and isolated angiitis of the CNS) [2].

Table 1
Summary of neurologic manifestations and reported frequency

General class	Subset	Frequency of manifestations of neurosarcoidosis (reported range)
Cranial neuropathy		50%–75%
	First	1%–10%
	Seventh	25%–50%
Meningeal		10%–20%
	Hydrocephalus	10%
Parenchymal brain lesions		50%
	Hypothalamic	10%–15%
	Mass lesions	5%–10%
	Encephalopathy	5%–10%
Spinal cord		5%–10%
	Intramedullary	Most frequent spinal lesion
Peripheral neuropathy		15%

Table 2
Criteria for neurosarcoidosis

	Zajicek et al [17]	Judson et al[a] [57]
Definite	Clinical presentation suggestive of neurosarcoidosis with exclusion of other possible diagnoses and the presence of positive nervous system histology	1. Positive MR imaging with uptake in meninges or brainstem 2. Cerebral spinal fluid with increased lymphocytes or protein 3. Diabetes insipidus 4. Seventh cranial nerve paralysis 5. Positive peripheral or central nerve biopsy
Probable	Clinical syndrome suggestive of neurosarcoidosis with laboratory support for CNS inflammation (elevated levels of CSF protein or cells, the presence of oligoclonal bands or MR imaging evidence compatible with neurosarcoidosis) and exclusion of alternative diagnoses together with evidence for systemic sarcoidosis (through positive histology, including Kveim test, or at least two indirect indicators from Gallium scan, chest imaging, and serum angiotensin-converting enzyme)	1. Other abnormalities on MR imaging 2. Unexplained neuropathy 3. Positive electromyelogram
Probable	Clinical presentation suggestive of neurosarcoidosis with exclusion of alternative diagnoses where the above criteria are not met	1. Unexplained headaches 2. Peripheral nerve radiculopathy

[a] Only applied to patients who had biopsy-confirmed sarcoidosis.

Because 50% of patients who have neurosarcoidosis have other systemic disease, patients should be evaluated for involvement of other organs, including lung, skin, lymph nodes, or eye. Although other clues, such as elevated serum angiotensin enzyme or serum immunoglobulins, hypercalcemia, or hypercalciuria, may suggest the diagnosis of sarcoidosis, none of these tests is confirmatory [2,4,62]. Diagnostic radiologic evaluation may include chest X ray and CT. Fig. 3 shows the chest X ray and CT scan of a patient who presented with weakness in her legs and was found to have a spinal cord lesion. Other imaging includes MR imaging, whole-body fluorodeoxyglucose positron emission tomography (PET), or gallium scan. Recently, Teirstein and colleagues [63] reported on the value of PET scan in identifying alternative areas to biopsy in patients who have possible sarcoidosis. Depending on clinical symptoms, pulmonary function tests or ophthalmologic and endoscopic nasal examinations may be rewarding.

Patients who have possible CNS sarcoidosis require a detailed examination related to

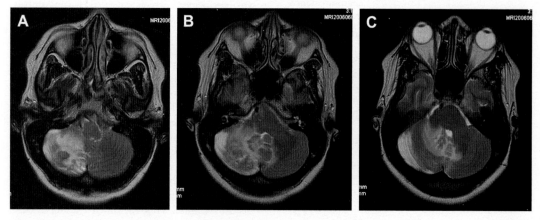

Fig. 2. (A–C) Axial T2-weighted images through cerebellum demonstrating nonspecific, ill-defined hyperintense T2 signal right hemispheric lesion with mass effect and edema. Biopsy proved toxoplasmosis.

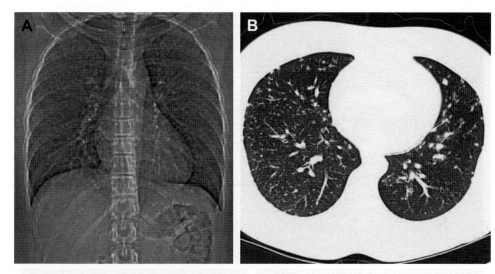

Fig. 3. (*A*) Posterior-anterior chest X ray demonstrating fine nodularity involving primarily mid- and lower lung fields. (*B*) Axial CT with lung windows demonstrating innumerable scattered 5 mm or less pulmonary nodules diffusely distributed in a subpleural, centrilobular, and perivascular distribution consistent with sarcoidosis.

neuroendocrinologic or hypothalamic dysfunction. This includes tests of thyroid function and tests for diabetes mellitus, diabetes insipidus, hypercalcemia, hypercalciuria, cortisol, prolactin, estradiol or testosterone, follicular stimulating hormone, and luteinizing hormone.

Tissue confirmation of noncaseating granulomas remains the gold standard for unconfirmed cases [17]. Patients who have known sarcoidosis who develop CNS masses may be treated empirically with corticosteroids if infection and malignancy are reasonably excluded. Biopsy may be necessary for patients who fail to respond to corticosteroids. Peripheral nerve or muscle biopsy can also be obtained to confirm histology. In patients who have neuropathic symptoms and unrevealing nerve conduction and electromyographic studies, skin biopsies can be pursued.

Diagnostic imaging

Magnetic resonance imaging: brain

MR imaging with gadolinium contrast enhancement remains the preferred imaging technique for neurosarcoidosis [64]. Leptomeningeal involvement is the most commonly reported imaging abnormality because it is seen in approximately 40% of neurosarcoidosis cases. This disease pattern usually appears as thickening with diffuse or focal/multifocal enhancement of the leptomeninges on contrast-enhanced

T1-weighted images (see Fig. 1). Sarcoidosis has a predilection for the basilar meninges [14]; however, involvement of the cortical sulci and perivascular space and cisterns around the base of the brain is indistinguishable from tuberculosis or lymphoma. Spread along the perivascular spaces can lead to parenchymal involvement (Fig. 4). Enhancing parenchymal lesions with contiguous meningeal enhancement on T2-weighted images may be indistinguishable from meningiomas [65]. Isolated contrast-enhanced T1-weighted images of the hypothalamus or pituitary infundibulum can mimic histiocytosis. Often these patients present with diabetes insipidus or amenorrhea.

Cranial nerve abnormalities may be associated with leptomeningeal disease, sinonasal disease, or an isolated finding. MR imaging hallmarks of cranial nerve abnormalities are enlargement and enhancement on T1-weighted contrast imaging (Fig. 5). Although facial nerve (VII) palsy is the most common cranial nerve involved clinically, the optic nerves are most commonly affected radiographically. The optic nerve and optic chiasm are best evaluated with T1-weighted images. Involvement may be bilateral or unilateral with the differential for isolated optic nerve involvement, including optic neuritis, optic nerve glioma, and optic nerve meningioma [17].

Neurosarcoidosis with dural involvement can present as diffuse thickening or focal masses (Fig. 6). These lesions typically enhance with T1-weighted imaging and are relatively hypointense

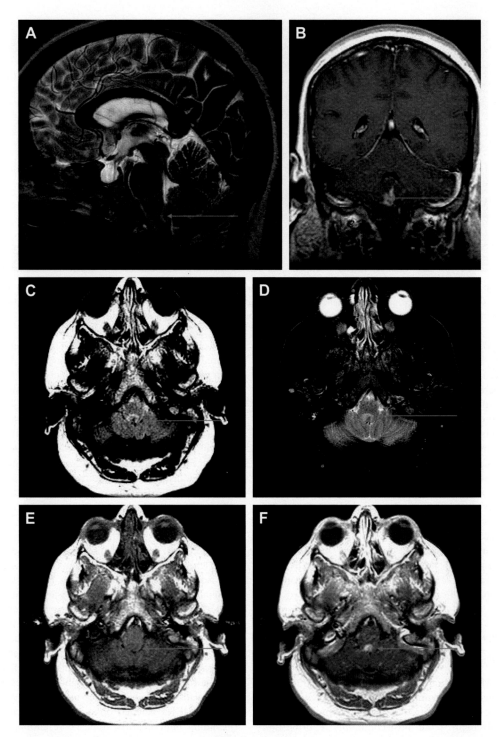

Fig. 4. (*A*) Sagittal T2-weighted image showing enlarged empty sella. (*B*) Coronal postcontrast T1-weighted images demonstrating neurosarcoid involvement of the posterior medulla and diffuse leptomeningeal enhancement throughout the posterior fossa (*red arrows*). Co-registered axial images: (*C*) FLAIR, (*D*) T2, (*E*) T1, and (*F*) T1-weighted postcontrast images demonstrating focal parenchymal involvement of the posterior medulla (*red arrows*). Panel *F* shows diffuse leptomeningeal enhancement throughout the posterior fossa.

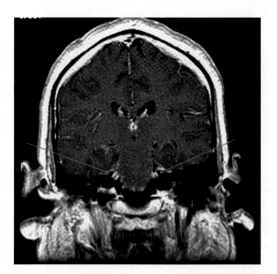

Fig. 5. T1-weighted postcontrast coronal MR image demonstrating thick enhancement surrounding the bilateral fifth cranial nerves (*red arrows*) and spotty coating of the adjacent brainstem.

on T2-weighted images. Differential considerations include calcified meningiomas, lymphoma, dural metastases, and hypertrophic cranial pachymeningitis. These patients usually present with headaches and symptoms related to cranial nerve involvement [64,65].

Parenchymal lesions in neurosarcoidosis may be nonenhancing or enhancing. Some series report multiple nonenhancing periventricular white matter lesions with high signal intensity of T2-weighted images (see Fig. 4). These lesions are commonly encountered in patients who have disease other than sarcoidosis, such as MS and vascular disease. Contrast-enhancing parenchymal lesions may be mistaken for primary or metastatic tumors [14,23,66]. Although central necrosis is frequently seen in tumors, it is uncommon in sarcoidosis. Often these patients may present with seizures, and frequently tissue confirmation is necessary.

Hydrocephalus is reported in 5% to 12% of patients who have neurosarcoidosis. Communicating hydrocephalus results from altered cerebrospinal fluid (CSF) resorption secondary to dural or leptomeningeal involvement. Adhesions or loculations in the ventricular system may cause obstructive hydrocephalus. Isolation of the fourth ventricle (ie, trapped fourth ventricle) may occur. Patients who have hydrocephalus often present with ataxia and altered gait, which can be improved with ventricular shunting (Figs. 7 and 8) [67].

Magnetic resonance imaging: spinal cord

Sarcoidosis can affect the spine in a variety of ways, including the cord or nerve roots, the intradural-extramedullarly space, the intracanalicular extradural space, or the vertebral bodies and disks [38]. Although intramedullary spinal disease is rare, the devastating clinical manifestations can include paralysis and severe pain. Contrast-enhanced spinal MR imaging can appear as an enhancing enlargement, focal or diffuse enhancement, or atrophy. These imaging findings are nonspecific, and the differential diagnosis includes tumors, MS, and fungal infections. This imaging modality may aid in the diagnosis of the rare neurosarcoid manifestation of cauda equina syndrome, which may be diagnosed as nodules, thickening, or matted nerve roots (Fig. 9).

Based on the histologic stages of the disease, Junger and colleagues [44] have proposed a MR imaging classification system for spinal sarcoidosis. In Phase 1, early inflammation is identified as contrast-imaged linear leptomeningeal enhancement. By Phase 2, secondary centripetal spread of the leptomeningeal inflammatory process occurs through Virchow spaces to the parenchyma with faint postcontrast enhancement and diffuse edema. By Phase 3, the swelling decreases, and the size of the spinal cord can be normal but associated with focal areas of enhancement, and this inflammatory process resolves into Phase 4 with normal size or atrophy of the spinal cord without enhancement. Phases 2 and 3 are more commonly reported.

Other imaging modalities

MR imaging may be nonspecific for sarcoidosis [64,68]. A recent study of 22 patients who had sarcoidosis with CNS symptoms revealed a diverse constellation of nonspecific MR imaging findings [69]. In 46% of these patients, the periventricular and white matter lesions identified on the T2-weighted images mimicked those seen in MS. Supratentorial and infratentorial mass lesions mimicked tumor metastases in 36%. Solitary intra-axial masses could not be differentiated from high-grade astrocytomas in 9% of patients, and solitary extra-axial masses mimicked meningiomas in 5%. MR imaging may also be negative because of small or peripheral lesions or the effect of therapy [16,17].

CT scan of the brain is less sensitive than MR imaging for neurosarcoidosis [17]. There are cases

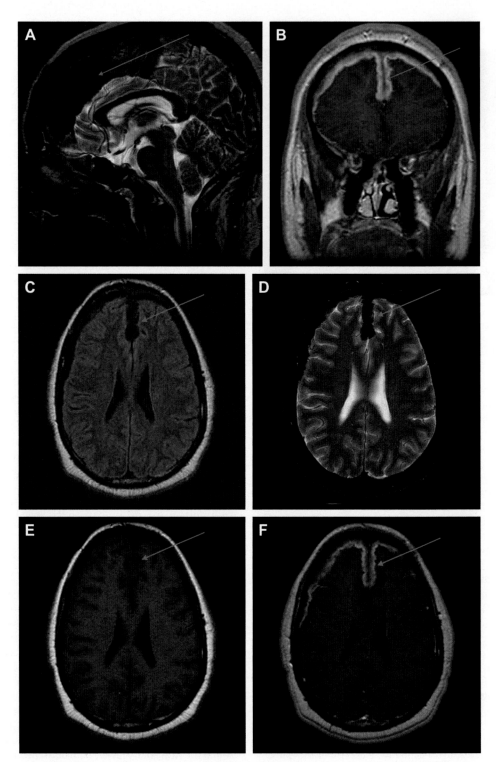

Fig. 6. (*A*) Sagittal T2-weighted and coronal postcontrast T1-weighted images demonstrating thick, hypointense T2, contrast-enhancing dural enhancement along the frontal lobes and falx cerebri (*red arrows*). Co-registered axial (*C*) FLAIR, (*D*) T2, (*E*) T1-weighted, and (*F*) T1-weighted postcontrast images demonstrating hypointense FLAIR/T2 thickening of the dura along the frontal lobes, right greater than left, and along the falx with prominent enhancement (*red arrows*).

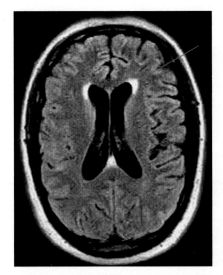

Fig. 7. Axial FLAIR image through the body of the lateral ventricles demonstrating mild hydrocephalus with hyperintense nonspecific periventricular signal changes (*red arrow*), which may represent a combination of white matter disease and transependymal CSF migration.

in which CT scan with contrast provides additional information. In a study of 14 patients who had CNS manifestations of neurosarcoidosis by MR imaging and CT, MR imaging detected

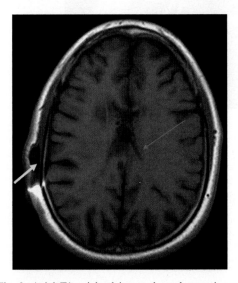

Fig. 8. Axial T1-weighted image through superior aspect of the lateral ventricles, demonstrating shunt catheter (*red arrow*) coursing through collapsed lateral ventricles in a patient with treated hydrocephalus related to neurosarcoidosis. Signal dropout (*yellow arrow*) in the right parietal scalp corresponds to extracranial course of the ventriculo-peritoneal shunt tubing.

lesions in all patients (100%) but was less accurate than CT in depicting disease in two patients. The CT detected lesions in 12 patients and was less accurate than MR imaging in delineating hypothalamic involvement in two patients and periventricular white-matter disease in three patients [70].

PET scanning with 18-F-fluorodeoxyglucose is a useful imaging modality in patients who have malignancy. Recent reports suggest that PET scanning can detect granulomatous involvement of multiple organs in sarcoidosis [63,71–73]. Alternative imaging with C-11 methionine and 18-F-fluorodeoxyglucose PET may improve localization of neurosarcoidosis [73].

A new MR imaging technique with the acronym IDEAL ASSIST (iterative decompositon of water and fat with echo asymmetric and least-squares estimation automated spine survey iterative scan technique) can provide rapid coverage of the entire spine with optimized fat–water separation (Fig. 10).

Cerebrospinal fluid analysis

Although neurosarcoidosis can be associated with an abnormal CSF analysis, no specific pattern is diagnostic [14,74]. Table 3 summarizes the CSF findings in sarcoidosis and other inflammatory disorders. In two large studies of neurosarcoidosis, increased protein, increased lymphocytes, or both were reported in 73% and 81% of patients [16,17]. Although an increased IgG index can be seen, the presence of oligoclonal bands is rare [9,75,76], with rare cases reported in patients who have neurosarcoidosis [77]. Where appropriate, cultures and special stains should be performed to exclude other granulomatous and infectious diseases, particularly tuberculosis and Cryptococcus. These diseases can also occur as complications of therapy for systemic sarcoidosis [60].

Special CSF studies, including angiotensin-converting enzyme and CD4:CD8 ratio, may be useful in detecting neurosarcoidosis in patients who have known sarcoidosis [78]. Increased CSF angiotensin-converting enzyme is relatively insensitive and nonspecific [75]. Elevated levels have been reported in approximately 50% of sarcoidosis cases and in many other diseases, including schizophrenia [76,79]. Increased CD4:CD8 ratio of CSF lymphocytes has also been noted in neurosarcoidosis [80,81]. Flow cytometry requires large numbers of viable lymphocytes, which are usually unavailable.

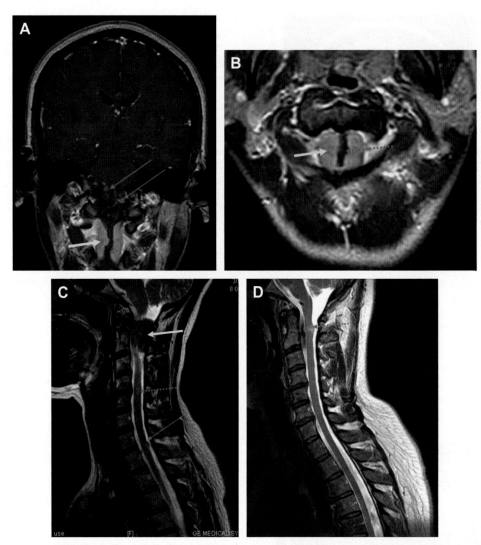

Fig. 9. (*A*) Coronal postcontrast T1 image of the head and upper cervical spine demonstrates small enhancing leptomeningeal nodules coating the medulla (*solid red arrows*) and marked circumferential dural and intradural involvement (*yellow arrow*) at the C1 and C2 levels severely compressing and deforming the cord (*dotted red arrow*). (*B*) Axial postcontrast T1 image at the C2 level redemonstrates marked transverse compression and flattening of the cord (*dotted red arrow*) by extensive intradural sarcoid involvement (*yellow arrow*). Sagittal midline T2 image of the cervical spine (*C*) redemonstrates the large relatively hypointense intradural mass (*yellow arrow*) markedly compressing and deforming the cord at the C1 and C2 levels. At C4–C5, there is hyperintense T2 signal intramedullary cord involvement (*dotted red arrow*), and at C7–T1 there is a small nodule along the dorsal cord surface (*solid red arrow*). Corresponding posttreatment sagittal T2 image (*D*) demonstrates marked regression of neurosarcoidosis with relatively mild deformity of the C1-C2 cervical cord and intramedullary increased T2 signal (*dotted red arrow*). The low signal ventral to the cord at this level reflects exaggerated CSF flow phenomena rather than hypointense intradural sarcoid.

Treatment of neurosarcoidosis

There are no randomized clinical trials defining the optimal treatment for neurosarcoidosis. In general, patients who have neurosarcoidosis present with a self-limited manifestation or a chronically progressive disease course [2,4,16]. Isolated cranial nerve abnormalities and aseptic meningitis are frequent monophasic presentations in two thirds of patients who have neurosarcoidosis. In particular, patients who have seventh nerve paralysis often have resolution of this symptom spontaneously or with a short course of corticosteroids

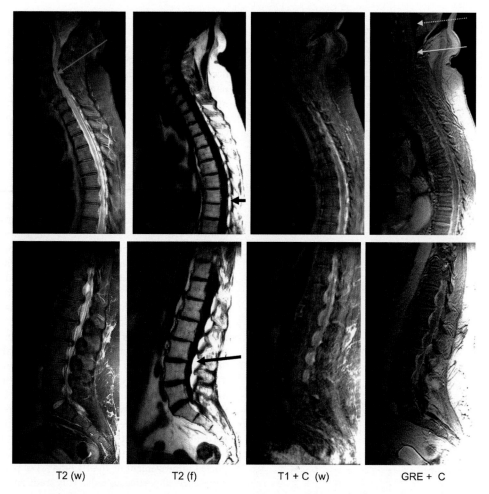

T2 (w)   T2 (f)   T1 + C (w)   GRE + C

Fig. 10. Rapid MR imaging screening of entire spine with IDEAL (iterative decomposition of water and fat with echo asymmetric and least-squares estimation) ASSIST (automated spine survey iterative technique) performed with two contiguous 35-cm field of view sagittal stations in a patient who has neurosarcoidosis. T2-weighted water (w) image (*first column*) demonstrates abnormal intramedullary cervical cord signal (*red arrow*). T2-weighted fat (f) image depicts steroid treatment–induced epidral lipomatosis in the thoracic (*short arrow*) and lumbar (*long arrow*) spine. T1-weighted, postcontrast (+C) water(w) image (*third column*) demonstrates thick abnormal dural and subdural enhancement throughout entire spinal canal (*dotted red arrow*), albeit degraded by motion artifact. Rapid postcontrast gradient echo sequence (GRE + C) is performed with breath holding, significantly reducing motion artifact (*fourth column*) and demonstrates fourth ventricular enlargement (*dotted yellow line*) as part of the patient's pan-hydrocephalus, atrophic upper cervical cord (*straight yellow arrow*) and redemonstrates thick dural and intradural enhancement throughout entire spinal canal (*dotted red arrow*).

[13,16]. Patients who have parenchymal, leptomeningeal disease with multiple cranial nerve abnormalities, myopathy, or spinal disease often experience a chronic remitting-relapsing course.

As in other forms of sarcoidosis, the goal of treatment is to palliate symptoms and to prevent irreversible fibrosis in target organs [4,82]. If certain manifestations of neurosarcoidosis, such as spinal cord disease or cauda equina syndrome [38,48–50], are not diagnosed and treated early,

life-threatening and devastating complications, including paraplegia, can develop.

Corticosteroids remain the mainstay of treatment for neurologic sarcoidosis. They are most useful early in treatment of the disease because they can lead to rapid reduction of the inflammation and the mass effect. Higher than usual doses of corticosteroids are often used to treat neurosarcoidosis [16,17,83,84]. One recommendation institutes daily treatment with as much as 1 mg/kg

Table 3
Comparison of cerebral spinal fluid findings

Disease	Cells	Increased protein	IgG index	Low glucose	Oligoclonal bands	Other features in CSF
Sarcoidosis	Lymphocytes common Increased CD4/CD4 ratio	Common	May be increased	Unusual	Rare	Elevated ACE
Multiple sclerosis	Mild increase lymphocytes	Normal	Almost always increased	Rare	Very common	—
Neuro lupus erythematosis	Usually acellular	Rare	Commonly increased	Rare	Common	—
Sjogren's syndrome	Lymphocytes, monocytes common	Common	Commonly increased	Common	Very common	—
Tuberculous meningitis	Lymphocyes common	Common	NA	Common	—	PCR for *M. tuberculosis*
Cryptococcal meningitis	Lymphocytes common	Common	NA	Common	—	Cryptococcal antigen
Leptomeningeal Carcinomatosis	Lymphocytes common	Common	NA	Common	—	Cytology

Abbreviations: NA, not available; PCR, polymerase chain reaction.
Data from Reske D, Petereit HF, Heiss WD. Difficulties in the differentiation of chronic inflammatory diseases of the central nervous system: value of cerebrospinal fluid analysis and immunological abnormalities in the diagnosis. Acta Neurol Scand 2005;112(4):207–13.

of prednisone or its equivalent [84]. Usually, isolated peripheral nerve palsies or myopathy can be successfully treated with short courses of prednisone; however, prolonged therapy may be necessary. Due to the chronic remitting-relapsing nature of severe neurologic disease, including mass lesions, leptomeningeal, and spinal cord disease, patients often require high-dose, prolonged courses of therapy [85]. Corticosteroid therapy has been the usual initial treatment strategy; however, many patients require alternative treatments due to intolerance of prednisone or persistent disease activity despite corticosteroids. Table 4 summarizes four series that reported on the response rate to corticosteroid therapy alone for neurosarcoidosis [16,17,83,85]. In three of these studies, less than 40% of the patients stabilized or improved with corticosteroid therapy alone. The report by Scott and colleagues [83] selected patients for early aggressive immunosuppressive therapy if they "presented with severe central nervous system …(intracranial lesions, hydrocephalus, myelopathy, seizures, or encephalopathy)." Of the patients selected to receive corticosteroids alone, 90% were stable or improved on this regimen. Table 4 shows the response to the use of cytotoxic agents with or without corticosteroids. The overall response rate was higher for patients treated with immunosuppressive agents than those treated with corticosteroids alone. Another study [9] of 32 patients who had neurosarcoidosis reported improvement in 16 of 19 (84%) of patients who received corticosteroids. This study included a variety of monophasic and chronic disease patients, and no immunosuppressive therapy was reported.

Because of the failure of corticosteroid therapy to control most cases of neurosarcoidosis, alternatives to corticosteroids have been sought [16,85,86]. Alternative therapies have included immunosuppressive drugs, including cyclophosphamide [16,87], methotrexate [16], azathioprine [83,85], mycophenolate mofetil [88], cyclosporine [85,89], and hydroxychloroquine [90]. None of these agents has been studied in a placebo-controlled trial in patients who have neurosarcoidosis, and there are no evidence-based guidelines for this disease process. Isolated series suggest clinical benefit when drugs such as cyclophosphamide are added to corticosteroids for the treatment of chronic neurosarcoidosis. The aggressive use of immunosuppressive agents for many cases of neurosarcoidosis seems to be supported by the data in Table 4. The cytotoxic

Table 4
Outcome of therapy for neurosarcoidosis

First author	Number treated	Improved/stable	Treatment	Number treated	Improved/stable
Agbogu [85]	26	38%	All[a]	19	79%
Lower [16]	48	29%	Methotrexate	28	61%
			Cyclophosphamide[b]	10	85%
Zajidek [17]	34	29%	—	—	—
Scott [83]	19[c]	90%	All	26	85%

[a] Cytotoxic agents ± corticosteroids.
[b] Only patients who failed methotrexate treatment were treated with cyclophosphamide.
[c] Treated with corticosteroids only in selected patients who had mild neurosarcoidosis.

agents methotrexate and azathioprine have reasonable response rates in about two thirds of the patients treated [16,83]. In one study of patients who failed methotrexate, 8 of 10 responded to intermittent, intravenous cyclophosphamide [16]. Similar results have been reported with cyclophosphamide for refractory neurosarcoidosis [87,91]. In addition, alternative immunosuppressive therapies have been beneficial in spinal cord sarcoidosis. In a small series of 14 evaluable patients who had spinal cord sarcoidosis, all patients were initially treated with corticosteroids. Subsequently, 5 of 10 patients who were treated with methotrexate alone responded, whereas all seven patients who were treated with cyclophosphamide (including some of the methotrexate failures) responded [38].

Newer targeted agents against tumor necrosis factor–alpha, including infliximab [92–94] and thalidomide [95], may be helpful. There have been some case reports indicating the benefit of infliximab for various manifestations of neurosarcoidosis [94,96–98], with a response seen within months of starting treatment. There is a recent report of successful treatment of spinal sarcoidosis with thalidomide [99]. As in other organ systems, careful monitoring for toxicity and side effects is mandatory (a more detailed discussion of drug therapy dosing and toxicity occurs elsewhere in this issue).

Neurosarcoidosis remains a relatively rare manifestation of the disease process without evidence-based treatment guidelines. Recommendations are based on case series and reports. The approach we use at our clinic is shown in Fig. 11. Patients are classified as "mild," "moderate," or "severe" based on initial presentation. Patients who have a monophasic disease, such as cranial neuropathy, alone are treated as "mild" and treated initially only with corticosteroids. Patients who have intracranial or spinal cord lesions, hydrocephalus, myelopathy, seizures, or encephalopathy are considered

"moderate" or "severe" and are treated initially with an immunosuppressive agent plus prednisone [16,83]. Patients who have "severe" disease are started on cyclophosphamide or infliximab. Patients who have milder disease or who respond well to corticosteroids may be started on methotrexate. Because cytotoxic agents may require up to 6 months for maximum benefit, patients may initially receive cyclophosphamide or infliximab to shorten the time to response and minimize excessive corticosteroid toxicity. Patients who have uncontrolled disease despite initial immunosuppressive agents are candidates for cyclophosphamide or infliximab.

Supportive, nonsystemic treatment of neurosarcoidosis

Although aggressive systemic treatment with corticosteroids and other immunosuppressive agents remains the mainstay of treatment for neurosarcoidosis, management of neurologic complications, including hydrocephalus, seizures, and dysfunction of the pituitary-hypothalmic axis, is important. Asymptomatic or mild hydrocephalus may not require therapy; however, this condition can rapidly deteriorate [100]. In some cases, this can be reversed by aggressive corticosteroid administration and ventricular shunt placement [101]. Granulomatous inflammation may lead to shunt obstruction, and careful monitoring is necessary to detect obstruction or infection [102]. Seizures, which may complicate hydrocephalus or mass lesions, are usually successfully treated by controlling the granulomatous inflammation along with antiepileptic medication [2]. Abnormal CSF findings do not always necessitate treatment, and therapy decisions are usually determined by clinical symptoms. Patients who have pituitary and hypothalamic disease require extensive hormone evaluation and replacement. Although corticosteroids may decrease mass lesions in the

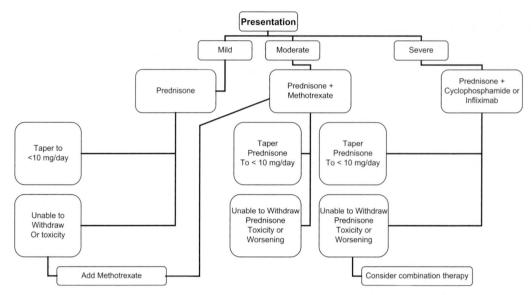

Fig. 11. Patients are classified as "mild," "moderate," or "severe" based on initial presentation. Patients who have monophasic disease or those who have cranial neuropathy alone are treated as "mild" with corticosteroids only. Patients who have intracranial or spinal cord lesions, hydrocephalus, myelopathy, seizures, or encephalopathy are considered "moderate" or "severe" depending on the extent of the disease and response to initial corticosteroids. Treatment options for the various presentations are shown. Therapy may be modified based on response and toxicity.

pituitary stalk or hypothalamus, polyuria secondary to diabetes insipidus can be chronic, necessitating desmopressin therapy [103]. Additional hormone replacement for hypopituitarism can include sex hormone replacement with estrogen or testosterone or thyroid replacement [21].

Surgery and radiation therapy have been advocated to ameliorate local symptoms. Because sarcoidosis remains a diagnosis of exclusion, providing tissue for diagnosis and culture is the main indication for surgery. In patients who have known sarcoidosis, additional surgical tissue may become necessary when additional diagnoses, including infection or malignancy, need to be excluded. There seems to be little role for routine complete surgical resection of granulomas. In fact, attempts to completely resect rather than debulk intramedullary lesions from sarcoidosis may worsen the prognosis [35,39,40]. Radiation therapy has been useful in limited cases, usually in the treatment of disease refractory to systemic therapies [104–107].

Painful neuropathy and myopathy may require additional treatment strategies [62]. Ipsilateral hemifacial spasms can be treated with periodic injections of botulinum toxin A [108]. After failure of standard medications, rhizotomy may effectively improve persistent trigeminal neuralgia.

Assessment of treatment response

Assessing clinical response in neurosarcoidosis can be difficult. Although treatment with corticosteroids can improve MR imaging [109], clinical responses may not correlate with roentgenographic improvement [38,110]. Studies suggest that clinical improvement is usually associated with improved MR image abnormalities, particularly contrast-enhancing lesions [85,109,111]. One case series of spinal cord sarcoidosis revealed improved MR image appearance without clinical improvement [110].

Because patients who have neurosarcoidosis may experience delayed relapses when treatment is discontinued [16], patients need to be followed for years after corticosteroids are withdrawn [112]. Because symptoms may recur before MR image changes, the clinician must be sensitive to new neurologic symptoms in a patient who has known neurosarcoidosis in whom treatment has been reduced or withdrawn.

Summary

The diagnosis and management of neurosarcoidosis remains one of the more difficult aspects of this disease. This manifestation remains challenging because of the diverse range of clinical presentations, difficulties encountered in identifying neurologic lesions, and the refractory nature that can occur with the disease process. Newer treatment options provide the treating physician better options to tailor therapy to the individual patient.

References

[1] Sharma OP. Neurosarcoidosis: a personal perspective based on the study of 37 patients. Chest 1997; 112:220–8.

[2] Stern BJ. Neurological complications of sarcoidosis. Curr Opin Neurol 2004;17(3):311–6.

[3] Stern BJ, Krumholz A, Johns C, et al. Sarcoidosis and its neurological manifestations. Arch Neurol 1985;42:909–17.

[4] Hoitsma E, Faber CG, Drent M, et al. Neurosarcoidosis: a clinical dilemma. Lancet Neurol 2004; 3(7):397–407.

[5] Baughman RP, du Bois RM, Lower EE. Sarcoidosis. Lancet 2003;361:1111–8.

[6] Gullapalli D, Phillips LH. Neurologic manifestations of sarcoidosis. Neurol Clin 2002;20(1): 59–83, vi.

[7] Burns TM. Neurosarcoidosis. Arch Neurol 2003; 60(8):1166–8.

[8] Delaney P. Neurologic manifestations in sarcoidosis: review of the literature, with a report of 23 cases. Ann Intern Med 1977;87(3):336–45.

[9] Allen RK, Sellars RE, Sandstrom PA. A prospective study of 32 patients with neurosarcoidosis. Sarcoidosis Vasc Diffuse Lung Dis 2003;20(2):118–25.

[10] Baughman RP, Teirstein AS, Judson MA, et al. Clinical characteristics of patients in a case control study of sarcoidosis. Am J Respir Crit Care Med 2001;164:1885–9.

[11] Ferriby D, de Seze J, Stojkovic T, et al. Long-term follow-up of neurosarcoidosis. Neurology 2001; 57(5):927–9.

[12] Chapelon C, Ziza JM, Piette JC, et al. Neurosarcoidosis: signs, course and treatment in 35 confirmed cases. Medicine (Baltimore) 1990;69:261–76.

[13] Winget D, O'Brien GM, Lower EE, et al. Bell's palsy as an unrecognized presentation for sarcoidosis. Sarcoidosis 1994;11:S368–70.

[14] Nowak DA, Widenka DC. Neurosarcoidosis: a review of its intracranial manifestation. J Neurol 2001;248(5):363–72.

[15] Palacios E, Rigby PL, Smith DL. Cranial neuropathy in neurosarcoidosis. Ear Nose Throat J 2003; 82(4):251–2.

[16] Lower EE, Broderick JP, Brott TG, et al. Diagnosis and management of neurologic sarcoidosis. Arch Intern Med 1997;157:1864–8.

[17] Zajicek JP, Scolding NJ, Foster O, et al. Central nervous system sarcoidosis: diagnosis and management. QJM 1999;92(2):103–17.

[18] Plotkin GR, Patel BR. Neurosarcoidosis presenting as chronic lymphocytic meningitis. Pa Med 1986;89(7):36–7.

[19] Mayer SA, Yim GK, Onesti ST, et al. Biopsy-proven isolated sarcoid meningitis: case report. J Neurosurg 1993;78:994–6.

[20] Akhondi H, Barochia S, Holmstrom B, et al. Hydrocephalus as a presenting manifestation of neurosarcoidosis. South Med J 2003;96(4):403–6.

[21] Murialdo G, Tamagno G. Endocrine aspects of neurosarcoidosis. J Endocrinol Invest 2002;25(7): 650–62.

[22] Veres L, Utz JP, Houser OW. Sarcoidosis presenting as a central nervous system mass lesion. Chest 1997;111(2):518–21.

[23] Powers WJ, Miller EM. Sarcoidosis mimicking glioma: case report and review of intracranial sarcoid mass lesions. Neurology 1981;31:907–10.

[24] Willigers H, Koehler PJ. Amnesic syndrome caused by neurosarcoidosis. Clin Neurol Neurosurg 1993; 95:131–5.

[25] O'Brien GM, Baughman RP, Broderick JP, et al. Paranoid psychosis due to neurosarcoidosis. Sarcoidosis 1994;11:34–6.

[26] Friedman SH, Gould DJ. Neurosarcoidosis presenting as psychosis and dementia: a case report. Int J Psychiatry Med 2002;32(4):401–3.

[27] Bona JR, Fackler SM, Fendley MJ, et al. Neurosarcoidosis as a cause of refractory psychosis: a complicated case report. Am J Psychiatry 1998; 155(8):1106–8.

[28] Sabaawi M, Gutierrez-Nunez J, Fragala MR. Neurosarcoidosis presenting as schizophreniform disorder. Int J Psychiatry Med 1992;22(3):269–74.

[29] Krumholz A, Stern BJ, Stern EG. Clinical implications of seizures in neurosarcoidosis. Arch Neurol 1991;48:842–4.

[30] Konrad D, Gartenmann M, Martin E, et al. Central diabetes insipidus as the first manifestation of neurosarcoidosis in a 10-year-old girl. Horm Res 2000;54(2):98–100.

[31] Tamagno G, Murialdo G. Amenorrhea-galactorrhea syndrome as an uncommon manifestation of isolated neurosarcoidosis. Ann Ital Med Int 2001; 16(4):260–6.

[32] Bullmann C, Faust M, Hoffmann A, et al. Five cases with central diabetes insipidus and hypogonadism as first presentation of neurosarcoidosis. Eur J Endocrinol 2000;142(4):365–72.

[33] Guoth MS, Kim J, de Lotbiniere AC, et al. Neurosarcoidosis presenting as hypopituitarism and a cystic pituitary mass. Am J Med Sci 1998;315(3): 220–4.

[34] Gleckman AM, Patalas ED, Joseph JT. Sudden unexpected death resulting from hypothalamic sarcoidosis. Am J Forensic Med Pathol 2002; 23(1):48–51.

[35] Day AL, Sypert GW. Spinal cord sarcoidosis. Ann Neurol 1977;1(1):79–85.

[36] Baruah JK, Glasauer FE, Sil R, et al. Sarcoidosis of the cervical spinal canal: case report. Neurosurgery 1978;3(2):216–8.

[37] Oksanen V. Neurosarcoidosis: clinical presentations and course in 50 patients. Acta Neurol Scand 1986;73:283–90.

[38] Bradley DA, Lower EE, Baughman RP. Diagnosis and management of spinal cord sarcoidosis. Sarcoidosis Vasc Diffuse Lung Dis 2006;23(1):58–65.

[39] Ayala L, Barber DB, Lomba MR, et al. Intramedullary sarcoidosis presenting as incomplete paraplegia: case report and literature review. J Spinal Cord Med 2000;23(2):96–9.

[40] Jallo GI, Zagzag D, Lee M, et al. Intraspinal sarcoidosis: diagnosis and management. Surg Neurol 1997;48(5):514–20.

[41] Rieger J, Hosten N. Spinal cord sarcoidosis. Neuroradiology 1994;36(8):627–8.

[42] Hayat GR, Walton TP, Smith K R Jr, et al. Solitary intramedullary neurosarcoidosis: role of MRI in early detection. J Neuroimaging 2001;11(1):66–70.

[43] Hashmi M, Kyritsis AP. Diagnosis and treatment of intramedullary spinal cord sarcoidosis. J Neurol 1998;245(3):178–80.

[44] Junger SS, Stern BJ, Levine SR, et al. Intramedullary spinal sarcoidosis: clinical and magnetic resonance imaging characteristics. Neurology 1993; 43(2):333–7.

[45] Connor SE, Marshman L, Al Sarraj S, et al. MRI of a spinal intradural extramedullary sarcoid mass. Neuroradiology 2001;43(12):1079–83.

[46] Prelog K, Blome S, Dennis C. Neurosarcoidosis of the conus medullaris and cauda equina. Australas Radiol 2003;47(3):295–7.

[47] Shah JR, Lewis RA. Sarcoidosis of the cauda equina mimicking guillain-barre syndrome. J Neurol Sci 2003;208(1-2):113–7.

[48] Abrey LE, Rosenblum MK, DeAngelis LM. Sarcoidosis of the cauda equina mimicking leptomeningeal malignancy. J Neurooncol 1998;39(3): 261–5.

[49] Ku A, Lachmann E, Tunkel R, et al. Neurosarcoidosis of the conus medullaris and cauda equina presenting as paraparesis: case report and literature review. Paraplegia 1996;34(2):116–20.

[50] Kaiboriboon K, Olsen TJ, Hayat GR. Cauda equina and conus medullaris syndrome in sarcoidosis. Neurologist 2005;11(3):179–83.

[51] Schaller B, Kruschat T, Schmidt H, et al. Intradural, extramedullary spinal sarcoidosis: report of a rare case and review of the literature. Spine J 2006;6(2):204–10.

[52] Colvin IB. Audiovestibular manifestations of sarcoidosis: a review of the literature. Laryngoscope 2006;116(1):75–82.

[53] Galassi G, Gibertoni M, Mancini A, et al. Sarcoidosis of the peripheral nerve: clinical, electrophysiological and histological study of two cases. Eur Neurol 1984;23(6):459–65.

[54] Said G, Lacroix C, Plante-Bordeneuve V, et al. Nerve granulomas and vasculitis in sarcoid peripheral neuropathy: a clinicopathological study of 11 patients. Brain 2002;125(Pt 2):264–75.

[55] Hoitsma E, Marziniak M, Faber CG, et al. Small fibre neuropathy in sarcoidosis. Lancet 2002; 359(9323):2085–6.

[56] Berger C, Sommer C, Meinck HM. Isolated sarcoid myopathy. Muscle Nerve 2002;26(4):553–6.

[57] Judson MA, Baughman RP, Teirstein AS, et al. Defining organ involvement in sarcoidosis: the ACCESS proposed instrument. Sarcoidosis Vasc Diffuse Lung Dis 1999;16:75–86.

[58] Marangoni S, Argentiero V, Tavolato B. Neurosarcoidosis: clinical description of 7 cases with a proposal for a new diagnostic strategy. J Neurol 2006;253(4):488–95.

[59] Baughman RP, Lower EE. Novel therapies for sarcoidosis. Semin Respir Crit Care Med 2007;28(1): 128–33.

[60] Baughman RP, Lower EE. Fungal infections as a complication of therapy for sarcoidosis. QJM 2005;98:451–6.

[61] Trojano M, Paolicelli D. The differential diagnosis of multiple sclerosis: classification and clinical features of relapsing and progressive neurological syndromes. Neurol Sci 2001;22(Suppl 2):S98–102.

[62] Spencer TS, Campellone JV, Maldonado I, et al. Clinical and magnetic resonance imaging manifestations of neurosarcoidosis. Semin Arthritis Rheum 2005;34(4):649–61.

[63] Teirstein AS, Machac J, Almeida O, et al. Results of 188 whole-body fluorodeoxyglucose positron emission tomography scans in 137 patients with sarcoidosis. Chest 2007;132(6):1949–53.

[64] Lury KM, Smith JK, Matheus MG, et al. Neurosarcoidosis: review of imaging findings. Semin Roentgenol 2004;39(4):495–504.

[65] Urbach H, Kristof R, Zentner J, et al. Sarcoidosis presenting as an intra– or extra-axial cranial mass: report of two cases. Neuroradiology 1997; 39(7):516–9.

[66] Krejchi D, Caldemeyer KS, Vakili ST, et al. Neurosarcoidosis resembling meningioma: MRI characteristics and pathologic correlation. J Neuroimaging 1998;8(3):177–9.

[67] Scott TF, Brillman J. Shunt-responsive dementia in sarcoid meningitis: role of magnetic resonance imaging and cisternography. J Neuroimaging 2000; 10(3):185–6.

[68] Smith JK, Matheus MG, Castillo M. Imaging manifestations of neurosarcoidosis. AJR Am J Roentgenol 2004;182(2):289–95.

[69] Pickuth D, Heywang-Kobrunner SH. Neurosarcoidosis: evaluation with MRI. J Neuroradiol 2000;27(3):185–8.

[70] Hayes WS, Sherman JL, Stern BJ, et al. MR and CT evaluation of intracranial sarcoidosis. AJR Am J Roentgenol 1987;149(5):1043–9.

[71] Aide N, Benayoun M, Kerrou K, et al. Impact of [18F]-fluorodeoxyglucose ([18F]-FDG) imaging in sarcoidosis: unsuspected neurosarcoidosis discovered by [18F]-FDG PET and early metabolic response to corticosteroid therapy. Br J Radiol 2007;80(951):e67–71.

[72] Dubey N, Miletich RS, Wasay M, et al. Role of fluorodeoxyglucose positron emission tomography in the diagnosis of neurosarcoidosis. J Neurol Sci 2002;205(1):77–81.

[73] Ng D, Jacobs M, Mantil J. Combined C-11 methionine and F-18 FDG PET imaging in a case of neurosarcoidosis. Clin Nucl Med 2006;31(7):373–5.

[74] Reske D, Petereit HF, Heiss WD. Difficulties in the differentiation of chronic inflammatory diseases of the central nervous system: value of cerebrospinal fluid analysis and immunological abnormalities in the diagnosis. Acta Neurol Scand 2005;112(4):207–13.

[75] Dale JC, O'Brien JF. Determination of angiotensin-converting enzyme levels in cerebrospinal fluid is not a useful test for the diagnosis of neurosarcoidosis. Mayo Clin Proc 1999;74(5):535.

[76] Tahmoush AJ, Amir MS, Connor WW, et al. CSF-ACE activity in probable CNS neurosarcoidosis. Sarcoidosis Vasc Diffuse Lung Dis 2002;19(3):191–7.

[77] Scott TF, Seay AR, Goust JM. Pattern and concentration of IgG in cerebrospinal fluid in neurosarcoidosis. Neurology 1989;39(12):1637–9.

[78] Oksanen V, Fyhrquist F, Somer H, et al. Angiotensin converting enzyme in cerebrospinal fluid: a new assay. Neurology 1985;35(8):1220–3.

[79] Oksanen V, Fyhrquist F, Gronhagen-Riska C, et al. CSF angiotensin-converting enzyme in neurosarcoidosis. Lancet 1985;1:1050–1.

[80] Juozevicius JL, Rynes RI. Increased helper/suppressor T-lymphocyte ratio in the cerebrospinal fluid of a patient with neurosarcoidosis. Ann Intern Med 1986;104:807–8.

[81] Stern BJ, Griffin DE, Luke RA, et al. Neurosarcoidosis: cerebrospinal fluid lymphocyte subpopulations. Neurology 1987;37:878–81.

[82] Luke RA, Stern BJ, Krumholz A, et al. Neurosarcoidosis: the long-term clinical course. Neurology 1987;37(3):461–3.

[83] Scott TF, Yandora K, Valeri A, et al. Aggressive therapy for neurosarcoidosis: long-term follow-up of 48 treated patients. Arch Neurol 2007;64(5):691–6.

[84] Hunninghake GW, Costabel U, Ando M, et al. ATS/ERS/WASOG statement on sarcoidosis. American thoracic society/European respiratory society/world association of sarcoidosis and other granulomatous disorders. Sarcoidosis Vasc Diffuse Lung Dis 1999;16(Sep):149–73.

[85] Agbogu BN, Stern BJ, Sewell C, et al. Therapeutic considerations in patients with refractory neurosarcoidosis. Arch Neurol 1995;52:875–9.

[86] Patel AV, Stickler DE, Tyor WR. Neurosarcoidosis. Curr Treat Options Neurol 2007;9(3):161–8.

[87] Doty JD, Mazur JE, Judson MA. Treatment of corticosteroid-resistant neurosarcoidosis with a short-course cyclophosphamide regimen. Chest 2003;124(5):2023–6.

[88] Kouba DJ, Mimouni D, Rencic A, et al. Mycophenolate mofetil may serve as a steroid-sparing agent for sarcoidosis. Br J Dermatol 2003;148(1):147–8.

[89] Stern BJ, Schonfeld SA, Sewell C, et al. The treatment of neurosarcoidosis with cyclosporine. Arch Neurol 1992;49:1065–72.

[90] Sharma OP. Effectiveness of chloroquine and hydroxychloroquine in treating selected patients with sarcoidosis with neurologic involvement. Arch Neurol 1998;55:1248–54.

[91] Zuber M, Defer G, Cesaro P, et al. Efficacy of cyclophosphamide in sarcoid radiculomyelitis. J Neurol Neurosurg Psychiatry 1992;55(2):166–7.

[92] Baughman RP, Lower EE. Infliximab for refractory sarcoidosis. Sarcoidosis Vasc Diffuse Lung Dis 2001;18:70–4.

[93] Baughman RP, Drent M, Kavuru M, et al. Infliximab therapy in patients with chronic sarcoidosis and pulmonary involvement. Am J Respir Crit Care Med 2006;174(7):795–802.

[94] Doty JD, Mazur JE, Judson MA. Treatment of sarcoidosis with infliximab. Chest 2005;127(3):1064–71.

[95] Baughman RP, Judson MA, Teirstein AS, et al. Thalidomide for chronic sarcoidosis. Chest 2002;122:227–32.

[96] Baughman RP, Bradley DA, Lower EE. Infliximab for chronic ocular inflammation. Int J Clin Pharmacol Ther 2005;43:7–11.

[97] Pettersen JA, Zochodne DW, Bell RB, et al. Refractory neurosarcoidosis responding to infliximab. Neurology 2002;59(10):1660–1.

[98] Toth C, Martin L, Morrish W, et al. Dramatic MRI improvement with refractory neurosarcoidosis treated with infliximab. Acta Neurol Scand 2007;116(4):259–62.

[99] Hammond ER, Kaplin AI, Kerr DA. Thalidomide for acute treatment of neurosarcoidosis. Spinal Cord 2007;45(12):802–3.

[100] Scott TF. Cerebral herniation after lumbar puncture in sarcoid meningitis. Clin Neurol Neurosurg 2000;102(1):26–8.

[101] Benzagmout M, Boujraf S, Gongora-Rivera F, et al. Neurosarcoidosis which manifested as acute hydrocephalus: diagnosis and treatment. Intern Med 2007;46(18):1601–4.

[102] Maniker AH, Cho ES, Schulder M. Neurosarcoid infiltration of the ventricular catheter causing shunt failure: a case report. Surg Neurol 1997;48(5):527–9.

[103] Tabuena RP, Nagai S, Handa T, et al. Diabetes insipidus from neurosarcoidosis: long-term

follow-up for more than eight years. Intern Med 2004;43(10):960–6.

[104] Kang S, Suh JH. Radiation therapy for neurosarcoidosis: report of three cases from a single institution. Radiat Oncol Investig 1999;7(5):309–12.

[105] Menninger MD, Amdur RJ, Marcus RB Jr. Role of radiotherapy in the treatment of neurosarcoidosis. Am J Clin Oncol 2003;26(4):e115–8.

[106] Bejar JM, Kerby GR, Ziegler DK, et al. Treatment of central nervous system sarcoidosis with radiotherapy. Ann Neurol 1985;18(2):258–60.

[107] Rubinstein I, Gray TA, Moldofsky H, et al. Neurosarcoidosis associated with hypersomnolence treated with corticosteroids and brain irradiation. Chest 1988;94(1):205–6.

[108] Frei K, Truong DD, Dressler D. Botulinum toxin therapy of hemifacial spasm: comparing different therapeutic preparations. Eur J Neurol 2006; 13(Suppl 1):30–5.

[109] Lexa FJ, Grossman RI. MR of sarcoidosis in the head and spine: spectrum of manifestations and radiographic response to steroid therapy. AJNR Am J Neuroradiol 1994;15(5):973–82.

[110] Koike H, Misu K, Yasui K, et al. Differential response to corticosteroid therapy of MRI findings and clinical manifestations in spinal cord sarcoidosis. J Neurol 2000;247(7):544–9.

[111] Christoforidis GA, Spickler EM, Recio MV, et al. MR of CNS sarcoidosis: correlation of imaging features to clinical symptoms and response to treatment. AJNR Am J Neuroradiol 1999;20(4):655–69.

[112] Gottlieb JE, Israel HL, Steiner RM, et al. Outcome in sarcoidosis: the relationship of relapse to corticosteroid therapy. Chest 1997;111(3):623–31.

ELSEVIER
SAUNDERS

Clin Chest Med 29 (2008) 493–508

CLINICS
IN CHEST
MEDICINE

Cardiac Sarcoidosis

Uma S. Ayyala, MD[a], Ajith P. Nair, MD[b], Maria L. Padilla, MD[a],*

[a]Division of Pulmonary and Critical Care Medicine, Mount Sinai Medical Center, One Gustave L. Levy Place,
New York, NY 10029, USA
[b]Cardiovascular Institute, Mount Sinai Medical Center, One Gustave L. Levy Place, New York, NY 10029, USA

Sarcoidosis is a multiorgan disease with good prognosis, high remission rate, and low mortality. Cardiac involvement alters this prognosis for those who are affected. Cardiac sarcoidosis represents a significant challenge both in its diagnosis and management. Clinical manifestations range from asymptomatic disease to life-threatening arrhythmias, conduction abnormalities, and congestive heart failure. Although endomyocardial biopsy is of limited yield in establishing histologic diagnosis of cardiac sarcoidosis, recent advances in imaging modalities have proved useful in detecting cardiac involvement. These modalities include thallium-201 radionuclide scintigraphy, MRI, and positron emission tomography (PET). Treatment includes aggressive immunosuppressant therapy in combination with insertion of permanent pacemakers or implantable cardioverter-defibrillators (ICD) when indicated. Early detection with a high index of suspicion is essential to prevent sudden death in otherwise asymptomatic patients.

Epidemiology

Myocardial involvement of sarcoidosis was described as early as 1929 by Bernstein and Sidlick [1]. The first large autopsy series reviewing cardiac sarcoidosis was published in 1952. Twenty percent of 92 autopsies in patients with sarcoidosis demonstrated noncaseating granulomas of the heart [2]. Although other clinicopathologic studies have shown a similar incidence of myocardial involvement on autopsy, clinical disease is present only in a minority of patients. There is geographic variation of cardiac involvement. Cardiac sarcoidosis is more common in Japan than in Europe or the United States. It is involved in as many as 85% of sarcoidosis-related deaths in Japan [3]. In Japan, cardiac sarcoidosis is more common in women over the age of 40 years and is the leading cause of death in this group of patients [4–6]. In contrast, there is no such gender or age predilection in the United States, where myocardial involvement is clinically apparent in only 5% of patients, but is detected at autopsy in at least 25% of patients [7]. In the ACCESS (A Case Control Etiologic Study of Sarcoidosis) report, among patients studied within 6 months of histologic diagnosis of sarcoidosis, the incidence of cardiac involvement was 2.3% [8]. Although clinical involvement is infrequent, cardiac disease remains the second most common cause of death in patients who have sarcoidosis in the Western hemisphere. [9].

Pathologic findings

Any structure of the heart can be involved by sarcoidosis, but the myocardium is the most common site. Granulomatous inflammation, fibrosis, hypertrophy, or thinning of cardiac structures can be seen on pathologic examination. The hallmark of sarcoidosis is the presence of noncaseating granulomas surrounded by lymphocytes and Langerhans giant cells that may contain Schaumann's or asteroid bodies (Fig. 1). These granulomas can heal leaving scarring, fibrosis, and thinning of ventricular walls. Commonly involved sites, in decreasing order of frequency, include the left ventricular free wall, basal aspect of the ventricular septum, right ventricular free walls, papillary muscles, and the atrial walls

* Corresponding author.
E-mail address: maria.padilla@mountsinai.org
(M.L. Padilla).

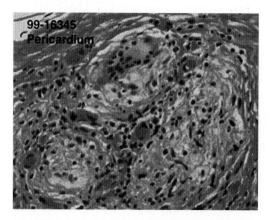

Fig. 1. Noncaseating, multinucleated granuloma on histologic specimen from the pericardium of a patient who has sarcoidosis (Hematoxylin and eosin stain, 40x original magnification.) (*Courtesy of* John Fallon, MD, PhD, New York, NY.).

(Fig. 2) [10]. Clinical consequences of involvement of these structures include arrhythmias and intraventricular conduction abnormalities (ventricular septal involvement); valvular abnormalities (mitral regurgitation from papillary muscle infiltration); dilated cardiomyopathy; and aneurysmal dilatation from scar tissue [10–13].

Cardiac granulomas have a wide differential including giant cell myocarditis, lymphocytic myocarditis, rheumatic fever, Chagas' disease, syphilis, fungal infections, tuberculosis, hypersensitivity myocarditis, rheumatoid arthritis, Takayasu's arteritis, and Wegener's granulomatosis. Giant cell myocarditis is frequently mistaken for cardiac sarcoidosis. Histologic factors to distinguish the two diseases include the presence of myocyte

necrosis in giant cell myocarditis (absent in sarcoidosis) and the loosely formed granulomas seen in giant cell myocarditis, in stark contrast to the well-organized granulomas of sarcoidosis.

Pathogenesis of cardiac sarcoidosis

The precise etiology of sarcoidosis remains unknown; the principal inciting event leads to granuloma formation, which can then either resolve or progress to fibrosis. Activated $CD4^+$ cells differentiate into type 1 helper T cells inducing secretion of interleukin (IL)-2 and interferon-γ leading to recruitment and activation of macrophages. In turn, macrophages secrete cytokines including IL-1, IL-6, and tumor necrosis factor-α (TNF-α), further augmenting the type 1 helper inflammatory cascade. The shift from inflammation to fibrosis may be caused by a predominant type 2 helper T-cell response stimulating fibroblast and collagen production.

Matrix metalloproteinases have been implicated to be involved with the progression to pulmonary fibrosis [14]. Tissue specimens from sarcoidosis patients have demonstrated increased immunoreactivity for matrix metalloproteinase-1, -2, and -9, and very low activity of inhibitors to matrix metalloproteinase leading to tissue destruction and remodeling [15].

Cytokines associated with cardiac sarcoidosis include IL-6, IL-10, brain natriuretic peptide, atrial natriuretic peptide, and adrenomedullin [16–18]. Increased serum IL-10 levels have been demonstrated in patients with cardiac sarcoidosis compared with controls [16].

Genetics of cardiac sarcoidosis

Both HLA and non-HLA genes have been associated with various forms of sarcoidosis. A significant overrepresentation of DQB1.0601 has been demonstrated in patients with cardiac involvement [19]. Recent phenotypic analysis of a large genome scan of black Americans with sarcoidosis found a linkage between cardiac and renal features of sarcoidosis and genes at the chromosome 18q22.20 locus [20]. Both genes for TNF-α and TNF-β have been studied for association with sarcoidosis; the less common TNF-a 2 allele was increased in a small group of Japanese patients with cardiac sarcoidosis, suggesting a predilection of this polymorphism for cardiac diseas [21].

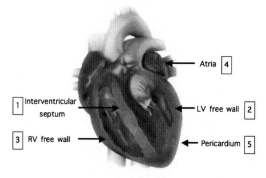

Fig. 2. Sites of cardiac involvement include in descending order the interventricular septum, left ventricular free wall, right ventricular free wall, the atria, and the pericardium.

Clinical manifestations

Clinical manifestations of cardiac sarcoidosis are dependent on the location, extent, and activity of disease. Cardiac signs and symptoms may be the first presentation of sarcoidosis [22]. Cardiac involvement can be unpredictable, ranging from clinically silent disease to the most feared consequence, sudden cardiac death from ventricular arrhythmia. The three principal sequelae of cardiac sarcoidosis are (1) conduction abnormalities, (2) arrhythmias, and (3) heart failure.

In addition to classic symptoms of systemic sarcoidosis (fevers, weight loss, malaise), common presenting cardiac symptoms include progressive dyspnea, fatigue, palpitations, and syncope. In one large case series, approximately 75% of patients were in class II New York Heart Association heart failure on presentation [23]. Syncope often indicates a significant electrophysiologic abnormality. Other reported symptoms include anginal chest pain mimicking acute coronary syndromes [24], and pleuritic chest pain from pericardial involvement. Acute pericarditis, pericardial effusions, and rarely tamponade have been reported as manifestations of cardiac sarcoidosis [25,26].

Conduction abnormalities

Conduction abnormalities ranging from first-degree atrioventricular block, bundle branch blocks, and complete heart block may be observed in cardiac sarcoidosis. On autopsy series, these conduction defects stem from granulomatous infiltration or scarring of the basal intraventricular septum containing the conduction system [10,27]. Complete heart block is the most common conduction abnormality found in cardiac sarcoidosis, described in 23% to 30% of patients [10]. Patients with cardiac sarcoidosis tend to present in complete heart block at a younger age than those with non–sarcoidosis-related heart disease [28]. In one study of Japanese patients with high degree A-V block, sarcoidosis was diagnosed in 11% of the group [29]. Clinical manifestations range from asymptomatic disease to syncope in as many as 68% of patients (Stokes-Adams attacks) [10]. Bundle branch block can occur in these patients, right bundle branch more commonly than left, and is documented in 12% to 61% of cases of cardiac sarcoidosis [10,30].

Ventricular arrhythmias

Nonsustained ventricular tachycardia (VT) is the second most common manifestation of cardiac sarcoidosis. In combination with complete heart block, VT accounted for 67% of sudden cardiac deaths in one large autopsy review [10]. The mechanism of VT in cardiac sarcoidosis is predominantly (68% in one study) caused by re-entry mechanisms [31,32]. These re-entry ventricular arrhythmias arise from both active granulomatous foci and healed or scarred granulomas. Unlike other cardiac manifestations of sarcoidosis, the inducibility of VT has been shown to have poor correlation with disease activity [33,34]. Lack of association between disease activity and ventricular arrhythmia has grave implications for treatment. Often, corticosteroids and antiarrhythmic drug therapy are futile, and patients experience recurrence of VT and even sudden death.

Atrial arrhythmias

Supraventricular arrhythmias (eg, atrial fibrillation and atrial flutter), although less common than ventricular arrhythmias, occur in approximately 19% of patients [27]. These arrhythmias may be secondary to atrial dilatation or caused by inflammatory atrial foci.

Sudden death

Sudden death is the most severe cardiac manifestation of sarcoidosis and is usually caused by either ventricular arrhythmia or complete heart block. In one large autopsy study of 113 patients, sudden death accounted for two thirds of the cases; in 35% of these patients, sudden death was the initial manifestation of sarcoidosis [10]. There are no factors that can predict sudden death from sarcoidosis and antemortem diagnosis is uncommon. Although sudden death can occur at any stage of sarcoidosis, it is more common in cases of extensive myocardial involvement [27].

Congestive heart failure

Sudden death has been considered the most common cause of mortality in sarcoidosis, but with increased recognition and earlier treatment including device implantation, the trend in mortality is shifting toward congestive heart failure. Congestive heart failure is becoming the leading cause of death in cardiac sarcoidosis. Yazaki and colleagues [35] prospectively studied 95 patients with cardiac sarcoidosis for an average follow-up of 68 months, and among 40 deaths, congestive heart failure was the principal cause in 73%. Cardiac sarcoidosis can manifest as either restrictive or dilated cardiomyopathy with diastolic or systolic ventricular dysfunction. Roberts and colleagues [10] described 23% of patients with cardiac sarcoidosis as having congestive heart failure. In a study of 50 patients with known pulmonary sarcoidosis but no clinical evidence of cardiac disease, 14% were diagnosed with diastolic dysfunction by echocardiography [36]. Other studies have documented up to 59% of a sarcoidosis cohort with diastolic dysfunction on echocardiography [37].

Patients with advanced fibrotic lung disease from sarcoidosis often develop secondary pulmonary hypertension and right ventricular hypertrophy leading to cor pulmonale. In addition, uncommon cases of right ventricular dominant cardiac involvement and cardiac sarcoidosis imitating right ventricular arrhythmogenic dysplasia have been reported [38,39].

Pericardial, valvular, and aneurysmal involvement

Pericardial involvement demonstrated by echocardiography has been described in as many as 19% of patients with sarcoidosis. Pericarditis secondary to sarcoidosis can present with pericardial effusions that are often large and either straw colored or serosanguinous in appearance. Massive pericardial effusions causing tamponade have been reported in the literature [26,40]. Of note, constrictive pericarditis is a rare manifestation of sarcoidosis [41].

Methods of diagnosing cardiac sarcoidosis

The definition of cardiac sarcoidosis varies. The American Thoracic Society and World Association for Sarcoidosis and Other Granulomatous Disorders consider cardiac dysfunction, ECG abnormalities, and thallium-201 imaging defects with or without endomyocardial biopsy in sarcoidosis patients as evidence of cardiac involvement [42]. ACCESS panel investigators defined criteria for "definite" cardiac involvement as treatment-responsive cardiomyopathy, ECGs with conduction defects, and positive cardiac gallium scans [43]. A positive thallium-201 scan was suggestive of "probable" cardiac involvement. One of the most widely used standards to establish the diagnosis of cardiac sarcoidosis is the Japanese Ministry of Health and Welfare criteria set forth in 1993 (Box 1). Cardiac sarcoidosis using these criteria is defined histologically through the presence of noncaseating granulomas on endomyocardial biopsy, or clinically in patients with

---

Box 1. Japanese Ministry of Health and Welfare criteria for the diagnosis of cardiac sarcoidosis

1. *Histologic diagnosis*
Cardiac sarcoidosis confirmed through histologic analysis of endomyocardial biopsy demonstrating epithelioid, noncaseating granulomas

2. *Clinical diagnosis group*
In patients who have histologic confirmation of extracardiac sarcoid, cardiac sarcoid is based on the presence of (a) and one or more of items (b) through (e)
   a. Complete right bundle branch block, left axis deviation, atrioventricular block, VT, premature ventricular contractions, or abnormal Q or ST-T wave changes on ECG
   b. Abnormal wall motion, regional wall thinning, or dilation of the ventricle
   c. Perfusion defect by thallium-201 scintigraphy or abnormal accumulation by gallium-67 or technetium-99m scintigraphy
   d. Depressed ejection fraction, low cardiac output
   e. Moderate-grade interstitial fibrosis or cellular infiltration on biopsy

---

extracardiac sarcoidosis through the presence of conduction system abnormalities and structural abnormalities seen by echocardiography, thallium or gallium imaging, or fibrosis seen by biopsy. These criteria do not use other imaging modalities including PET or cardiac MRI, both of which have proved useful in the diagnosis of cardiac and extracardiac sarcoidosis [44]. A combination of noninvasive methods and possibly endomyocardial biopsy, despite its low yield and invasive nature, are necessary to establish the diagnosis of cardiac sarcoidosis and periodic re-evaluation is necessary to assess disease activity. Lack of biopsy or negative findings do not exclude the diagnosis of cardiac sarcoidosis in patients with suspected involvement.

Electrocardiography

ECG manifestations may occur in up to 20% to 50% of who have sarcoidosis patients and typically include first- and second-degree atrioventricular block, complete atrioventricular dissociation, and nonspecific T wave abnormalities [45–47]. The first reports of conduction abnormalities in sarcoidosis patients described primarily atrioventricular block and VT as presenting symptoms [45,46,48,49]. In a study of Japanese and Swedish patients, the prevalence of ECG abnormalities was similar among both ethnic backgrounds [50]. The incidence of first-degree atrioventricular block and ST-T segment abnormalities was similar among the groups, although the appearance of right bundle branch block and left anterior hemi-block was noted to occur in patients with longer-standing disease. In a separate study of 89 Japanese patients presenting with high-degree atrioventricular block, 11.2% of patients were eventually diagnosed with cardiac sarcoidosis, most of whom were middle-aged women [51]. A small study of 40 patients with cardiac sarcoidosis and preserved left ventricular function found that atrioventricular block resolved in 57.1% of patients treated with long-term corticosteroids (79.4 ± 39.9 months) with no resolution in those who were not treated.

QT dispersion, the maximal interlead difference in QT interval on surface 12-lead ECG, is increased in cardiac disease and can be a predictor of sudden cardiac death. In a limited study of 35 patients with systemic sarcoidosis, QT dispersion was prolonged in patients with cardiac involvement compared with those without, correlating with increased frequency of premature ventricular contractions in limited follow-up [52].

In conjunction with ECG, Holter monitoring provides a simple, noninvasive method for screening patients with sarcoidosis for cardiac involvement. Holter abnormalities may include atrioventricular block, atrial and ventricular ectopy, and arrhythmias [53]. Frequent ventricular ectopic beats (≥100 beats per day) or nonsustained VT on Holter can provide evidence of possible myocardial involvement necessitating further noninvasive imaging and consideration for invasive risk stratification [54]. One prospective Japanese study of 38 patients with sarcoidosis reported that Holter monitoring had a sensitivity and specificity of 67% and 80%, respectively, for the detection of cardiac involvement [54]. Heart rate variability analysis may also be assessed by Holter monitoring and may serve as a measure of autonomic activity and as a predictor of sudden cardiac death. Patients with cardiac sarcoidosis, defined by the presence of systemic sarcoidosis and abnormal thallium-201 single-photon emission CT (SPECT) imaging, were observed to have decreased heart rate variability compared with those without cardiac involvement in a study of 35 patients with biopsy-proved systemic sarcoidosis [55]. The incidence of ventricular arrhythmias, however, was not characterized.

Signal-averaged ECG has additional use for the diagnosis of cardiac sarcoidosis. In a study of 114 patients, conduction abnormalities manifested by late potentials on signal-averaged ECG were found in 80% of patients with a history of cardiac sarcoidosis, 46.2% of patients with pulmonary sarcoidosis, and in only 5.8% of controls [56]. Abnormal Holter results and plasma brain natriuretic peptide levels were only evident in patients with cardiac sarcoidosis. The occurrence of late potentials in patients with pulmonary sarcoidosis may be indicative of minute conduction system abnormalities and latent myocardial fibrosis that merits further investigation and follow-up.

Noninvasive imaging

Noninvasive imaging methods useful in the diagnosis and evaluation of cardiac sarcoid include echocardiography, MRI, nuclear myocardial perfusion imaging, and PET (Table 1). Echocardiography can be used for the assessment of biventricular systolic function, diastolic function, and regional wall motion abnormalities. Although limited in its specificity for the detection of myocardial granulomatous infiltration, echocardiography has use in detecting gross myocardial dysfunction and diastolic filling abnormalities that may be indicative of early infiltrative disease [57].

Cardiac sarcoidosis involvement may result in segmental myocardial hypokinesis that can progress to global hypokinesis with diffuse infiltration [58]. Symptoms of congestive heart failure and conduction abnormalities are common in such patients. In other cases, ECG features of myocardial sarcoidosis can mimic other disorders, such as arrhythmogenic right ventricular dysplasia, because of primarily right-sided disease [59] or hypertrophic cardiomyopathy (Fig. 3). In a Japanese study of sarcoidosis patients referred for echocardiography, asymmetric septal hypertrophy and apical hypertrophy were noted in a minority of patients who also had histologic evidence of cellular infiltration [60].

Echocardiography is the most comprehensive noninvasive method to demonstrate evidence of

Table 1
Imaging modalities in the diagnosis of cardiac sarcoidosis

Imaging method	Findings	Advantages	Disadvantages
Echocardiography	Abnormal left ventricular or right ventricular function; wall thickening or thinning; atypical hypertrophic cardiomyopathy and aneurysms	Effective methods to follow ventricular function	Nonspecific findings with low sensitivity and specificity for disease
	Diastolic dysfunction	Ability to evaluate diastolic function comprehensively	
Thallium-201 and technetium 99m myocardial perfusion imaging	Reverse distribution, which likely correlates to microvascular obstruction at rest that improves with dipyridamole infusion	May be used to evaluate for ischemic heart disease	Findings are nonspecific
	Scarring may result in hypoperfusion at rest and with stress		Other nuclear imaging modalities have proved superior
Gallium-67 scintigraphy	Abnormal accumulation of gallium corresponds to areas of active inflammation	Correlates to active inflammation	Less sensitive than PET imaging for detecting myocardial sarcoidosis
		May be used to assess treatment response	
PET	Increased FDG uptake correlates with active inflammation	Sensitive in detecting active cardiac sarcoidosis and myocardial scarring	Limited information on myocardial structure and function
	Rb-82 images with hypoperfusion and FDG images with hypermetabolism correlate to granulomatous cardiomyopathy	May be used to follow treatment response	
	Rb-82 hypoperfusion and FDG hypometabolism indicate myocardial scarring		
Cardiac MRI	Sarcoid infiltration may be visualized as areas of increased signal intensity on T2-weighted black blood images and gadolinium-enhanced images	May be used to detect active granulomatous disease and myocardial scarring	Lower sensitivity in detecting myocardial sarcoidosis in asymptomatic patients
	Delayed hyperenhancement may be seen in areas of scarring	Right and left ventricular structure and function can be assessed	Cannot be used in patients with pacemakers and defibrillators
		High sensitivity in detecting active disease in symptomatic patients	
		May guide EMB	

Abbreviations: EMB, endomyocardial biopsy; FDG, fluorodeoxyglucose; MIBG, 123I-metaiodobenzylguanidine (MIBG) scintigraphy; PET, positron emission tomography; Rb-82, rubidium-82.

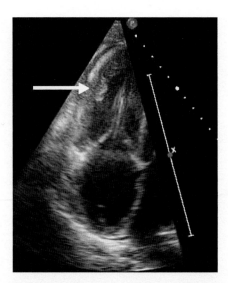

Fig. 3. Granuloma present in right ventricular (*arrow*) in a patient with known cardiac sarcoidosis. PET imaging demonstrated increased uptake in the same area confirming active sarcoidosis.

diastolic filling abnormalities that may be secondary to infiltrative disease. Doppler interrogation can reveal abnormal mitral inflow E wave and A wave patterns reflective of impaired relaxation in mild disease to restriction in severe disease. Other indices of diastolic dysfunction include short E wave deceleration times associated with impaired compliance, left atrial enlargement, and pulmonary vein inflow abnormalities. In a study of 50 patients with pulmonary sarcoidosis and no suspected cardiac involvement, 14% were found to have evidence of diastolic dysfunction that may have reflected subclinical sarcoid cardiomyopathy [36]. Patients with diastolic dysfunction were significantly older and hypertensive, however, risk factors that are typically associated with diastolic filling abnormalities in the absence of cardiac sarcoidosis. In another study of 18 consecutive patients with sarcoidosis, 11 patients had ECG abnormalities suggestive of cardiac involvement and seven of those patients had diastolic dysfunction by ECG [61]. Only two of these patients had cardiac MRIs with evidence of active disease. Other ECG methods for the early detection of cardiac sarcoidosis involvement have included cycle-dependent variation of myocardial integrated backscatter analysis, which can differentiate damaged and normal myocardial by measuring acoustic properties of the myocardium [51].

Nuclear imaging modalities to evaluate the presence and activity of cardiac sarcoidosis include thallium-201 and technetium-99m myocardial SPECT, gallium-67 scintigraphy, and PET. Myocardial perfusion imaging may demonstrate perfusion abnormalities of both the left and right ventricles, although the presence of these defects may not consistently correlate with active cardiac disease in sarcoidosis patients [25,62]. Abnormalities in the left ventricle may correlate with atrioventricular block and arrhythmias and those in the right ventricle to ventricular tachyarrhythmias of right ventricular origin [63]. A pattern of "reverse distribution" has been demonstrated during dipyridamole infusion on both thallium-201 and technetium-99m imaging, where focal defects in the resting phase of perfusion scanning decrease in size during stress imaging [64,65]. This redistribution likely correlates with reversible microvascular constriction in coronary arterioles and not with scarring from granulomatous involvement [66–69]. Reverse distribution is not specific for cardiac sarcoidosis, and it may occur in obese patients because of soft tissue attenuation and in patients with microvascular ischemia [70].

Gallium-67 scintigraphy has been used alone and in combination with thallium or technetium to detect myocardial involvement. Gallium accumulates in areas of active inflammation, and correlates with active sarcoid disease. Defects seen on thallium-201 SPECT can show gallium-67 accumulation indicative of active disease and may predict response to corticosteroid (CS) therapy [61,69]. Moreover, lack of gallium-67 uptake in a region of thallium-201 defect correlates with myocardial scarring and poor steroid responsiveness [68]. Dual gallium-67 and technetium-99m has also been proved to improve the accuracy and spatial resolution of nuclear scanning in the diagnosis of sarcoidosis [71]. In a study of 25 patients with cardiac sarcoidosis, active inflammation detected by gallium-67 scintigraphy was more common in patients with VT than those without [72]. Five of six patients with VT who had decreased gallium-67 uptake after CS treatment demonstrated resolution of arrhythmias. In another study of 15 patients with sarcoidosis-associated arrhythmias, however, increased gallium-67 uptake was noted in 8 out of 10 patients with complete atrioventricular block versus only one of seven patients with sustained VT [34]. Abolishment of gallium-67 uptake occurred in all patients after CS treatment, and resolution of atrioventricular block occurred in most patients. Gallium-67 may be used in conjunction with other imaging tests to establish the presence of myocardial sarcoidosis and to evaluate the efficacy of treatment. Its use in predicting ventricular arrhythmias remains limited.

PET scanning using 18F-fluorodeoxyglucose (FDG) has been used to detect areas of active inflammation. The premise of 18-FDG PET imaging is that inflammatory cells have increased uptake or accumulation of FDG. Uptake of radiotracer correlates with disease activity and correspondingly, a decrease in uptake of FDG may be seen with CS therapy (Fig. 4). Simultaneous cardiac perfusion stress testing is conducted to exclude significant obstructive coronary artery disease. The use of total body 18F-FDG PET was shown in a retrospective review performed on 137 patients with biopsy-proved sarcoidosis [44]. Of the 188 studies performed, 139 demonstrated extracardiac hypermetabolism. In 15% of patients, 18F-FDG PET scans found areas of active disease that were not detected by physical examination or other imaging modalities. In addition, a reduction in radiotracer uptake was seen in 11 repeat scans following CS therapy. In another study of 17 patients with histologic evidence of sarcoidosis and cardiac involvement, a minority of patients demonstrated abnormal gallium-67 or thallium-201 scans, whereas 14 patients had abnormalities on cardiac $(13)N-NH(3)/(18)F$-FDG PET [73]. Most patients treated with steroids demonstrated decreased 18F-FDG uptake. 18F-FDG PET may detect the early stages of cardiac sarcoidosis, where there are fewer perfusion abnormalities yet significant inflammatory activity, providing a tool for evaluating treatment response. In a study of 22 patients with systemic sarcoidosis, 18F-FDG PET, (99 m) Tc-methoxyisobutylisonitrile SPECT, and gallium-67 scintigraphy were performed in all patients, half of whom had cardiac sarcoid by the Japanese Ministry of Health and Welfare guidelines [74]. The sensitivity of PET in detecting cardiac sarcoidosis was 100% versus 63.6% for SPECT and 36.3% for gallium scanning, supporting previous evidence that 18F-FDG PET can detect earlier stages of cardiac sarcoidosis before advanced myocardial dysfunction. When compared with normal subjects, 18F-FDG PET imaging typically shows focal areas of activity versus diffuse involvement. This was demonstrated in a study of 32 patients with cardiac sarcoidosis who underwent 18F-FDG PET imaging and were compared with 30 control patients [75]. Those patients with abnormal 18F-FDG PET

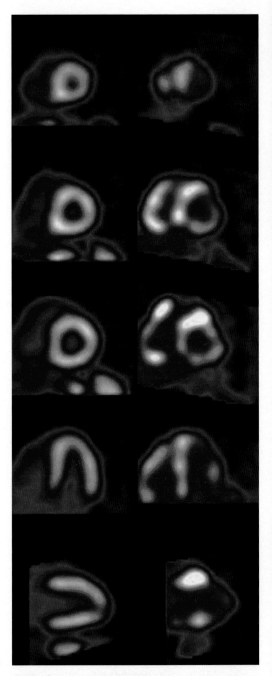

Fig. 4. Myocardial PET study of a patient with biopsy-proved cardiac sarcoidosis shows area of increased metabolism in both the right and left ventricles on FDG images (*right images*).

scans had either focal disease or focal on diffuse disease patterns.

Cardiac MRI with gadolinium-diethylenetriamine pentaacetic acid enhancement has proved to be valuable in the detection of myocardial sarcoidosis. In addition to presenting with regional wall motion abnormalities and areas of thinning, sarcoidal infiltration may be visible on MRI as focal, intramyocardial areas with increased signal intensity on T2-weighted and gadolinium-enhanced images caused by inflammation and associated edema (Fig. 5) [76]. Increased myocardial thickness, which can mimic hypertrophy, may result from edema or granulomatous involvement. Inflammation can be localized to the basal septum, left ventricular free wall, and less commonly the apex and right ventricle, and enhancement typically occurs in the epicardium and the mid-myocardial segments rather than the endocardium as seen in ischemic heart disease. Granulomas may also be apparent on T2-weighted images and are characterized by a central, low-intensity signal from hyaline fibrotic tissue and peripheral high-signal intensity secondary to inflammation [77]. Delayed gadolinium enhancement may occur because of accumulation of gadolinium in areas of scarring. In advanced stages of the disease, delayed enhancement is more commonly observed secondary to diffuse fibrosis with little inflammatory activity. Images may demonstrate typical features of dilated cardiomyopathy. Cardiac MRI is superior to other imaging modalities in the assessment of right ventricular dysfunction. It is limited in its use in patients with pacemaker, defibrillators, and mechanical valves.

Cardiac MRI with gadolinium enhancement has demonstrated greater use than echocardiography and thallium-201 scintigraphy in diagnosing myocardial sarcoidosis. A Netherlands study of 58 patients with sarcoidosis demonstrated a sensitivity of 100%, specificity of 78%, and positive and negative predictive values of 55%

and 100%, respectively, for cardiac MRI when using modified Japanese Ministry of Health and Welfare Guidelines as a gold standard [78]. Cardiac MRI was able to detect myocardial fibrosis, scarring, and impaired ventricular function more frequently than echocardiography and thallium-201 perfusion imaging. In asymptomatic sarcoidosis patients, cardiac MRI may be able to detect subclinical disease, and the extent of delayed enhancement with gadolinium has been correlated with the severity of ventricular dysfunction and potential for ventricular arrhythmias [79,80].

In addition to diagnosing subclinical cardiac disease, MRI has also been useful in assessing the efficacy of therapy similar to PET imaging. Resolution of MRI findings seen after immunosuppressive therapy correlates with clinical improvement, whereas worsening MRI abnormalities equates to clinical deterioration [76,81]. Cardiac MRI may additionally aid in directing endomyocardial biopsy when the diagnosis of cardiac sarcoidosis is otherwise unclear through noninvasive and clinical methodology [82].

Endomyocardial biopsy

Endomyocardial biopsy serves as a gold standard for the detection of cardiac sarcoidosis. Granulomatous involvement of the myocardium with fibrosis, few eosinophils, and little myocyte necrosis may be seen in patients with active disease. In patients with suspected cardiac sarcoidosis, the yield of endomyocardial biopsy may be low because of the predilection of left ventricular involvement and heterogeneous distribution of granulomatous involvement. Right ventricular biopsy performed in 26 Japanese patients who fulfilled diagnostic criteria for cardiac sarcoidosis yielded noncaseating granulomas in only five

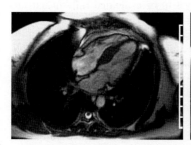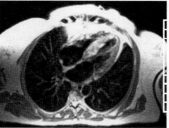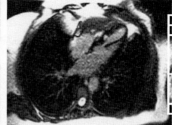

Fig. 5. Cardiac MRI with gadolinium enhancement demonstrates thickened interventricular septum. On T2-weighted black images there is patchy, hyperintensity in the hypertrophic segments suggestive of myocardial edema (*center image*). Delayed hyperenhancement is seen in these areas on postcontrast images (*right image*). These findings are highly suggestive of myocardial sarcoidosis.

(19.2%) patients, four of whom had dilated cardiomyopathy and another patient who had primarily conduction disturbances [83]. Likewise, in an analysis of 1235 patients who underwent endomyocardial biopsy at the Johns Hopkins Hospital, only 7 of 28 patients with presumed cardiac sarcoidosis had positive biopsy results [84]. This was in contrast to early reports suggesting that endomyocardial biopsy may diagnose cardiac sarcoidosis in up to half of suspected patients [85]. Nonetheless, guidelines set forth by the American Heart Association and European Society of Cardiology give endomyocardial biopsy a class IIa, level of evidence C recommendation in patients with unexplained heart failure of greater than 3 months duration with a dilated ventricle and new ventricular arrhythmias or second- or third-degree heart block [86]. Endomyocardial biopsy may be able to distinguish cardiac sarcoidosis from idiopathic giant cell myocarditis, both of which have giant cells and are associated with VT and heart block. The prognosis, however, is worse with giant cell myocarditis. In the multicenter idiopathic giant cell myocarditis registry, the 5-year transplant-free survival in patents with cardiomyopathy from sarcoidosis was 69.8% versus 21.9% for patients with idiopathic giant cell myocarditis ($P < .0001$) [87].

In addition to endomyocardial biopsy, the Kveim test has proved useful at the authors' institution in patients presenting with ventricular arrhythmias or conduction system abnormalities where the diagnosis of cardiac sarcoidosis in suspected. The test requires the subcutaneous injection of validated spleen or lymph node extracts. A skin biopsy performed 4 to 6 weeks subsequently is considered confirmatory for sarcoidosis if noncaseating granulomas are present. Further noninvasive imaging studies may be performed to evaluate for cardiac and extracardiac involvement.

Ventricular arrhythmias and methods of risk assessment

Once the diagnosis of cardiac sarcoidosis has been established, risk stratification for sudden cardiac death is mandated. The use of programmed ventricular stimulation in the risk stratification of patients with cardiac sarcoidosis was assessed in a study of 32 consecutive patients with cardiac sarcoidosis [88]. All patients underwent programmed ventricular stimulation, and those

patients with spontaneous or inducible sustained ventricular arrhythmias subsequently had placement of ICDs. Over a mean follow-up of 32 months, 83% of patients with spontaneous sustained ventricular arrhythmias and 67% of patients with inducible sustained ventricular arrhythmias but not spontaneous arrhythmias received appropriate ICD therapy. Only 10% of patients without either spontaneous or inducible sustained ventricular arrhythmias had sudden death or sustained ventricular arrhythmias. A positive electrophysiology study predicted future arrhythmic events in the entire population (hazard ratio 4.47; 95% confidence interval, 1.30–15.39), and in those patients without spontaneous ventricular arrhythmias a positive study proved effective in identifying those patients at risk for subsequent arrhythmic events (hazard ratio 6.97; 95% confidence interval, 1.27–38.27). This study was limited, however, in the determination of cardiac sarcoidosis; patients were diagnosed on the basis of biopsy-proven sarcoidosis in any organ as opposed to use of Japanese Ministry of Health and Welfare guidelines. Furthermore, it is unknown whether results of programmed ventricular stimulation differed in patients with active versus quiescent disease. In a limited study of eight patients, transient entrainment was documented in VTs by ventricular pacing and VT could also be initiated by programmed stimulation and terminated by rapid pacing [31]. The inducibility of VT varied with the active and inactive phases of disease, limiting therapy and making risk assessment difficult. A number of small, retrospective studies have failed to demonstrate that immunosuppressive therapy leads to resolution of ventricular arrhythmias, however, and the activity of disease likely does not make an impact on the need for ICDs [33,34,89]. Use of other methods of risk stratification, namely microvolt T wave alternans, has yet to be evaluated fully in patients with cardiac sarcoidosis.

Another method that may prove useful in the detection of cardiac sarcoidosis and risk stratification for sudden cardiac death involves the assessment of cardiac sympathetic dysfunction. Cardiovascular autonomic dysfunction has been associated with morbidity and mortality, and 123I-metaiodobenzylguanidine (MIBG) scintigraphy has been used to assess cardiac autonomic function. In patients with heart failure, abnormal 123I-MIBG scans have been useful in predicting future cardiac events [90]. Small-fiber neuropathy occurs in patients with sarcoidosis and may be associated with sympathetic denervation. In a study of 45 consecutive sarcoidosis patients, up to 37.8% of patients were found to have reductions in 123I-MIBG regional myocardial uptake significant for heterogeneous sympathetic nerve denervation [91]. 123I-MIBG uptake defects correlated with small fiber neuropathy as determined by abnormal thermal threshold testing. In addition to myocyte damage, sympathetic nerve damage may also occur with sarcoidosis. The diagnostic and prognostic value of 123I-MIBG imaging in cardiac sarcoidosis requires clarification through additional studies.

Treatment

Immunosuppressive therapy

CS is the cornerstone of treatment for cardiac sarcoidosis despite the lack of confirmatory randomized trials to confirm this treatment. It is known that early initiation of CS therapy can improve and possibly reverse cardiac disease secondary to sarcoidosis. Anecdotal accounts of response to CS have been reported as evaluated by imaging studies, clinical symptoms, and histopathologic improvement [61,68,76,81,92–95]. In one large retrospective study of 95 patients with cardiac sarcoidosis, patients treated with CS had a 5-year survival of 75% versus 10% for patients treated without CS [35]. In addition, patients with left ventricular ejection fraction greater than or equal to 50% treated with CS had a 10-year survival rate of 89% compared with 27% for those with left ventricular ejection fraction less than 50% [35].

The dose and duration of CS therapy has not been established. Because the consequences of cardiac sarcoidosis can be fatal, if myocardial disease is suspected treatment should be initiated. The standard recommendation for initial CS therapy has been to use high doses (prednisone, 60–80 mg/day) [96]. When patients were treated with high initial daily dose of CS (prednisone >40 mg) compared with low dose (prednisone <30 mg), however, there was no difference in outcome [35]. Given the lethal consequences of cardiac sarcoidosis, long-term maintenance therapy is often necessary. There are the adverse effects of CS including the development of ventricular aneurysms [10]. CS-sparing agents including methotrexate, azathioprine, hydroxychloroquine, and cyclophosphamide have been used with varying efficacy [23,97]. Use of

infliximab, a TNF-α inhibitor, has also been described in the literature as a successful treatment for cardiac sarcoidosis [98]. The duration of immunosuppressant therapy is poorly defined and recurrence has been described with tapering or cessation of medication [23,99]. Although there are no randomized trials, a sensible approach to cardiac sarcoidosis is initial therapy with CS in combination with other immunomodulating medications, especially for refractory cases or when CS is contraindicated.

Permanent pacemakers, antiarrhythmic therapy, radiofrequency ablation, implantable cardioverter defibrillators

The indication for permanent pacemakers in cardiac sarcoidosis is the presence of high degree atrioventricular block. Vaughn-Williams class Ia, Ib, Ic, and III agents have been used in patients with cardiac sarcoidosis for the prevention of ventricular arrhythmias. Despite early reports that programmed electrical stimulation could be effective in guiding antiarrhythmic therapy [100], subsequent studies demonstrated the high risk associated with spontaneous VT and the need for implantable defibrillators in these patients. In a study of seven patients with spontaneous sustained VT associated with sarcoidosis, sustained VT was easily induced on electrophysiology study in all patients [32]. CS therapy failed to prevent spontaneous VT. Despite antiarrhythmic therapy that included a combination of quinidine, lidocaine, mexilitine, procainamide, flecainide, or sotalol, two patients experienced sudden cardiac death and four others had recurrent VT. Four patients who received ICDs received appropriate shocks. CS and antiarrhythmic therapy may be ineffective in suppressing arrhythmias, necessitating the implantation of ICDs.

The effectiveness of radiofrequency ablation in the prevention of recurrent arrhythmias in cardiac sarcoidosis is limited. In a single-center study of patients with recurrent monomorphic VT who were referred for radiofrequency ablation over a 7-year period, eight were found to have cardiac sarcoidosis [101]. Electrophysiologic evaluation demonstrated scar-related re-entry as the mechanisms of ventricular arrhythmias, which were characterized by multiple monomorphic VTs of both left and right bundle patterns. Ablation therapy was only effective in controlling a minority (two of eight patients) of arrhythmias in 6-month follow-up. Half were arrhythmia free in long-term follow-up (6 months to 7 years) after receiving additional ablation. The arrhythmias were speculated to be difficult to control because of diffuse and heterogeneous granulomatous involvement of ventricles producing a robust substrate for re-entrant circuits and midmyocardium and epicardial scars that were not amenable to radiofrequency ablation.

Although radiofrequency ablation and antiarrhythmic medications may be effective in transiently suppressing ventricular arrhythmias, patients presenting after near sudden death or ventricular arrhythmias and those who are inducible on electrophysiologic evaluation are at high risk for subsequent cardiac events and warrant ICD therapy. ICDs have been shown effectively to terminate potentially lethal arrhythmias in high-risk patients, and among patients with defibrillators, mean survival time from first appropriate ICD therapy to death or transplant was determined to be 60 months [88].

Cardiac failure and transplantation

Congestive heart failure may result from progressive ventricular dysfunction resulting from fibrosis and scarring. Treatment of patients with congestive heart failure should include angiotensin-converting enzyme inhibitors or angiotensin receptor blockers, β-blocker therapy, diuretic therapy, and possibly aldosterone antagonists. Ultimately, patients progressing to World Health Organization Stage D cardiac failure should be considered for cardiac transplantation evaluation. Additionally, recalcitrant ventricular arrhythmias not amenable to ablation merit consideration of transplantation. Among patients undergoing transplantation for sarcoidosis cardiomyopathy, short and intermediate survival has been demonstrated to be better than most transplant recipients. Retrospective analysis of pooled data from 38 United States transplant centers identified 65 patients who received orthotopic heart

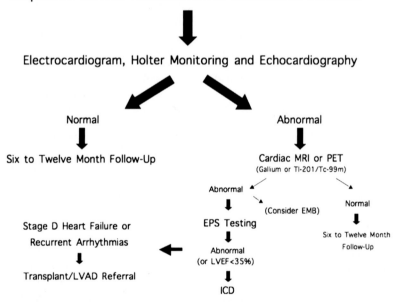

Fig. 6. Algorithm for the diagnosis and management of cardiac sarcoidosis. In all patients with sarcoidosis, electrocardiograms, Holter monitoring, and echocardiography should be performed to evaluate for conduction abnormalities, arrhythmias, or structural heart disease. Abnormal results mandate imaging tests, primarily MRI or PET, to evaluate for granulomatous involvement. Gallium, thallium-201 (Tl-201), or technetium-99m (Tc-99m) may also be used to image patients but are inferior to PET and MRI. Endomyocardial biopsy may be performed when the diagnosis remains questionable or to distinguish between other infiltrative processes. Patients with evidence of cardiac sarcoidosis should undergo electrophysiology testing for risk stratification for sudden cardiac death. Patients that are inducible on EP testing or who have severe left ventricular dysfunction should undergo ICD placement. Refractory arrhythmias or end-stage heart failure should prompt consideration for ventricular assist device therapy and cardiac transplantation. EMB, endomyocardial biopsy; EPS, electrophysiology study; ICD, implantable cardioverter-defibrillators; LVEF, left ventricular ejection fraction; LVAD, left ventricular assist device.

transplantations for cardiac sarcoidosis between 1987 and 2005 [102]. Over a mean follow-up period of 40 months, 4 operative deaths and 12 late deaths occurred. One-year posttransplantation survival time was significantly better for sarcoidosis patients versus patients with other diagnoses (87.7% versus 84.5%, $P = .03$). Despite case reports of recurrence of cardiac sarcoidosis as early as 24 weeks [103] and as late as 19 months [104] posttransplantation and the possibility of transmission of sarcoidosis from donor to recipient [105], cardiac transplantation remains a viable option in patients with end-stage heart failure.

Prognosis

The mortality from sarcoidosis is low at 1% to 5% per year, usually secondary to progressive lung disease. With the addition of cardiac involvement, the prognosis is adversely impacted. In an early autopsy study of 113 patients, the median survival was less than 2 years following development of cardiac signs and symptoms [10]. A decade later, a United Kingdom study observed a 5-year survival rate in a cohort of patients with cardiac sarcoidosis of 40% [106]. With the increased recognition of cardiac sarcoidosis and use of CS therapy and device implantation, the prognosis is improving. Yazaki and colleagues [35] evaluated 95 patients with cardiac sarcoidosis to determine mortality predictors and effect of CS therapy. Significant independent predictors of mortality were New York Heart Association functional class, left ventricular end-diastolic diameter, and sustained VT. Pulmonary involvement was associated with improved survival likely secondary to earlier recognition of cardiac disease.

Summary

Sarcoidosis is a disease with grave consequences when there is cardiac involvement. This article reviews the protean manifestations of cardiac involvement in patients known to have sarcoidosis. Also reviewed is the initial manifestations in patients whose sarcoidosis was detected only after first presentation with a cardiac event. A high degree of suspicion and systematic evaluation to uncover the involvement is warranted to improve outcome of patients with sarcoidosis and cardiac involvement (Fig. 6). To clarify the natural history of cardiac involvement in sarcoidosis, the incidence, and the response to therapy, establishment of an international registry is strongly advocated.

References

[1] Berstein M, Konzelmann FW, Sidlick DM. Boeck's sarcoid. Arch Intern Med 1929;44:721–34.

[2] Longcope WT, Freiman DG. A study of sarcoidosis: based on a combined investigation of 160 cases including 30 autopsies from The Johns Hopkins Hospital and Massachusetts General Hospital. Medicine (Baltimore) 1952;31(1):1–132.

[3] Doughan AR, Williams BR. Cardiac sarcoidosis. Heart 2006;92(2):282–8.

[4] Iwai K, Tachibana T, Takemura T, et al. Pathological studies on sarcoidosis autopsy. I. Epidemiological features of 320 cases in Japan. Acta Pathol Jpn 1993;43(7–8):372–6.

[5] Iwai K, Tachibana T, Hosoda Y, et al. Sarcoidosis autopsies in Japan: frequency and trend in the last 28 years. Sarcoidosis 1988;5(1):60–5.

[6] Iwai K, Sekiguti M, Hosoda Y, et al. Racial difference in cardiac sarcoidosis incidence observed at autopsy. Sarcoidosis 1994;11(1):26–31.

[7] Sharma OP, Maheshwari A, Thaker K. Myocardial sarcoidosis. Chest 1993;103(1):253–8.

[8] Freemer M, King TE Jr. The ACCESS study: characterization of sarcoidosis in the United States. Am J Respir Crit Care Med 2001;164(10 Pt 1):1754–5.

[9] Gideon NM, Mannino DM. Sarcoidosis mortality in the United States 1979–1991: an analysis of multiple-cause mortality data. Am J Med 1996;100(4): 423–7.

[10] Roberts WC, McAllister HA Jr, Ferrans VJ. Sarcoidosis of the heart: a clinicopathologic study of 35 necropsy patients (group 1) and review of 78 previously described necropsy patients (group 11). Am J Med 1977;63(1):86–108.

[11] Bharati S, Lev M, Denes P, et al. Infiltrative cardiomyopathy with conduction disease and ventricular arrhythmia: electrophysiologic and pathologic correlations. Am J Cardiol 1980;45(1):163–73.

[12] Kosuge H, Noda M, Kakuta T, et al. Left ventricular apical aneurysm in cardiac sarcoidosis. Jpn Heart J 2001;42(2):265–9.

[13] Haraki T, Ueda K, Shintani H, et al. Spontaneous development of left ventricular aneurysm in a patient with untreated cardiac sarcoidosis. Circ J 2002;66(5):519–21.

[14] Henry MT, McMahon K, Mackarel AJ, et al. Matrix metalloproteinases and tissue inhibitor of metalloproteinase-1 in sarcoidosis and IPF. Eur Respir J 2002;20(5):1220–7.

[15] Gonzalez AA, Segura AM, Horiba K, et al. Matrix metalloproteinases and their tissue inhibitors in the lesions of cardiac and pulmonary sarcoidosis: an immunohistochemical study. Hum Pathol 2002; 33(12):1158–64.

[16] Fuse K, Kodama M, Okura Y, et al. Levels of serum interleukin-10 reflect disease activity in patients with cardiac sarcoidosis. Jpn Circ J 2000; 64(10):755–9.

[17] Schoppet M, Pankuweit S, Maisch B. Cardiac sarcoidosis: cytokine patterns in the course of the disease. Arch Pathol Lab Med 2003;127(9):1207–10.

[18] Date T, Shinozaki T, Yamakawa M, et al. Elevated plasma brain natriuretic peptide level in cardiac sarcoidosis patients with preserved ejection fraction. Cardiology 2007;107(4):277–80.

[19] Naruse TK, Matsuzawa Y, Ota M, et al. HLA-DQB1*0601 is primarily associated with the susceptibility to cardiac sarcoidosis. Tissue Antigens 2000;56(1):52–7.

[20] Rybicki BA, Sinha R, Iyengar S, et al. Genetic linkage analysis of sarcoidosis phenotypes: the sarcoidosis genetic analysis (SAGA) study. Genes Immun 2007;8(5):379–86.

[21] Takashige N, Naruse TK, Matsumori A, et al. Genetic polymorphisms at the tumour necrosis factor loci (TNFA and TNFB) in cardiac sarcoidosis. Tissue Antigens 1999;54(2):191–3.

[22] Nelson JE, Kirschner PA, Teirstein AS. Sarcoidosis presenting as heart disease. Sarcoidosis Vasc Diffuse Lung Dis 1996;13(2):178–82.

[23] Chapelon-Abric C, de Zuttere D, Duhaut P, et al. Cardiac sarcoidosis: a retrospective study of 41 cases. Medicine (Baltimore) 2004;83(6):315–34.

[24] Wait JL, Movahed A. Anginal chest pain in sarcoidosis. Thorax 1989;44(5):391–5.

[25] Kinney E, Murthy R, Ascunce G, et al. Pericardial effusions in sarcoidosis. Chest 1979;76(4):476–8.

[26] Verkleeren JL, Glover MU, Bloor C, et al. Cardiac tamponade secondary to sarcoidosis. Am Heart J 1983;106(3):601–3.

[27] Silverman KJ, Hutchins GM, Bulkley BH. Cardiac sarcoid: a clinicopathologic study of 84 unselected patients with systemic sarcoidosis. Circulation 1978;58(6):1204–11.

[28] Fleming HA. Cardiac sarcoidosis. Seminars in Respiratory Medicine 1986;8:65–71.

[29] Yoshida Y, Morimoto S, Hiramitsu S, et al. Incidence of cardiac sarcoidosis in Japanese patients with high-degree atrioventricular block. Am Heart J 1997;134(3):382–6.

[30] Fleming HA, Bailey SM. Sarcoid heart disease. J R Coll Physicians Lond 1981;15(4):245–53.

[31] Furushima H, Chinushi M, Sugiura H, et al. Ventricular tachyarrhythmia associated with cardiac sarcoidosis: its mechanisms and outcome. Clin Cardiol 2004;27(4):217–22.

[32] Winters SL, Cohen M, Greenberg S, et al. Sustained ventricular tachycardia associated with sarcoidosis: assessment of the underlying cardiac anatomy and the prospective utility of programmed ventricular stimulation, drug therapy and an implantable antitachycardia device. J Am Coll Cardiol 1991;18(4):937–43.

[33] Mezaki T, Chinushi M, Washizuka T, et al. Discrepancy between inducibility of ventricular tachycardia and activity of cardiac sarcoidosis: requirement of defibrillator implantation for the inactive stage of cardiac sarcoidosis. Intern Med 2001;40(8):731–5.

[34] Banba K, Kusano KF, Nakamura K, et al. Relationship between arrhythmogenesis and disease activity in cardiac sarcoidosis. Heart Rhythm 2007; 4(10):1292–9.

[35] Yazaki Y, Isobe M, Hiroe M, et al. Prognostic determinants of long-term survival in Japanese patients with cardiac sarcoidosis treated with prednisone. Am J Cardiol 2001;88(9):1006–10.

[36] Fahy GJ, Marwick T, McCreery CJ, et al. Doppler echocardiographic detection of left ventricular diastolic dysfunction in patients with pulmonary sarcoidosis. Chest 1996;109(1):62–6.

[37] Skold CM, Larsen FF, Rasmussen E, et al. Determination of cardiac involvement in sarcoidosis by magnetic resonance imaging and Doppler echocardiography. J Intern Med 2002;252(5):465–71.

[38] Halushka MK, Yuh DD, Russell SD. Right ventricle-dominant cardiac sarcoidosis with sparing of the left ventricle. J Heart Lung Transplant 2006;25(4):479–82.

[39] Shiraishi J, Tatsumi T, Shimoo K, et al. Cardiac sarcoidosis mimicking right ventricular dysplasia. Circ J 2003;67(2):169–71.

[40] Zelcer AA, LeJemtel TH, Jones J, et al. Pericardial tamponade in sarcoidosis. Can J Cardiol 1987;3(1): 12–3.

[41] Garrett J, O'Neill H, Blake S. Constrictive pericarditis associated with sarcoidosis. Am Heart J 1984; 107(2):394.

[42] Hunninghake GW, Costabel U, Ando M, et al. ATS/ERS/WASOG statement on sarcoidosis. American Thoracic Society/European Respiratory Society/World Association of Sarcoidosis and other Granulomatous Disorders. Sarcoidosis Vasc Diffuse Lung Dis 1999;16(2):149–73.

[43] Judson MA, Baughman RP, Teirstein AS, et al. Defining organ involvement in sarcoidosis: the AC-CESS proposed instrument. ACCESS Research Group. A case control etiologic study of sarcoidosis. Sarcoidosis Vasc Diffuse Lung Dis 1999;16(1): 75–86.

[44] Teirstein AS, Machac J, Almeida O, et al. Results of 188 whole-body fluorodeoxyglucose positron emission tomography scans in 137 patients with sarcoidosis. Chest 2007;132(6):1949–53.

[45] Duvernoy WF, Garcia R. Sarcoidosis of the heart presenting with ventricular tachycardia and atrioventricular block. Am J Cardiol 1971;28(2):348–52.

[46] Fawcett FJ, Goldberg MJ. Heart block resulting from myocardial sarcoidosis. Br Heart J 1974; 36(2):220–3.

[47] Stein E, Jackler I, Stimmel B, et al. Asymptomatic electrocardiographic alterations in sarcoidosis. Am Heart J 1973;86(4):474–7.

[48] Lie JT, Hunt D, Valentine PA. Sudden death from cardiac sarcoidosis with involvement of conduction system. Am J Med Sci 1974;267(2):123–8.

[49] Numao Y, Sekiguchi M, Hirosawa K, et al [Evaluation of cardiac involvement through electrocardiogram in patients with sarcoidosis (author's transl)]. Kokyu To Junkan 1981;29(4):421–8 [in Japanese].

[50] Larsen F, Pehrsson SK, Hammar N, et al. ECG-abnormalities in Japanese and Swedish patients with sarcoidosis: a comparison. Sarcoidosis Vasc Diffuse Lung Dis 2001;18(3):284–8.

[51] Hyodo E, Hozumi T, Takemoto Y, et al. Early detection of cardiac involvement in patients with sarcoidosis by a non-invasive method with ultrasonic tissue characterisation. Heart 2004; 90(11):1275–80.

[52] Uyarel H, Uslu N, Okmen E, et al. QT dispersion in sarcoidosis. Chest 2005;128(4):2619–25.

[53] Tachibana T, Ohmori F, Ueda E. Clinical study on cardiac sarcoidosis. Ann N Y Acad Sci 1986;465: 530–42.

[54] Suzuki T, Kanda T, Kubota S, et al. Holter monitoring as a noninvasive indicator of cardiac involvement in sarcoidosis. Chest 1994;106(4): 1021–4.

[55] Uslu N, Akyol A, Gorgulu S, et al. Heart rate variability in patients with systemic sarcoidosis. Ann Noninvasive Electrocardiol 2006;11(1):38–42.

[56] Yodogawa K, Seino Y, Ohara T, et al. Non-invasive detection of latent cardiac conduction abnormalities in patients with pulmonary sarcoidosis. Circ J 2007;71(4):540–5.

[57] Tan LB, Dickie S, McKenna WJ. Left ventricular diastolic characteristics of cardiac sarcoidosis. Am J Cardiol 1986;58(11):1126–7.

[58] Burstow DJ, Tajik AJ, Bailey KR, et al. Two-dimensional echocardiographic findings in systemic sarcoidosis. Am J Cardiol 1989;63(7):478–82.

[59] Ott P, Marcus FI, Sobonya RE, et al. Cardiac sarcoidosis masquerading as right ventricular dysplasia. Pacing Clin Electrophysiol 2003;26(7 Pt 1): 1498–503.

[60] Matsumori A, Hara M, Nagai S, et al. Hypertrophic cardiomyopathy as a manifestation of cardiac sarcoidosis. Jpn Circ J 2000;64(9):679–83.

[61] Taki J, Nakajima K, Bunko H, et al. Cardiac sarcoidosis demonstrated by Tl-201 and Ga-67 SPECT imaging. Clin Nucl Med 1990;15(9):636–9.

[62] Kinney EL, Caldwell JW. Do thallium myocardial perfusion scan abnormalities predict survival in sarcoid patients without cardiac symptoms? Angiology 1990;41(7):573–6.

[63] Eguchi M, Tsuchihashi K, Hotta D, et al. Technetium-99m sestamibi/tetrofosmin myocardial perfusion scanning in cardiac and noncardiac sarcoidosis. Cardiology 2000;94(3):193–9.

[64] Tellier P, Paycha F, Antony I, et al. Reversibility by dipyridamole of thallium-201 myocardial scan

defects in patients with sarcoidosis. Am J Med 1988;85(2):189–93.

[65] Tellier P, Valeyre D, Nitenberg A, et al. Cardiac sarcoidosis: reversion of myocardial perfusion abnormalities by dipyridamole. Eur J Nucl Med 1985;11(6–7):201–4.

[66] Hirose Y, Ishida Y, Hayashida K, et al. Myocardial involvement in patients with sarcoidosis: an analysis of 75 patients. Clin Nucl Med 1994; 19(6):522–6.

[67] Mana J. Nuclear imaging: 67Gallium, 201thallium, 18F-labeled fluoro-2-deoxy-D-glucose positron emission tomography. Clin Chest Med 1997; 18(4):799–811.

[68] Okayama K, Kurata C, Tawarahara K, et al. Diagnostic and prognostic value of myocardial scintigraphy with thallium-201 and gallium-67 in cardiac sarcoidosis. Chest 1995;107(2):330–4.

[69] Tawarahara K, Kurata C, Okayama K, et al. Thallium-201 and gallium 67 single photon emission computed tomographic imaging in cardiac sarcoidosis. Am Heart J 1992;124(5):1383–4.

[70] Araujo W, DePuey EG, Kamran M, et al. Artifactual reverse distribution pattern in myocardial perfusion SPECT with technetium-99m sestamibi. J Nucl Cardiol 2000;7(6):633–8.

[71] Nakazawa A, Ikeda K, Ito Y, et al. Usefulness of dual 67Ga and 99mTc-sestamibi single-photon-emission CT scanning in the diagnosis of cardiac sarcoidosis. Chest 2004;126(4):1372–6.

[72] Futamatsu H, Suzuki J, Adachi S, et al. Utility of gallium-67 scintigraphy for evaluation of cardiac sarcoidosis with ventricular tachycardia. Int J Cardiovasc Imaging 2006;22(3–4):443–8.

[73] Yamagishi H, Shirai N, Takagi M, et al. Identification of cardiac sarcoidosis with (13)N-NH(3)/ (18)F-FDG PET. J Nucl Med 2003;44(7):1030–6.

[74] Okumura W, Iwasaki T, Toyama T, et al. Usefulness of fasting 18F-FDG PET in identification of cardiac sarcoidosis. J Nucl Med 2004;45(12): 1989–98.

[75] Ishimaru S, Tsujino I, Takei T, et al. Focal uptake on 18F-fluoro-2-deoxyglucose positron emission tomography images indicates cardiac involvement of sarcoidosis. Eur Heart J 2005;26(15):1538–43.

[76] Vignaux O, Dhote R, Duboc D, et al. Detection of myocardial involvement in patients with sarcoidosis applying T2-weighted, contrast-enhanced, and cine magnetic resonance imaging: initial results of a prospective study. J Comput Assist Tomogr 2002;26(5):762–7.

[77] Vignaux O. Cardiac sarcoidosis: spectrum of MRI features. AJR Am J Roentgenol 2005;184(1): 249–54.

[78] Smedema JP, Snoep G, van Kroonenburgh MP, et al. Evaluation of the accuracy of gadolinium-enhanced cardiovascular magnetic resonance in the diagnosis of cardiac sarcoidosis. J Am Coll Cardiol 2005;45(10):1683–90.

[79] Smedema JP, Snoep G, van Kroonenburgh MP, et al. The additional value of gadolinium-enhanced MRI to standard assessment for cardiac involvement in patients with pulmonary sarcoidosis. Chest 2005;128(3):1629–37.

[80] Smedema JP, Truter R, de Klerk PA, et al. Cardiac sarcoidosis evaluated with gadolinium-enhanced magnetic resonance and contrast-enhanced 64-slice computed tomography. Int J Cardiol 2006;112(2): 261–3.

[81] Vignaux O, Dhote R, Duboc D, et al. Clinical significance of myocardial magnetic resonance abnormalities in patients with sarcoidosis: a 1-year follow-up study. Chest 2002;122(6):1895–901.

[82] Borchert B, Lawrenz T, Bartelsmeier M, et al. Utility of endomyocardial biopsy guided by delayed enhancement areas on magnetic resonance imaging in the diagnosis of cardiac sarcoidosis. Clin Res Cardiol 2007;96(10):759–62.

[83] Uemura A, Morimoto S, Hiramitsu S, et al. Histologic diagnostic rate of cardiac sarcoidosis: evaluation of endomyocardial biopsies. Am Heart J 1999; 138(2 Pt 1):299–302.

[84] Ardehali H, Howard DL, Hariri A, et al. A positive endomyocardial biopsy result for sarcoid is associated with poor prognosis in patients with initially unexplained cardiomyopathy. Am Heart J 2005; 150(3):459–63.

[85] Ratner SJ, Fenoglio JJ Jr, Ursell PC. Utility of endomyocardial biopsy in the diagnosis of cardiac sarcoidosis. Chest 1986;90(4):528–33.

[86] Cooper LT, Baughman KL, Feldman AM, et al. The role of endomyocardial biopsy in the management of cardiovascular disease: a scientific statement from the American Heart Association, the American College of Cardiology, and the European Society of Cardiology. Endorsed by the Heart Failure Society of America and the Heart Failure Association of the European Society of Cardiology. J Am Coll Cardiol 2007;50(19):1914–31.

[87] Okura Y, Dec GW, Hare JM, et al. A clinical and histopathologic comparison of cardiac sarcoidosis and idiopathic giant cell myocarditis. J Am Coll Cardiol 2003;41(2):322–9.

[88] Aizer A, Stern EH, Gomes JA, et al. Usefulness of programmed ventricular stimulation in predicting future arrhythmic events in patients with cardiac sarcoidosis. Am J Cardiol 2005;96(2):276–82.

[89] Belhassen B, Pines A, Laniado S. Failure of corticosteroid therapy to prevent induction of ventricular tachycardia in sarcoidosis. Chest 1989;95(4):918–20.

[90] Agostini D, Verberne HJ, Burchert W, et al. I-123-mIBG myocardial imaging for assessment of risk for a major cardiac event in heart failure patients: insights from a retrospective European multicenter study. Eur J Nucl Med Mol Imaging 2008;35(3): 535–46.

[91] Hoitsma E, Faber CG, van Kroonenburgh MJ, et al. Association of small fiber neuropathy with cardiac sympathetic dysfunction in sarcoidosis. Sarcoidosis Vasc Diffuse Lung Dis 2005;22(1): 43–50.

[92] Sekiguchi M, Numao Y, Imai M, et al. Clinical and histopathological profile of sarcoidosis of the heart and acute idiopathic myocarditis: concepts through a study employing endomyocardial biopsy. I. Sarcoidosis. Jpn Circ J 1980;44(4):249–63.

[93] Yazaki Y, Isobe M, Hiramitsu S, et al. Comparison of clinical features and prognosis of cardiac sarcoidosis and idiopathic dilated cardiomyopathy. Am J Cardiol 1998;82(4):537–40.

[94] Ishikawa T, Kondoh H, Nakagawa S, et al. Steroid therapy in cardiac sarcoidosis: increased left ventricular contractility concomitant with electrocardiographic improvement after prednisolone. Chest 1984;85(3):445–7.

[95] Stein E, Stimmel B, Siltzbach LE. Clinical course of cardiac sarcoidosis. Ann N Y Acad Sci 1976;278: 470–4.

[96] Shabetai R. Sarcoidosis and the heart. Curr Treat Options Cardiovasc Med 2000;2(5):385–98.

[97] Demeter SL. Myocardial sarcoidosis unresponsive to steroids: treatment with cyclophosphamide. Chest 1988;94(1):202–3.

[98] Uthman I, Touma Z, Khoury M. Cardiac sarcoidosis responding to monotherapy with infliximab. Clin Rheumatol 2007;26(11):2001–3.

[99] Sekiguchi M, Yazaki Y, Isobe M, et al. Cardiac sarcoidosis: diagnostic, prognostic, and therapeutic considerations. Cardiovasc Drugs Ther 1996; 10(5):495–510.

[100] Huang PL, Brooks R, Carpenter C, et al. Antiarrhythmic therapy guided by programmed electrical stimulation in cardiac sarcoidosis with ventricular tachycardia. Am Heart J 1991;121(2 Pt 1):599–601.

[101] Koplan BA, Soejima K, Baughman K, et al. Refractory ventricular tachycardia secondary to cardiac sarcoid: electrophysiologic characteristics, mapping, and ablation. Heart Rhythm 2006;3(8): 924–9.

[102] Zaidi AR, Zaidi A, Vaitkus PT. Outcome of heart transplantation in patients with sarcoid cardiomyopathy. J Heart Lung Transplant 2007;26(7): 714–7.

[103] Oni AA, Hershberger RE, Norman DJ, et al. Recurrence of sarcoidosis in a cardiac allograft: control with augmented corticosteroids. J Heart Lung Transplant 1992;11(2 Pt 1):367–9.

[104] Yager JE, Hernandez AF, Steenbergen C, et al. Recurrence of cardiac sarcoidosis in a heart transplant recipient. J Heart Lung Transplant 2005;24(11): 1988–90.

[105] Burke WM, Keogh A, Maloney PS, et al. Transmission of sarcoidosis via cardiac transplantation. Lancet 1990;336(8730):1579.

[106] Fleming HA, Bailey SM. The prognosis of sarcoid heart disease in the United Kingdom. Ann N Y Acad Sci 1986;465:543–50.

ELSEVIER
SAUNDERS

Clin Chest Med 29 (2008) 509–524

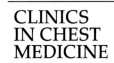

CLINICS
IN CHEST
MEDICINE

Hepatic, Ocular, and Cutaneous Sarcoidosis

Anthony S. Rose, MD, Marcus A. Tielker, MD, Kenneth S. Knox, MD*

Division of Pulmonary and Critical Care Medicine, Indiana University, Richard L. Roudebush VA Medical Center, 1481 W. 10th Street, VA111P-IU, Indianapolis, IN 46202, USA

Sarcoid affecting the skin, eye, or liver can cause significant morbidity. These are almost exclusively nonfatal manifestations of the disease, however. An extensive literature with a rich history details ocular and skin involvement in sarcoid patients. Interest in sarcoid of the liver has emerged as it is increasingly recognized as a common (albeit often asymptomatic) manifestation that requires further study.

Hepatic sarcoid

The incidence of hepatic sarcoid likely is underestimated, as patients are frequently asymptomatic, and other clinical manifestations (ie, pulmonary, ocular, cardiac) tend to overshadow the clinical course. Additionally, symptoms are often nonspecific and therefore not attributed to hepatobiliary involvement. The spleen, abdominal lymph nodes, and visceral organs also can cause similar nonspecific symptoms. Nevertheless, hepatic sarcoidosis can be severe, leading to cirrhosis and requiring liver transplantation. The 1999 American Thoracic Society (ATS) guidelines recommend testing liver function at the time of diagnosis, but further evaluation often is guided by clinical scenario with information derived from small case series and retrospective reports. The relationship between hepatitis C infection, granuloma formation, and sarcoidosis has sparked interest in the liver as an important organ of study in this disease. Finally, as medications used to treat sarcoidosis can cause liver injury, it is important to distinguish drug toxicity from sarcoid involvement.

Epidemiology

Sarcoidosis of the liver can mimic other primary hepatic conditions and infections, particularly when classic features of systemic sarcoidosis are absent [1–5]. Depending on the methods used to define hepatic sarcoidosis, the frequency of hepatobiliary involvement varies. It is estimated that liver biopsy specimens demonstrate granulomas in over 75% of patients who have systemic sarcoidosis [5,6], far more than those who have liver function test abnormalities or clinical symptoms [3,7]. A Case Controlled Study of Sarcoidosis (ACCESS) reported 11.5% of the study population had liver involvement and supported previous observations that hepatic sarcoid is twice as common in blacks than whites [3,8,9]. Recent data from the Sarcoidosis Genetic Analysis (SAGA) study showed for the 16% of patients who had liver manifestations, the other affected sibling was three times more likely to also have liver involvement [10]. Treatment for hepatitis C viral infection (HCV) with recombinant interferon-alfa appears to be a risk factor for development of sarcoidosis [11–13]. The clinical picture can be confusing, as patients who have HCV infection often have constitutional symptoms, abnormal liver function, and abnormal abdominal imaging. Clinical manifestations of interferon-related sarcoid are diverse, with the lung being the most commonly involved organ.

Signs and symptoms

Most patients who have hepatic sarcoid are asymptomatic [8]. When symptoms are present,

---

* Corresponding author.
E-mail address: kknox1@iupui.edu (K.S. Knox).

they most commonly are nonspecific and include fever, fatigue, weight loss, and abdominal pain [3,14]. Hepatosplenomegaly is common [15]. In a recent retrospective study from the authors' institution, male gender, hepatomegaly, splenomegaly, and a normal chest radiograph were associated with sarcoid-related liver disease [16]. Patients may present with jaundice and a clinical picture of chronic cholestasis mimicking primary sclerosing cholangitis or primary biliary cirrhosis [1,2,17]. Cirrhosis (biliary and nonbiliary), portal hypertension, Budd-Chiari syndrome, and variceal bleeding occur uncommonly (less than 1% of cases) but can be life-threatening complications of hepatic sarcoidosis [3,18,19].

Laboratory tests

Liver function tests are abnormal in approximately one third of patients, with an increased alkaline phosphatase being the most common abnormality. Sarcoidosis patients who have symptomatic liver disease almost always have an elevated alkaline phosphatase. The alkaline phosphatase can be several-fold over normal values and can be accompanied by transaminase elevations. Transaminase elevations occur in approximately 50% of patients who have clinical evidence of hepatic sarcoidosis. In advanced disease, hyperbilirubinemia can develop [3,8,15,16,20]. Liver function test abnormalities should prompt abdominal imagining and an evaluation for concomitant hepatitis viral infection in a patient who has known sarcoidosis. A patient who does not carry a definitive diagnosis of sarcoidosis likely would require imaging and biopsy of the liver or other affected organ.

Imaging

Several retrospective studies have examined the radiographic findings of hepatic sarcoidosis. The frequency of hepatic abnormalities detected by abdominal CT scan in patients who have sarcoidosis is surprisingly low. Currently, no imaging modalities or radiographic findings are sufficiently specific to obviate the need for further evaluation. Hepatomegaly and splenomegaly are the most common abdominal CT findings [21–23], but sarcoidosis also can mimic the classic findings of cirrhosis [24]. Recent improvements in techniques such as intravenous contrast delivery, CT resolution, and rapid scanner times have improved detection of hepatic and splenic nodules in abdominal sarcoidosis [25]. The most characteristic nodules are low attenuation lesions with variability in size (1 mm to 3 cm); they are often innumerable (Fig. 1). Intravenous contrast is usually necessary to see these hypodense nodules on CT. The liver uncommonly is involved in isolation of the spleen [25]. Ultrasound also can detect hyperechoic nodules and organ heterogeneity [26]. On MRI, nodules are seen most clearly on T2 weighted and gadolinium-enhanced images [26,27]. Fluorodeoxyglucose (FDG) uptake also has been reported in the liver of hepatic sarcoidosis [28]. These radiographic findings can pose a diagnostic dilemma if the patient is not known to have sarcoidosis. The differential diagnosis often includes abscess, tuberculosis (TB), metastatic

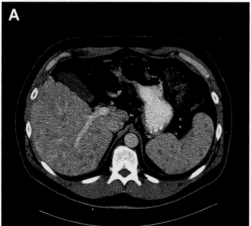 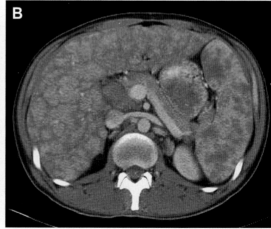

Fig. 1. (*A*) Hypodense liver and spleen lesions of sarcoidosis. (*B*) Nodular infiltration of liver.

malignancy, cysts, or lymphoma. In a patient who has known, biopsy-supported chronic sarcoidosis, these lesions often are followed serially, as they may improve spontaneously.

Biopsy

When granulomas are discovered on biopsy and in the absence of other etiologies, a diagnosis of sarcoidosis is entertained. Sarcoidosis is a diagnosis of exclusion, however, and other causes, particularly infectious, must be sought rigorously when granulomas are found [5,14,29,30]. In several large retrospective series, granulomas are recognized in 2% to 15% of liver biopsies [4,31–38]. In countries where TB is not prevalent, hepatic granulomas most often are caused by primary biliary cirrhosis (PBC), sarcoidosis, and idiopathic granulomatous hepatitis [39]. Granulomas caused by viral hepatitis and treatment of HCV with recombinant interferon-alfa are recognized and increasingly noted in more recent studies [4,40–42].

Granulomas are the main histologic abnormality noted on sarcoid liver biopsies. The granulomas are indistinguishable from lung granulomas in sarcoid patients, with multinucleated giant cells noted in 72% of cases [3]. Lesions in hepatic sarcoidosis are typically very small in size and many in number. The granulomas can coalesce and form larger lesions and areas of scar and fibrosis. Granulomas can be found throughout the liver parenchyma with associated mononuclear inflammation, but have a predilection for the portal zones [3,6,43,44]. Other histologic features of hepatic sarcoidosis include hepatocellular degeneration with necrosis, cholestasis, and reduction in interlobular bile ducts [1,2]. This reduction in interlobular ducts, termed ductopenia, is a characteristic finding in many hepatic sarcoid studies [16]. Although major hepatic complications are rare, chronic intrahepatic cholestasis resembles PBC and can lead to cirrhosis with ascites, variceal bleeding, and death [17]. Portal hypertension can be a result of chronic cholestasis or may occur independently of cholestasis by various mechanisms [19,43].

Clinical diagnosis

When granulomas are noted on a liver biopsy for any reason, an extensive clinical evaluation is warranted. In addition to excluding granulomatous infections, this evaluation must include a detailed history of medications, chemicals, and other potential exposures [5]. Once these causes are excluded, systemic inflammatory diseases can be considered. The diagnosis of sarcoidosis requires involvement of a second organ or other evidence such as a hypercalcemia, a CD4 alveolitis, or an elevated angiotensin-converting enzyme (ACE) or lysozyme level. When hepatic granulomas are found in isolation, in the absence of other evidence of sarcoidosis, granulomatous hepatitis is the preferred diagnosis [14,29]. On the other hand, when a patient carries a clinical diagnosis of sarcoidosis, usually supported by biopsy of an extrahepatic organ, the diagnosis of hepatic sarcoidosis can be made clinically without biopsy confirmation. An elevated alkaline phosphatase or abdominal CT findings suggesting sarcoidosis typically are required to make the diagnosis noninvasively. Importantly, no other clinical explanation for the liver abnormalities can exist [45]. Patients who have ongoing symptoms or evidence of progressive disease often require frequent monitoring of liver function tests and may require serial liver biopsies.

Treatment

Most patients who have hepatic sarcoidosis do not require any therapy. Most patients who have elevated liver function tests do not require therapy and have spontaneous resolution of their biochemical abnormality. Those patients who have asymptomatic elevation in their liver function tests but receive therapy for an extrahepatic indication often show biochemical improvement also [8,46]. When symptoms such as fever, fatigue, weight loss, or abdominal pain persist, treatment is warranted. Corticosteroids frequently are used to treat hepatic sarcoidosis and are effective in relieving symptoms. Lower doses are often sufficient (ie, 10 to 20 mg/d) treatment for constitutional symptoms associated with hepatic sarcoid. Higher doses (ie, up to 60 mg/d) may be necessary to treat more severe cases (ie, jaundice or pruritus) with more variable effect on symptoms. Once bile duct depletion and fibrosis have occurred, therapy is predictably ineffective. Even when patients have symptom relief, progression of disease commonly occurs, particularly when chronic cholestasis or portal hypertension is present [1,2,17,43,47–49]. Use of alternative immunosuppressive agents also has been reported and includes azathioprine, methotrexate, and infliximab [46,49,50]. Methotrexate can be hepatotoxic, and close evaluation is warranted [51]. Ursodeoxycholic acid dosed at 10 mg/kg/d appears to be useful for managing symptoms related to intrahepatic cholestasis [52]. Although rare, patients who progress to end-stage liver disease require liver transplantation and have 1-year and 5-year survival rates, comparable with patients transplanted for other indications [53,54]. Sarcoidosis can recur following liver transplantation [55,56]. Hepatic granulomas can be seen (0.24%) in biopsies of liver transplant recipients treated with pegylated interferon for recurrent HCV infection [57]. Whether granulomas found on post-transplant liver biopsies require further clinical evaluation depends on the severity of organ dysfunction and the index of suspicion for infection in these immunocompromised patients.

Summary

Most patients who have hepatic sarcoidosis are asymptomatic, have normal or mildly elevated alkaline phosphatase, and require no therapy. When symptoms occur, a liver biopsy shows significant inflammation/fibrosis, or disease progresses, however, a treatment trial of corticosteroids is warranted. Disease may progress despite improvement of liver function tests and symptoms. Although rare, severe disease requiring liver transplantation is a potentially life-threatening complication of sarcoidosis.

Ocular sarcoidosis

Sarcoidosis is an important etiology of inflammatory eye disease and has a myriad of manifestations. Ocular manifestations of systemic sarcoidosis have significant impact on visual prognosis; 45% of patients with sarcoid uveitis have been observed to lose vision during long-term follow-up [58]. In one study, 10% of patients were blind in at least one eye [59]. The 1999 ATS consensus guidelines recommend all patients undergo an ophthalmologic examination at the time of their initial evaluation [60,61]. This recommendation is noteworthy given many patients who have sarcoidosis can have silent or asymptomatic uveitis. and no specific extraocular manifestation of sarcoidosis reliably predicts eye involvement [60,61].

Epidemiology

The reported incidence of ocular sarcoidosis varies greatly because of geographic, racial, and gender differences. Other confounders such as referral bias and lack of a supporting biopsy predominate in the literature. The Japanese population has a high rate of ocular sarcoidosis. A study of 110 university hospitals in Japan reported 3060 patients in whom sarcoidosis was the most common disease causing intraocular inflammation [62]. In a second Japanese study, 50% of all tissue-proven sarcoid patients with ophthalmologic evaluations were found to have uveitis [63], notably higher than the 11.8% eye involvement reported in the ACCESS trial. The ACCESS trial confirmed previous observations that United States blacks and women have a higher incidence of ocular sarcoidosis. Additional analysis of the ACCESS database showed that ocular involvement in black siblings showed some phenotypic concordance, but clinical outcomes differed [10]. Anterior uveitis is more common in blacks and posterior uveitis more common in whites [61]. Both blacks and whites with the HLADRB1*0401 genetic polymorphism seem to be at higher risk for ocular sarcoidosis based on analysis of the ACCESS database [64]. A single nucleotide polymorphism in the HSP-70/Hom gene, which encodes for a constitutively expressed heat shock protein, recently was reported to have a strong association with ocular sarcoidosis in white patients [65]. Another investigation has shown increased serum CXCL9 and CXCL10 cytokines in patients who have ocular sarcoidosis as compared with other etiologies of uveitis, which may explain TH1 lymphocyte migration to the eye [66]. Uveitis rarely is the presenting symptom of sarcoidosis, but can precede the diagnosis of sarcoidosis by several years [61,67,68].

Specific manifestations

Anterior uveitis and conjunctiva

Sarcoid inflammation can affect any portion of the eye and its surrounding structures. Intraocular inflammation or uveitis can manifest as anterior, intermediate, posterior, or panuveitis depending on the affected portion of the uveal tract [69]. Sarcoidosis may begin in one anatomic compartment of the eye and spill over into adjacent structures; significant overlap occurs. Anterior uveitis, or inflammation of the iris and/or ciliary body, is the most common manifestation of ocular sarcoidosis and typically presents subacutely, early in the course of systemic disease [70]. Acute anterior uveitis can occur in conjunction with Lofgren's syndrome (LS) (hilar adenopathy, erythema nodosum, and polyarthralgias) and generally has a favorable prognosis [71]. The combination of parotitis, uveitis, and cranial nerve palsy is termed Heerfordt's syndrome [72]. Symptoms, when present, may include blurry vision, photophobia, pain, or excessive lacrimation. Inflammation involving the anterior uvea traditionally has been classified as granulomatous inflammation when medium-to-large keratic mutton fat precipitates, or iris nodules are observed. Keratic precipitates are not specific to uveitis caused by sarcoidosis. Iris nodules may be found at the papillary margin (Koeppe nodules) or on the surface of the iris (Busacca's nodules). When keratic precipitates are small or absent, inflammation is described as nongranulomatous. In a recent retrospective review of 81 biopsy-proven sarcoidosis patients at an ophthalmologic referral center, uveitis was the most common ocular manifestation, and most of these patients had nongranulomatous inflammation [73]. In contrast, chronic anterior uveitis is more notable for causing ocular morbidity including synechiae formation and glaucoma, band keratopathy, and cystoid macular edema (Fig. 2) [70,74]. Corneal involvement in ocular sarcoidosis rarely is reported but may be found in association with chronic anterior uveitis [74].

Granulomatous inflammation of the conjunctiva is a common manifestation of ocular sarcoidosis [74], resulting in small yellow nodule formations, which are typically asymptomatic. Conjunctival biopsy for tissue diagnosis in sarcoidosis holds many advantages; it is simple, safe, less costly, and less invasive than other procedures used to obtain tissue samples [75]. The yield of conjunctival biopsy increases with clinically apparent involvement [76] in a fashion similar to that of endobronchial biopsy [77]. Overall, yields of 10% to 55% have been reported [78]. In a recent series from Taiwan, bilateral biopsies resulted in diagnostic yield of 38% in sarcoid patients who did not have visible conjunctival nodules [79]. Nevertheless, blind conjunctival biopsies are not recommended. In the future, in vivo confocal microscopy may provide an entirely noninvasive manner by which to examine the conjunctiva for granulomatous inflammation [80].

Posterior and intermediate uveitis

The posterior segment of the eye consists of the vitreous, retina, choroid, and optic nerve. Twenty-five percent to 94% of patients who have sarcoidosis may suffer from posterior segment disease [81–83]. Inflammatory patterns can be further classified as posterior (retina, choroid) or intermediate (vitreous) uveitis according to accepted nomenclature recommendations [69]. Affected patients can be asymptomatic or experience vision loss because of various complications such as macular scarring, cystoid macular edema, retinal vasculitis, vitreous inflammation or hemorrhage, optic nerve inflammation, and neovascularization. Dilated fundus examination is fundamental in detecting posterior segment involvement. Two common findings include retinal periphlebitis and vitritis. Retinal and choroidal infiltrates (Fig. 3) surrounding retinal veins with a waxy, yellow appearance have been described as candle wax drippings. Rounded, variably sized opacities found in the dependent region of the vitreous are called

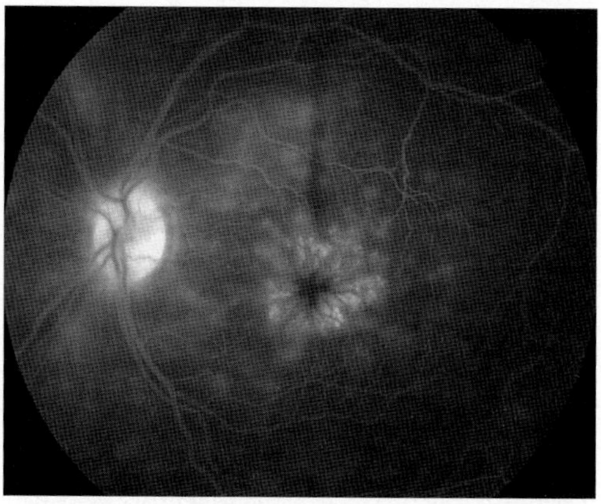

Fig. 2. Black-and-white photo of cystoid macular edema in a patient with chronic anterior uveitis from sarcoid.

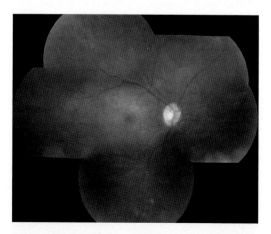

Fig. 3. Mosaicized digital fundus photograph of the right eye of a patient with sarcoid panuveitis. Note venous sheathing and multiple choroidal granulomas (*white lesions*) inferiorly.

snowballs and are indicative of vitritis (intermediate uveitis). Both findings are suggestive but not diagnostic of posterior segment sarcoidosis. Fluorescein angiography can be used to thoroughly evaluate retinal vessel vasculitis and chorioretinal neovascularization and may detect subclinical posterior uveal involvement in patients thought to have limited anterior uveitis [84]. Posterior uveitis should be considered vision-threatening and has been observed to accompany central nervous system (CNS) sarcoidosis in a minority of patients [74]. The optic nerve can be affected secondarily by posterior uveitis or directly as an optic. Such effects may cause visual field deficits and present a diagnostic challenge when no apparent optic disk abnormalities are seen on funduscopic examination [85]. Inflammation of all three ocular compartments (anterior, intermediate, and posterior), or panuveitis, is quite common and is a poor prognostic risk factor [59].

Lacrimal gland and other extraocular structures

Lacrimal gland inflammation, or dacrocystitis, is recognized as a common occurrence in sarcoidosis based on gallium scanning [86], but rarely results in physically obvious lacrimal gland enlargement. When it does, patients may experience bilateral upper eyelid pain and swelling (Fig. 4). Exposure keratopathy also can occur. Keratoconjunctivitis sicca (KC) also may result, but most often is found in the absence of clinically obvious lacrimal gland enlargement [73]. KC can be confirmed by the Schirmer's test. The eyelid and orbital soft tissues can be involved in sarcoidosis. Periocular soft tissue inflammation has been described to result in both exopthalmosis [87] and enopthalmosis [88] and may mimic that of Grave's ophthalmopathy.

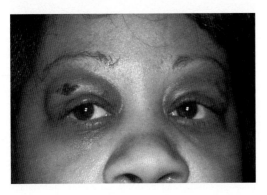

Fig. 4. Profound sarcoid lacrimal gland involvement.

Diagnostics

No extraocular manifestation of sarcoidosis reliably predicts ocular involvement. Thus, ophthalmologic examination is important as a screening tool and at routine intervals during follow-up, even in the absence of specific symptoms. Physical examination by nonophthalmologists, including outer eye inspection and funduscopy, can detect evidence of ocular sarcoidosis readily. The ophthalmologic examination, however, routinely includes measurement of ocular pressures, slit lamp examination, and possibly fluorescein angiography.

Normal serum ACE levels do not exclude the presence of ocular sarcoidosis and do not correlate with ocular disease [73]. ACE levels in the vitreous [89] and tears [90] appear to be elevated in ocular sarcoidosis and can be useful as an adjunct to diagnosis. Like ACE in the cerebrospinal fluid (CSF), it is not clear that increased levels are not caused by increased permeability and higher serum levels. Serum lysozyme (a product of stimulated mononuclear phagocytes) has been studied as an adjunctive test for ocular sarcoidosis. Lysozyme is generally less specific and sensitive than serum ACE for ocular involvement [91], but has been observed to correlate well with increasing pulmonary stage and total organ involvement [92]. Although alveolar lymphocytosis with a high CD4:CD8 ratio can be clinically useful in the diagnosis of sarcoidosis, this finding is not specific for sarcoid-related uveitis and has been found in other uveal inflammatory diseases [93]. The panda sign (symmetric, bilateral lacrimal and parotid inflammation) is a nonspecific finding of sarcoidosis on [67] gallium scanning [94]. Gallium scintigraphy is nonspecific, and should not be used routinely in the diagnosis of sarcoidosis. CT and MRI can characterize lacrimal, orbital, and CNS involvement with specific regard to the optic nerve and can be useful when visual symptoms are present without readily identifiable funduscopic abnormalities [95]. As mentioned previously, in the appropriate clinical setting when conjunctival lesions are visible, directed biopsy may be useful.

Differential diagnosis

The exclusion of granulomatous infectious diseases is essential when the diagnosis of ocular sarcoidosis is considered. TB can affect the eyelids and conjunctiva and is a common cause of infectious uveitis outside the United States.

Similar to ocular sarcoidosis, iris nodules and mutton fat keratic precipitates can be observed with tuberculous anterior segment involvement. Histoplasmosis can affect the eye with manifestations of disciform macular lesions and white atrophic choroidal scars (histospots), typically in the absence of vitreal inflammation. Similarly, additional endemic fungi such as blastomycosis and coccidioidomycosis can cause granulomatous uveitis. Other important infectious causes of uveitis include syphilis and toxoplasmosis. Systemic diseases including Behcet's disease and Wegener's granulomatosis can affect the eye in a similar fashion to sarcoidosis. Ocular Wegener's granulomatosis has a myriad of manifestations ranging from conjunctivitis and orbital soft tissue inflammation to necrotizing scleritis and retinal vasculitis. The effect of systemic inflammatory diseases on the eye was reviewed recently [96].

Treatment

Corticosteroids are considered first-line therapy for treating sarcoidosis, but evidence for their long-term benefit in pulmonary disease is lacking [97]. Similarly, corticosteroid therapy should not be considered curative in ocular sarcoidosis, as relapses often occur [70]. The ocular complications of steroid therapy (ie, cataract formation and glaucoma) make long-term steroid therapy problematic [98]. Treatment of uveitis begins with topical and/or periocular steroid administration (depending on the sites of inflammation) and a cycloplegic agent to help prevent formation of synechiae and secondary glaucoma. Systemic steroids are used in the treatment of uveitis (recurrent, chronic, posterior, or poorly responsive to topical steroids), symptomatic orbital or lacrimal inflammation, and in high doses for optic nerve involvement. Disease refractory to steroids may necessitate the use of alternative immunomodulatory therapies. Methotrexate has been investigated as a steroid-sparing agent for treating symptomatic sarcoidosis and showed efficacy in a retrospective study of 11 patients who had sarcoid panuveitis requiring dose reduction in systemic corticosteroid therapy [99]. For patients who cannot tolerate methotrexate, leflunomide was shown to have similar efficacy in ocular sarcoid improvement in a study of 32 patients who had chronic sarcoidosis [100]. The literature is devoid of randomized, controlled trials specifically focused on the treatment of ocular sarcoidosis with immunomodulatory agents. Agents such as azathioprine and mycophenolate mofetil, however, have been used in other forms of inflammatory ocular diseases and may serve as adjunctive therapies to corticosteroids in sarcoidosis. Evidence suggests infliximab therapy for refractory inflammatory eye disease is useful [49,101–104]. In contrast, etanercept, another biologic tumor necrosis factor (TNF) antagonist, had disappointing results in chronic ocular sarcoidosis [105]. Glaucoma and cataracts may warrant surgical intervention, and uncontrolled preoperative inflammation is related to a worse visual prognosis [106]. Surgical interventions, such as vitrectomy for vitreous opacities, have been reported as beneficial for small numbers of patients with refractory ocular disease [107].

Summary

Sarcoidosis is a systemic inflammatory disease that commonly affects the eye and can cause significant ocular morbidity and potentially blindness. Any structure within or adjacent to the eye can be affected, and routine ophthalmologic examination is crucial to the care of patients who have sarcoidosis. Corticosteroids are the mainstay of treatment, but various immunomodulatory agents are available and are used often to avoid the long-term ocular complications of steroid use.

Cutaneous sarcoidosis

Introduction

Cutaneous lesions were the first recognized manifestations of sarcoidosis. Jonathan Hutchinson is credited for his initial description of a patient who had cutaneous sarcoidosis in 1877 [108]. Hutchinson later reported a second patient who had skin lesions involving the nose, ears, and upper extremities, defining characteristics of lupus pernio [60,109]. Carl Wilhelm Boeck and Ernest Besnier were the first to characterize the histology of sarcoidosis. Finally, the Kveim skin test has improved the understanding of the immunology of this enigmatic disease [110–114].

Sarcoid skin involvement is the second most common manifestation of sarcoidosis. Lesions are divided into two types based on classic characteristics and histology: specific lesions and nonspecific lesions. The classic specific lesion is lupus pernio, but all specific lesions demonstrate evidence of noncaseating granulomas on biopsy. The classic nonspecific lesion is erythema nodosum

(EN), a lesion that is inflammatory, but not granulomatous. The diagnosis of sarcoidosis is established when clinical and radiological evidence is supported by a biopsy showing non-caseating granulomas [60]. The presence of cutaneous sarcoidosis can aid in a more rapid diagnosis, because the lesions are obvious and easily biopsied. In one study of 189 patients, the presence of skin manifestations significantly decreased the time to diagnosis (less than 6 months versus greater than 6 months, $P = .02$) [115].

Epidemiology and clinical findings

Nonspecific lesions

Cutaneous manifestations were observed in 24.2% of patients who had sarcoidosis in ACCESS, with EN noted in 8.3% of patients [9]. In contrast, European cohorts often report EN in up to 48% of patients [116–119]. Women from Puerto Rico frequently present with EN [120]. Approximately 15% of Middle Easterners have EN as a sign of systemic sarcoidosis [121]. EN is found infrequently in Japan [122]. ACCESS found a significantly higher percentage of women (10.5%) who present with erythema nodosum than men (4.5%). The study, however, did not demonstrate a significant difference in erythema nodosum between United States black and white subjects. Sarcoidosis-related EN worldwide preferentially affects females [9,60,123–125].

EN in the presence of bilateral hilar lymphadenopathy is referred to as LS and first was recognized by Lofgren and Lundback in the 1950s [126]. LS can be associated with numerous clinical symptoms. In one trial of 186 Spanish patients diagnosed with LS, arthralgias (68%), fever (38%), granulomatous skin lesions (13%), and ocular involvement (5%) were present at diagnosis [124]. The prevalence of LS varies greatly over different geographic areas, race, and gender, and mirrors that of EN. Young women of childbearing age and northern European descent appear to present most commonly with LS. A recent study, however, has shown that manifestations of LS differ between men and women, with classic EN found predominantly in women. In contrast, when marked periarticular inflammation of the ankles is removed from a broader definition of EN, LS without EN was seen preferentially in men [127,128].

EN and LS sarcoid patients carry a very good prognosis, and the disease is usually self-limiting. Based on genetic studies [129] and immunologic basis of disease [110,130,131], it is reasonable to speculate LS may represent a different disease entity from non-LS sarcoidosis. Some patients who have LS, however, experience clinical progression. A northern European study recently reported HLA-DRB1*0301 positivity portends a better overall prognosis in the setting of LS, and this may be related to a reduced Th1 cytokine response [132,133]. In this same population, AV2S3(+) T cells are expanded preferentially and reacting to various autoantigens [130,134]. This homogenous group of patients with HLA-DRB1*0301-associated LS provides unprecedented mechanistic insight into this form of sarcoidosis. Other studies characterizing the genetics of LS have been reviewed recently [135].

EN is distinguished from other sarcoid lesions based on its clinical appearance. Lesions are painful, red, often raised, and nonulcerative subcutaneous nodules [136]. EN usually occurs on the anterior tibial surface but can occur anywhere on the limbs or trunk. Importantly, EN is not specific to sarcoidosis and can be present in a myriad of systemic diseases. Bechet's disease, inflammatory bowel disease, TB, streptococcal infection, fungal infections (histoplasmosis, coccidioidomycosis, blastomycosis), leprosy, drugs, and certain malignancies have been associated with EN [137]. Histologic appearances of EN do not differentiate the various etiologies, and they usually are seen as a panniculitis involving the deep dermis and subcutaneous tissue [138]. Thus, biopsies of EN are not clinically useful for diagnosing sarcoidosis. The exact mechanisms responsible for the inflammatory response in EN remain unclear, but previous reports have demonstrated a possible role of circulating immune complexes [139,140]. Other nonspecific lesions, including Sweets syndrome, are uncommon [141,142].

Specific lesions

In ACCESS, 15.9% of patients suffered from specific sarcoid skin lesions. This manifestation often is associated with a chronic and aggressive disease course [9]. Lupus pernio is perhaps the best characterized chronic lesion of sarcoidosis and refers to relatively symmetric, red-violaceous, indurated or smooth plaques on the nose, cheeks, ears, and digits (Fig. 5). The epidermis is classically undisturbed. Lupus pernio is more common in blacks and Puerto Ricans and has been associated with granulomatous lesions involving the upper airway, nasal mucosa, pulmonary infiltrates or fibrosis, and bone cysts [60,78,115,143–146]. In contrast to EN, chronic sarcoidosis skin lesions

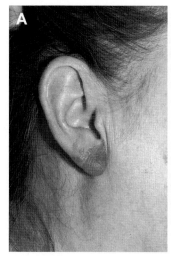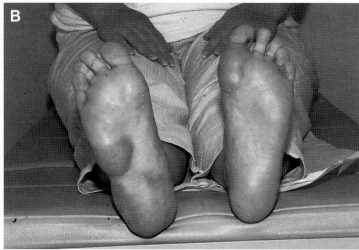

Fig. 5. (*A, B*) Lupus pernio ear and feet.

are not painful. Truly classic lupus pernio lesions are diagnostic and may not require biopsy. Cutaneous manifestations of sarcoidosis, when present, are often present at the time of diagnosis and can aid in a timely diagnosis.

When grouped together, papules, nodules, and maculopapular eruptions are the most frequently observed sarcoidosis skin lesions. Papules (Fig. 6) are often smooth-surfaced, soft, yellow-brown, with an erythematous background and may progress into plaques [141,145,147]. These lesions can occur anywhere on the body. Sarcoid plaques (Figs. 7 and 8) are more likely to leave scar, require treatment, and have worse systemic disease [148]. Darier-Roussy sarcoid refers to multiple subcutaneous nodules and is associated with systemic disease [123,148,149]. Cutaneous sarcoidosis may develop around previous traumatized skin or imbedded foreign material and is referred to as scar sarcoid or tattoo sarcoid. Paying particular attention to traumatized areas of the skin may provide further supportive evidence toward a diagnosis of sarcoidosis in difficult cases. The lesions usually are raised, purplish brown, and can develop over weeks [148,150].

Noncaseating granulomas have been observed in many additional sarcoid-associated skin lesions. These recently have been reviewed and include: plaques, angiolupoid plaques, psoriasiform plaques, ulcerative lesions, discoid lupus-like lesions with alopecia, nail dystrophy, pustular lesions, palmar erythema, hyper- and hypopigmented plaques and macules, and erythrodermic and icthyosiform lesions [145,147]. Skin lesions of sarcoidosis can resemble numerous primary dermatologic conditions and cutaneous

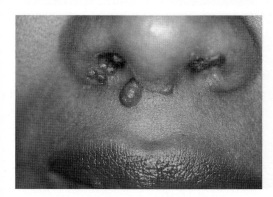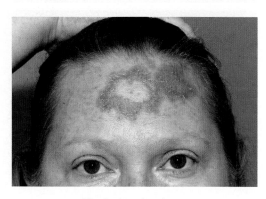

Fig. 6. Nasal sarcoid papules.

Fig. 7. Annular plaque.

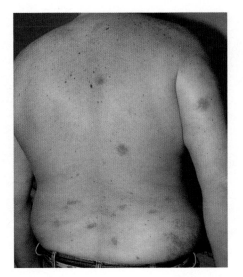

Fig. 8. Multiple sarcoid lesions resembling lupus pernio.

manifestations of other serious systemic conditions (malignancies), necessitating biopsy and detailed clinical evaluation in many cases [151,152]. Foreign body granulomas need to be excluded in limited disease, but foreign bodies also can be seen in sarcoid granulomas [153]. Additionally, numerous infectious diseases can mimic features of sarcoidosis and make the diagnosis problematic. Fungal pathogens, mycobacterial species, leishmaniasis, and syphilis infections can mimic cutaneous and systemic sarcoid and must be excluded before diagnosis [60,154].

Treatment

Nonspecific lesions erythema nodosum

Nonsarcoid causes of EN, such as TB, must be excluded and treated if present. Treatment of sarcoid-related EN is targeted to symptoms. EN is typically a self-limited disease and lasts up to 6 weeks in most cases [136]. Rest, analgesics, nonsteroidal anti-inflammatory medications, and occasionally a short course of low-dose corticosteroids may be used [155].

Specific lesions

Because cutaneous sarcoidosis is not life-threatening, treatment strategies often are geared to patient concern and cosmesis. When concomitant pulmonary or other serious manifestations of sarcoidosis are present, treatment is dictated by organ involvement. Corticosteroids remain the

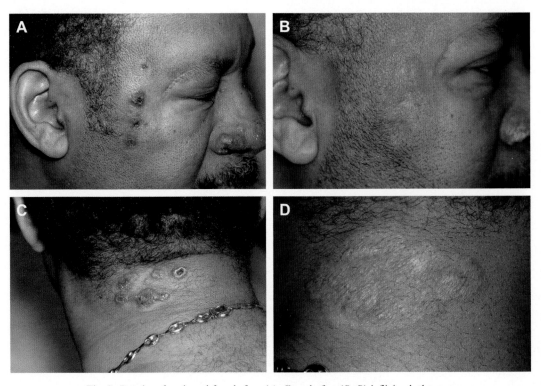

Fig. 9. Papules of neck and face before (A, C) and after (B, D) infliximab therapy.

cornerstone of therapy. Topical corticosteroids and local injections are used for isolated lesions. Systemic corticosteroid therapy should be reserved for unresponsive lesions or diffuse disease. By convention, a starting dose of 20 to 40 mg weaned to the lowest effective dose to avoid potential adverse effects, for 6 months to 2 years is recommended for most nonlife-threatening sarcoid organ involvement. If adverse effects develop or disease is recalcitrant, additional immunomodulatory agents may be required.

The traditionally used steroid sparing agents for cutaneous sarcoidosis include methotrexate, hydroxychloroquine, azathioprine, and cyclophosphamide [60]. All drugs are teratogenic. Methotrexate is a well-studied alternative to systemic glucocorticoids and is relatively safe, according to long-term studies [156,157]. Liver function monitoring and biopsy for hepatotoxicity are controversial [51,158]. Effectiveness of methotrexate therapy for skin lesions is estimated at 80% [159]. Hydroxychloroquine has been used in for treating cutaneous sarcoidosis, with significant response rates in small case series [160]. Thalidomide also demonstrated subjective improvement in 14 of 14 patients treated for chronic cutaneous sarcoidosis [161]. Interestingly, infliximab was given to 10 treatment refractory sarcoid patients, 5 with lupus pernio. All five patients treated with infliximab had dramatic improvement [50]. Other reports, including the authors' own experience (Fig. 9), have documented successes with infliximab for cutaneous sarcoid [101,162]. Of note, almost all cytotoxic (ie, mycophenolate and leflunomide) and biological agents (ie, rituximab, adalimumab and abatacept) used for other inflammatory conditions (ie, rheumatoid arthritis and Crohn's disease) are likely to be tried in chronic sarcoidosis, but little data exist to guide therapy [159,163].

Summary

Sarcoidosis is a systemic granulomatous disease with numerous skin manifestations. Cutaneous sarcoidosis can mimic infections and malignancies. The recognition of specific lesions often hastens diagnosis. EN is associated with a good prognosis, while lupus pernio and other chronic skin manifestations are associated with more severe disease. Treatment strategies range from no treatment when the course is benign or not cosmetically displeasing, to specific topical or systemic therapy.

Acknowledgments

The authors thank Dr. Ramana S. Moorthy for the critical review of this article and providing ocular photographs. We thank Dr. Marc D. Kohli for providing the radiographs in this article.

References

[1] Rudzki C, Ishak KG, Zimmerman HJ. Chronic intrahepatic cholestasis of sarcoidosis. Am J Med 1975;59(3):373–87.

[2] Murphy JR, Sjogren MH, Kikendall JW, et al. Small bile duct abnormalities in sarcoidosis. J Clin Gastroenterol 1990;12(5):555–61.

[3] Devaney K, Goodman ZD, Epstein MS, et al. Hepatic sarcoidosis. Clinicopathologic features in 100 patients. Am J Surg Pathol 1993;17(12):1272–80.

[4] Dourakis SP, Saramadou R, Alexopoulou A, et al. Hepatic granulomas: a 6-year experience in a single center in Greece. Eur J Gastroenterol Hepatol 2007;19(2):101–4.

[5] Judson MA. Hepatic, splenic, and gastrointestinal involvement with sarcoidosis. Semin Respir Crit Care Med 2002;23(6):529–41.

[6] Hercules HD, Bethlem NM. Value of liver biopsy in sarcoidosis. Arch Pathol Lab Med 1984; 108(10):831–4.

[7] Rizzato G, Palmieri G, Agrati AM, et al. The organ-specific extrapulmonary presentation of sarcoidosis: a frequent occurrence but a challenge to an early diagnosis. A 3-year-long prospective observational study. Sarcoidosis Vasc Diffuse Lung Dis 2004;21(2):119–26.

[8] Vatti R, Sharma OP. Course of asymptomatic liver involvement in sarcoidosis: role of therapy in selected cases. Sarcoidosis Vasc Diffuse Lung Dis 1997;14(1):73–6.

[9] Baughman RP, Teirstein AS, Judson MA, et al. Clinical characteristics of patients in a case–control study of sarcoidosis. Am J Respir Crit Care Med 2001;164(10 Pt 1):1885–9.

[10] Judson MA, Hirst K, Iyengar SK, et al. Comparison of sarcoidosis phenotypes among affected African American siblings. Chest 2006;130(3):855–62.

[11] Ramos-Casals M, Mana J, Nardi N, et al. Sarcoidosis in patients with chronic hepatitis C virus infection: analysis of 68 cases. Medicine (Baltimore) 2005;84(2):69–80.

[12] Goldberg H, Fiedler D, Webb A, et al. Sarcoidosis after treatment with interferon-alfa: a case series and review of literature. Respir Med 2006; 100(11):2063–8.

[13] Weyer P, Cummings OW, Knox KS. A 49-year-old woman with hepatitis, confusion, and abnormal chest radiograph findings. Chest 2005;128(4): 3076–9.

[14] Sartin JS, Walker RC. Granulomatous hepatitis: a retrospective review of 88 cases at the Mayo Clinic. Mayo Clin Proc 1991;66(9):914–8.

[15] Maddrey WC, Johns CJ, Boitnott JK, et al. Sarcoidosis and chronic hepatic disease: a clinical and pathologic study of 20 patients. Medicine (Baltimore) 1970;49(5):375–95.

[16] Kahi CJ, Saxena R, Temkit M, et al. Hepatobiliary disease in sarcoidosis. Sarcoidosis Vasc Diffuse Lung Dis 2006;23(2):117–23.

[17] Pereira-Lima J, Schaffner F. Chronic cholestasis in hepatic sarcoidosis with clinical features resembling primary biliary cirrhosis. Report of two cases. Am J Med 1987;83(1):144–8.

[18] Judson MA. Extrapulmonary sarcoidosis. Semin Respir Crit Care Med 2007;28(1):83–101.

[19] Blich M, Edoute Y. Clinical manifestations of sarcoid liver disease. J Gastroenterol Hepatol 2004; 19(7):732–7.

[20] Israel HL, Margolis ML, Rose LJ. Hepatic granulomatosis and sarcoidosis. Further observations. Dig Dis Sci 1984;29(4):353–6.

[21] Britt AR, Francis IR, Glazer GM, et al. Sarcoidosis: abdominal manifestations at CT. Radiology 1991;178(1):91–4.

[22] Warshauer DM, Dumbleton SA, Molina PL, et al. Abdominal CT findings in sarcoidosis: radiologic and clinical correlation. Radiology 1994;192(1): 93–8.

[23] Warshauer DM, Molina PL, Hamman SM, et al. Nodular sarcoidosis of the liver and spleen: analysis of 32 cases. Radiology 1995;195(3):757–62.

[24] Brancatelli G, Federle MP, Ambrosini R, et al. Cirrhosis: CT and MR imaging evaluation. Eur J Radiol 2007;61(1):57–69.

[25] Scott GC, Berman JM, Higgins JL Jr. CT patterns of nodular hepatic and splenic sarcoidosis: a review of the literature. J Comput Assist Tomogr 1997; 21(3):369–72.

[26] Warshauer DM, Lee JK. Imaging manifestations of abdominal sarcoidosis. AJR Am J Roentgenol 2004;182(1):15–28.

[27] Kessler A, Mitchell DG, Israel HL, et al. Hepatic and splenic sarcoidosis: ultrasound and MR imaging. Abdom Imaging 1993;18(2):159–63.

[28] Guglielmi AN, Kim BY, Bybel B, et al. False-positive uptake of FDG in hepatic sarcoidosis. Clin Nucl Med 2006;31(3):175.

[29] Irani SK, Dobbins WO 3rd. Hepatic granulomas: review of 73 patients from one hospital and survey of the literature. J Clin Gastroenterol 1979;1(2): 131–43.

[30] Zoutman DE, Ralph ED, Frei JV. Granulomatous hepatitis and fever of unknown origin. An 11-year experience of 23 cases with three years' follow-up. J Clin Gastroenterol 1991;13(1):69–75.

[31] Lefkowitch JH. Hepatic granulomas. J Hepatol 1999;30(Suppl 1):40–5.

[32] Guckian JC, Perry JE. Granulomatous hepatitis. An analysis of 63 cases and review of the literature. Ann Intern Med 1966;65(5):1081–100.

[33] Wagoner G, Freiman DG, Schiff L. An unusual case of jaundice in a patient with sarcoidosis. Gastroenterology 1953;25(4):574–81.

[34] Mir-Madjlessi SH, Farmer RG, Hawk WA. Granulomatous hepatitis. A review of 50 cases. Am J Gastroenterol 1973;60(2):122–34.

[35] McCluggage WG, Sloan JM. Hepatic granulomas in Northern Ireland: a thirteen-year review. Histopathology 1994;25(3):219–28.

[36] Satti MB, al-Freihi H, Ibrahim EM, et al. Hepatic granuloma in Saudi Arabia: a clinicopathological study of 59 cases. Am J Gastroenterol 1990;85(6): 669–74.

[37] Hughes M, Fox H. A histological analysis of granulomatous hepatitis. J Clin Pathol 1972;25(9): 817–20.

[38] Klatskin G. Hepatic granulomata: problems in interpretation. Ann N Y Acad Sci 1976;278: 427–32.

[39] Wainwright H. Hepatic granulomas. Eur J Gastroenterol Hepatol 2007;19(2):93–5.

[40] Gaya DR, Thorburn D, Oien KA, et al. Hepatic granulomas: a 10-year single-centre experience. J Clin Pathol 2003;56(11):850–3.

[41] Ozaras R, Tahan V, Mert A, et al. The prevalence of hepatic granulomas in chronic hepatitis C. J Clin Gastroenterol 2004;38(5):449–52.

[42] Tahan V, Ozaras R, Lacevic N, et al. Prevalence of hepatic granulomas in chronic hepatitis B. Dig Dis Sci 2004;49(10):1575–7.

[43] Valla D, Pessegueiro-Miranda H, Degott C, et al. Hepatic sarcoidosis with portal hypertension. A report of seven cases with a review of the literature. Q J Med 1987;63(242):531–44.

[44] Karagiannidis A, Karavalaki M, Koulaouzidis A. Hepatic sarcoidosis. Ann Hepatol 2006;5(4):251–6.

[45] Judson MA, Baughman RP, Teirstein AS, et al. Defining organ involvement in sarcoidosis: the ACCESS proposed instrument. ACCESS Research Group. A case–control etiologic study of sarcoidosis. Sarcoidosis Vasc Diffuse Lung Dis 1999;16(1): 75–86.

[46] Kennedy PT, Zakaria N, Modawi SB, et al. Natural history of hepatic sarcoidosis and its response to treatment. Eur J Gastroenterol Hepatol 2006;18(7): 721–6.

[47] Bass NM, Burroughs AK, Scheuer PJ, et al. Chronic intrahepatic cholestasis due to sarcoidosis. Gut 1982;23(5):417–21.

[48] Israel HL, Goldstein RA. Hepatic granulomatosis and sarcoidosis. Ann Intern Med 1973;79(5): 669–78.

[49] Ayyala US, Padilla ML. Diagnosis and treatment of hepatic sarcoidosis. Curr Treat Options Gastroenterol 2006;9(6):475–83.

[50] Doty JD, Mazur JE, Judson MA. Treatment of sarcoidosis with infliximab. Chest 2005;127(3): 1064–71.

[51] Baughman RP, Koehler A, Bejarano PA, et al. Role of liver function tests in detecting methotrexate-induced liver damage in sarcoidosis. Arch Intern Med 2003;163(5):615–20.

[52] Becheur H, Dall'osto H, Chatellier G, et al. Effect of ursodeoxycholic acid on chronic intrahepatic cholestasis due to sarcoidosis. Dig Dis Sci 1997; 42(4):789–91.

[53] Lipson EJ, Fiel MI, Florman SS, et al. Patient and graft outcomes following liver transplantation for sarcoidosis. Clin Transplant 2005;19(4):487–91.

[54] Casavilla FA, Gordon R, Wright HI, et al. Clinical course after liver transplantation in patients with sarcoidosis. Ann Intern Med 1993;118(11):865–6.

[55] Gur C, Lalazar G, Doviner V, et al. Late-onset sarcoidosis after liver transplantation for primary biliary cirrhosis. J Clin Gastroenterol 2007;41(3): 329–32.

[56] Hunt J, Gordon FD, Jenkins RL, et al. Sarcoidosis with selective involvement of a second liver allograft: report of a case and review of the literature. Mod Pathol 1999;12(3):325–8.

[57] Fiel M, Shukla D, Saraf N, et al. Development of hepatic granulomas in patients receiving pegylated interferon therapy for recurrent hepatitis C virus post-liver transplantation. Transpl Infect Dis 2007. doi:10.1111/j.1399-3062.2007.00258.x.

[58] Edelsten C, Pearson A, Joynes E, et al. The ocular and systemic prognosis of patients presenting with sarcoid uveitis. Eye 1999;13(Pt 6):748–53.

[59] Rothova A, Suttorp-Van Schulten MS, Frits Treffers W, et al. Causes and frequency of blindness in patients with intraocular inflammatory disease. Br J Ophthalmol 1996;80(4):332–6.

[60] Hunninghake GW, Costabel U, Ando M, et al. Statement on sarcoidosis. Joint Statement of the American Thoracic Society (ATS), the European Respiratory Society (ERS), and the World Association of Sarcoidosis and Other Granulomatous Disorders (WASOG) adopted by the ATS Board of Directors and by the ERS Executive Committee, February 1999. Am J Respir Crit Care Med 1999; 160(2):736–55.

[61] Rothova A, Alberts C, Glasius E, et al. Risk factors for ocular sarcoidosis. Doc Ophthalmol 1989; 72(3–4):287–96.

[62] Goto H, Mochizuki M, Yamaki K, et al. Epidemiological survey of intraocular inflammation in Japan. Jpn J Ophthalmol 2007;51(1):41–4.

[63] Matsuo T, Fujiwara N, Nakata Y. First presenting signs or symptoms of sarcoidosis in a Japanese population. Jpn J Ophthalmol 2005;49(2):149–52.

[64] Rossman MD, Thompson B, Frederick M, et al. HLA-DRB1*1101: a significant risk factor for sarcoidosis in blacks and whites. Am J Hum Genet 2003;73(4):720–35.

[65] Spagnolo P, Sato H, Marshall SE, et al. Association between heat shock protein 70/Hom genetic polymorphisms and uveitis in patients with sarcoidosis. Invest Ophthalmol Vis Sci 2007;48(7): 3019–25.

[66] Takeuchi M, Oh IK, Suzuki J, et al. Elevated serum levels of CXCL9/monokine induced by interferon-gamma and CXCL10/interferon-gamma-inducible protein-10 in ocular sarcoidosis. Invest Ophthalmol Vis Sci 2006;47(3):1063–8.

[67] Rizzato G, Angi M, Fraioli P, et al. Uveitis as a presenting feature of chronic sarcoidosis. Eur Respir J 1996;9(6):1201–5.

[68] Foster S. Ocular manifestations of sarcoidosis preceding systemic manifestations. Presented at the XI World Congress on Sarcoidosis and other Granulomatous Disorders. Milan, Italy, September 6–11, 1988.

[69] Jabs DA, Nussenblatt RB, Rosenbaum JT. Standardization of uveitis nomenclature for reporting clinical data. Results of the First International Workshop. Am J Ophthalmol 2005;140(3):509–16.

[70] Cowan CL. Sarcoidosis. In: Yanoff M, Augsburger JJ, editors. Ophthalmology. 2nd edition. St. Louis (MO): Mosby; 2004. p. 1185–90.

[71] Newman LS, Rose CS, Maier LA. Sarcoidosis. N Engl J Med 1997;336(17):1224–34.

[72] Heerfordt CF. Uveoparotid fever. Albrecht Von Graefes Arch Ophthalmol 1909;70:254 [in German].

[73] Evans M, Sharma O, LaBree L, et al. Differences in clinical findings between Caucasians and African Americans with biopsy-proven sarcoidosis. Ophthalmology 2007;114(2):325–33.

[74] Rothova A. Ocular involvement in sarcoidosis. Br J Ophthalmol 2000;84(1):110–6.

[75] Leavitt JA, Campbell RJ. Cost-effectiveness in the diagnosis of sarcoidosis: the conjunctival biopsy. Eye 1998;12(Pt 6):959–62.

[76] Spaide RF, Ward DL. Conjunctival biopsy in the diagnosis of sarcoidosis. Br J Ophthalmol 1990; 74(8):469–71.

[77] Shorr AF, Torrington KG, Hnatiuk OW. Endobronchial biopsy for sarcoidosis: a prospective study. Chest 2001;120(1):109–14.

[78] Lynch JP 3rd, Sharma OP, Baughman RP. Extrapulmonary sarcoidosis. Semin Respir Infect 1998; 13(3):229–54.

[79] Chung YM, Lin YC, Huang DF, et al. Conjunctival biopsy in sarcoidosis. J Chin Med Assoc 2006; 69(10):472–7.

[80] Wertheim MS, Mathers WD, Lim L, et al. Noninvasive detection of multinucleated giant cells in the conjunctiva of patients with sarcoidosis by in vivo confocal microscopy. Ocul Immunol Inflamm 2006;14(4):203–6.

[81] Obenauf CD, Shaw HE, Sydnor CF, et al. Sarcoidosis and its ophthalmic manifestations. Am J Ophthalmol 1978;86(5):648–55.

[82] Khalatbari D, Stinnett S, McCallum RM, et al. Demographic-related variations in posterior segment ocular sarcoidosis. Ophthalmology 2004;111(2): 357–62.

[83] Lobo A, Barton K, Minassian D, et al. Visual loss in sarcoid-related uveitis. Clin Experiment Ophthalmol 2003;31(4):310–6.

[84] Ciardella AP, Prall FR, Borodoker N, et al. Imaging techniques for posterior uveitis. Curr Opin Ophthalmol 2004;15(6):519–30.

[85] Mafee MF, Dorodi S, Pai E. Sarcoidosis of the eye, orbit, and central nervous system. Role of MR imaging. Radiol Clin North Am 1999;37(1):73–87, x.

[86] Usui Y, Kaiser ED, See RF, et al. Update of ocular manifestations in sarcoidosis. Sarcoidosis Vasc Diffuse Lung Dis 2002;19(3):167–75.

[87] Astudillo L, Soler V, Sailler L, et al. Bilateral exophthalmos revealing a case of husband and wife sarcoidosis. Am J Med 2006;119(5):e7–8.

[88] Attia S, Zaouali S, Jeguirim H, et al. Orbital sarcoidosis manifesting with enophthalmos. Ocul Immunol Inflamm 2006;14(6):379–81.

[89] Weinreb RN, Sandman R, Ryder MI, et al. Angiotensin-converting enzyme activity in human aqueous humor. Arch Ophthalmol 1985;103(1):34–6.

[90] Sharma OP, Vita JB. Determination of angiotensin-converting enzyme activity in tears. A noninvasive test for evaluation of ocular sarcoidosis. Arch Ophthalmol 1983;101(4):559–61.

[91] Baarsma GS, La Hey E, Glasius E, et al. The predictive value of serum angiotensin converting enzyme and lysozyme levels in the diagnosis of ocular sarcoidosis. Am J Ophthalmol 1987;104(3): 211–7.

[92] Tomita H, Sato S, Matsuda R, et al. Serum lysozyme levels and clinical features of sarcoidosis. Lung 1999;177(3):161–7.

[93] Jouveshomme S, Fardeau C, Finet JF, et al. Alveolar lymphocytosis in patients with chronic uveitis: relationship to sarcoidosis. Lung 2001;179(5): 305–17.

[94] Kurdziel KA. The panda sign. Radiology 2000; 215(3):884–5.

[95] Frohman LP, Guirgis M, Turbin RE, et al. Sarcoidosis of the anterior visual pathway: 24 new cases. J Neuroophthalmol 2003;23(3):190–7.

[96] McCluskey P, Powell RJ. The eye in systemic inflammatory diseases. Lancet 2004;364(9451): 2125–33.

[97] Paramothayan S, Jones PW. Corticosteroid therapy in pulmonary sarcoidosis: a systematic review. JAMA 2002;287(10):1301–7.

[98] Carnahan MC, Goldstein DA. Ocular complications of topical, peri-ocular, and systemic corticosteroids. Curr Opin Ophthalmol 2000;11(6):478–83.

[99] Dev S, McCallum RM, Jaffe GJ. Methotrexate treatment for sarcoid-associated panuveitis. Ophthalmology 1999;106(1):111–8.

[100] Baughman RP, Lower EE. Leflunomide for chronic sarcoidosis. Sarcoidosis Vasc Diffuse Lung Dis 2004;21(1):43–8.

[101] Roberts SD, Wilkes DS, Burgett RA, et al. Refractory sarcoidosis responding to infliximab. Chest 2003;124(5):2028–31.

[102] Pritchard C, Nadarajah K. Tumour necrosis factor alpha inhibitor treatment for sarcoidosis refractory to conventional treatments: a report of five patients. Ann Rheum Dis 2004;63(3):318–20.

[103] Baughman RP, Lower EE, Bradley DA, et al. Etanercept for refractory ocular sarcoidosis: results of a double-blind randomized trial. Chest 2005; 128(2):1062–7.

[104] Suhler EB, Smith JR, Wertheim MS, et al. A prospective trial of infliximab therapy for refractory uveitis: preliminary safety and efficacy outcomes. Arch Ophthalmol 2005;123(7):903–12.

[105] Baughman RP, Bradley DA, Lower EE. Infliximab in chronic ocular inflammation. Int J Clin Pharmacol Ther 2005;43(1):7–11.

[106] Akova YA, Foster CS. Cataract surgery in patients with sarcoidosis-associated uveitis. Ophthalmology 1994;101(3):473–9.

[107] Ieki Y, Kiryu J, Kita M, et al. Pars plana vitrectomy for vitreous opacity associated with ocular sarcoidosis resistant to medical treatment. Ocul Immunol Inflamm 2004;12(1):35–43.

[108] Hutchison J. Case of livid papillary psoriasis. In: Hutchison J, editor. Illustrations of clinical surgery, vol. 1. London: J & A Churchill; 1877. p. 42.

[109] Sharma OP. Sarcoidosis: a historical perspective. Clin Dermatol 2007;25(3):232–41.

[110] Noor A, Knox KS. Immunopathogenesis of sarcoidosis. Clin Dermatol 2007;25(3):250–8.

[111] Kataria YP, Park HK. Dynamics and mechanism of the sarcoidal granuloma. Detecting T cell subsets, non-T cells, and immunoglobulins in biopsies at varying intervals of Kveim-Siltzbach test sites. Ann N Y Acad Sci 1986;465:221–32.

[112] Teirstein AS. Kveim antigen: what does it tell us about causation of sarcoidosis? Semin Respir Infect 1998;13(3):206–11.

[113] Kveim A. Em ny og specifikk kutans-reaksjon ved Boecks sarcoid, en forelogiv meddelse. Nordic Medicine 1941;9:169–72.

[114] Siltzbach LE, Ehrlich JC. The Nickerson-Kveim reaction in sarcoidosis. Am J Med 1954;16(6): 790–803.

[115] Judson MA, Thompson BW, Rabin DL, et al. The diagnostic pathway to sarcoidosis. Chest 2003; 123(2):406–12.

[116] Fite E, Alsina JM, Mana J, et al. Epidemiology of sarcoidosis in Catalonia: 1979–1989. Sarcoidosis Vasc Diffuse Lung Dis 1996;13(2):153–8.

[117] Siltzbach LE, James DG, Neville E, et al. Course and prognosis of sarcoidosis around the world. Am J Med 1974;57(6):847–52.

[118] Garcia-Porrua C, Gonzalez-Gay MA, Vazquez-Caruncho M, et al. Erythema nodosum: etiologic and predictive factors in a defined population. Arthritis Rheum 2000;43(3):584–92.

[119] Milman N, Selroos O. Pulmonary sarcoidosis in the Nordic countries 1950–1982. II. Course and prognosis. Sarcoidosis 1990;7(2):113–8.

[120] Teirstein AS, Chuang M, Miller A, et al. Flexible-bronchoscope biopsy of lung and bronchial wall in intrathoracic sarcoidosis. Ann N Y Acad Sci 1976;278:522–7.

[121] Behbehani N, JayKrishnan B, Khadadah M, et al. Clinical presentation of sarcoidosis in a mixed population in the Middle East. Respir Med 2007; 101(11):2284–8.

[122] Pietinalho A, Ohmichi M, Hiraga Y, et al. The mode of presentation of sarcoidosis in Finland and Hokkaido, Japan. A comparative analysis of 571 Finnish and 686 Japanese patients. Sarcoidosis Vasc Diffuse Lung Dis 1996;13(2): 159–66.

[123] Yanardag H, Pamuk ON, Karayel T. Cutaneous involvement in sarcoidosis: analysis of the features in 170 patients. Respir Med 2003;97(8):978–82.

[124] Mana J, Gomez-Vaquero C, Montero A, et al. Lofgren's syndrome revisited: a study of 186 patients. Am J Med 1999;107(3):240–5.

[125] Honeybourne D. Ethnic differences in the clinical features of sarcoidosis in southeast London. Br J Dis Chest 1980;74(1):63–9.

[126] Lofgren S, Lundback H. The bilateral hilar lymphoma syndrome; a study of the relation to tuberculosis and sarcoidosis in 212 cases. Acta Med Scand 1952;142(4):265–73.

[127] Grunewald J, Eklund A. Sex-specific manifestations of Lofgren's syndrome. Am J Respir Crit Care Med 2007;175(1):40–4.

[128] Mana J, Gomez-Vaquero C, Salazar A, et al. Periarticular ankle sarcoidosis: a variant of Lofgren's syndrome. J Rheumatol 1996;23(5):874–7.

[129] Spagnolo P, Renzoni EA, Wells AU, et al. C-C chemokine receptor 2 and sarcoidosis: association with Lofgren's syndrome. Am J Respir Crit Care Med 2003;168(10):1162–6.

[130] Wahlstrom J, Dengjel J, Persson B, et al. Identification of HLA–DR-bound peptides presented by human bronchoalveolar lavage cells in sarcoidosis. J Clin Invest 2007;117(11):3576–82.

[131] Ho LP, Urban BC, Thickett DR, et al. Deficiency of a subset of T cells with immunoregulatory properties in sarcoidosis. Lancet 2005;365(9464): 1062–72.

[132] Berlin M, Fogdell-Hahn A, Olerup O, et al. HLA–DR predicts the prognosis in Scandinavian patients with pulmonary sarcoidosis. Am J Respir Crit Care Med 1997;156(5):1601–5.

[133] Idali F, Wiken M, Wahlstrom J, et al. Reduced Th1 response in the lungs of HLA-DRB1*0301 patients with pulmonary sarcoidosis. Eur Respir J 2006; 27(3):451–9.

[134] Katchar K, Wahlstrom J, Eklund A, et al. Highly activated T cell receptor AV2S3(+) CD4(+) lung T-cell expansions in pulmonary sarcoidosis. Am J Respir Crit Care Med 2001;163(7):1540–5.

[135] Mana J, Marcoval J. Erythema nodosum. Clin Dermatol 2007;25(3):288–94.

[136] James DG. Erythema nodosum. Br Med J 1961; 1(5229):853–7.

[137] Requena L, Requena C. Erythema nodosum. Dermatol Online J 2002;8(1):4.

[138] Hannuksela M. Erythema nodosum. Clin Dermatol 1986;4(4):88–95.

[139] Hedfors E, Norberg R. Evidence for circulating immune complexes in sarcoidosis. Clin Exp Immunol 1974;16(3):493–6.

[140] Jones JV, Cumming RH, Asplin CM, et al. Letter: circulating immune complexes in erythema nodosum and early sarcoidosis. Lancet 1976;1(7951): 153.

[141] Elgart ML. Cutaneous sarcoidosis: definitions and types of lesions. Clin Dermatol 1986;4(4):35–45.

[142] Saliba WR, Habib GS, Elias M. Sweet's syndrome and sarcoidosis. Eur J Intern Med 2005;16(8):545–50.

[143] Edmondstone WM, Wilson AG. Sarcoidosis in Caucasians, blacks and Asians in London. Br J Dis Chest 1985;79(1):27–36.

[144] Neville E, Walker AN, James DG. Prognostic factors predicting the outcome of sarcoidosis: an analysis of 818 patients. Q J Med 1983;52(208): 525–33.

[145] Marchell RM, Judson MA. Chronic cutaneous lesions of sarcoidosis. Clin Dermatol 2007;25(3): 295–302.

[146] Sharma OP. Cutaneous sarcoidosis: clinical features and management. Chest 1972;61(4):320–5.

[147] Fernandez-Faith E, McDonnell J. Cutaneous sarcoidosis: differential diagnosis. Clin Dermatol 2007;25(3):276–87.

[148] Mana J, Marcoval J, Graells J, et al. Cutaneous involvement in sarcoidosis. Relationship to systemic disease. Arch Dermatol 1997;133(7):882–8.

[149] Ahmed I, Harshad SR. Subcutaneous sarcoidosis: is it a specific subset of cutaneous sarcoidosis frequently associated with systemic disease? J Am Acad Dermatol 2006;54(1):55–60.

[150] Epstein WL. Cutaneous sarcoidosis. Semin Respir Crit Care Med 2002;23(6):571–7.

[151] Cather JC, Cohen PR. Ichthyosiform sarcoidosis. J Am Acad Dermatol 1999;40(5 Pt 2):862–5.

[152] Gregg PJ, Kantor GR, Telang GH, et al. Sarcoidal tissue reaction in Sezary syndrome. J Am Acad Dermatol 2000;43(2 Pt 2):372–6.

[153] Marcoval J, Mana J, Moreno A, et al. Foreign bodies in granulomatous cutaneous lesions of patients with systemic sarcoidosis. Arch Dermatol 2001; 137(4):427–30.

[154] Ezzie ME, Crouser ED. Considering an infectious etiology of sarcoidosis. Clin Dermatol 2007;25(3): 259–66.

[155] Schwartz RA, Nervi SJ. Erythema nodosum: a sign of systemic disease. Am Fam Physician 2007;75(5): 695–700.

[156] Lower EE, Baughman RP. Prolonged use of methotrexate for sarcoidosis. Arch Intern Med 1995; 155(8):846–51.

[157] Veien NK, Brodthagen H. Cutaneous sarcoidosis treated with methotrexate. Br J Dermatol 1977; 97(2):213–6.

[158] Kremer JM, Alarcon GS, Lightfoot RW Jr, et al. Methotrexate for rheumatoid arthritis. Suggested guidelines for monitoring liver toxicity. American College of Rheumatology. Arthritis Rheum 1994; 37(3):316–28.

[159] Baughman RP, Lower EE. Evidence-based therapy for cutaneous sarcoidosis. Clin Dermatol 2007; 25(3):334–40.

[160] Jones E, Callen JP. Hydroxychloroquine is effective therapy for control of cutaneous sarcoidal granulomas. J Am Acad Dermatol 1990;23(3 Pt 1):487–9.

[161] Baughman RP, Judson MA, Teirstein AS, et al. Thalidomide for chronic sarcoidosis. Chest 2002; 122(1):227–32.

[162] Baughman RP, Drent M, Kavuru M, et al. Infliximab therapy in patients with chronic sarcoidosis and pulmonary involvement. Am J Respir Crit Care Med 2006;174(7):795–802.

[163] Sweiss NJ, Curran J, Baughman RP. Sarcoidosis, role of tumor necrosis factor inhibitors and other biologic agents, past, present, and future concepts. Clin Dermatol 2007;25(3):341–6.

ELSEVIER
SAUNDERS

Clin Chest Med 29 (2008) 525–532

CLINICS
IN CHEST
MEDICINE

Quality of Life and Health Status in Sarcoidosis: A Review of the Literature

Jolanda De Vries, PhD, MSc[a,b,c,*], Marjolein Drent, MD, PhD[d]

[a]Department of Medical Psychology and Neuropsychology, Tilburg University, PO Box 90153,
5000 LE, Tilburg, The Netherlands
[b]Department of Medical Psychology, St Elisabeth Hospital, PO Box 90153, 5000 LE, Tilburg, The Netherlands
[c]Sarcoidosis Management Center, University Hospital Maastricht, PO Box 5800,
6202 AZ, Maastricht, The Netherlands
[d]Department of Respiratory Medicine, Sarcoidosis Management Center, University Hospital Maastricht,
PO Box 5800, 6202 AZ, Maastricht, The Netherlands

Sarcoidosis is a disease associated with a wide range of symptoms, such as cough, dyspnea on exertion, chest pain, wheezing, fever, weight loss, arthralgia, and general weakness [1,2]. An increasing number of studies have shown that fatigue is a major problem for patients [2–6]. These symptoms may negatively influence patients' quality of life (QOL) [6]. QOL is an important outcome measure of treatment, especially with regard to chronic diseases. It is a concept that concerns patients' evaluation of their functioning in a wide range of domains, but always the physical, psychologic, and social domain [7]. When only these three domains are assessed, one measures health-related QOL. QOL is often confused with health status (HS), which concerns patients' physical, psychologic, and social functioning [8,9]. This article focuses on what is known about the QOL and HS of sarcoidosis patients. For the purpose of clarity, studies on QOL and HS are presented separately.

Methods

A search using the PubMed database was performed with the key words "sarcoidosis and health status," "sarcoidosis and quality of life,"

and "sarcoidosis and fatigue" for the time period until November 2007. This resulted in 22, 68, and 105 papers, respectively. Only 15 of the papers with the key words "fatigue" and "sarcoidosis" seemed to be relevant studies; the others mainly were case reports or reviews. Fifteen papers found with the key words "sarcoidosis" and "health status" and 14 of "fatigue" and "sarcoidosis" overlapped with the other search. From the remaining 76 papers, 17 were reviews and not included in this article, resulting in 59 papers. These papers were further reduced to 35 based on the title or abstract. Reasons for excluding papers were language (ie, not written in English, German, or Dutch; N = 11); no pulmonary sarcoidosis (N = 4); guidelines (N = 1); focus is on development or validation of questionnaires (N = 2); HS or QOL were not examined (N = 5); or not by means of questionnaires (N = 1). Finally, 24 studies resulted that directly assessed QOL, HS, or fatigue.

Results

Sarcoidosis quality of life and fatigue

The greatest impact on QOL in sarcoidosis, as seen in clinical practice, is caused by rather nonspecific symptoms hard to objectify, such as fatigue and sleeping disorders [4]. For instance, in one study there seemed to be a number of QOL areas in which sarcoidosis patients, particularly

---

* Corresponding author. Department of Medical Psychology and Neuropsychology, Tilburg University, PO Box 90153, 5000 LE, The Netherlands.
  E-mail address: j.devries@uvt.nl (J. De Vries).

those with current symptoms, experienced problems. Patients either with or without current symptoms suffered from fatigue, sleeping problems, and impaired general QOL compared with a healthy control group. Besides the physical problems mentioned previously, patients with current symptoms suffered from impaired QOL with regard to their mobility, working capacity, and activities of daily living. This was also shown in a different way in a study among Croatian sarcoidosis patients that examined the predictive value of the most frequently reported symptoms on patients QOL [7]. Fatigue, breathlessness, reduced exercise capacity, and arthralgia were the most frequently reported symptoms. Women scored lower on the domains Physical health, Psychologic health, Social relationships, and Environment, and the general facet Overall QOL. Using corticosteroids predicted a lower QOL in all domains except Spirituality. Having a partner was associated with the QOL domains Psychologic health and Level of independence, whereas a low educational level and arthralgia predicted scores on the domain Social relationships in a positive and negative way, respectively. Fatigue had a negative effect on patients' QOL domain scores for Physical health, Psychologic health, and Level of independence. Finally, diffusing capacity of lung for carbon monoxide was positively related to Spirituality [7]. In a study that focused exclusively on the relationship between fatigue and QOL, fatigue seemed to have a negative impact on all domains of QOL. In addition, the diffusing capacity for carbon monoxide was positively related to the QOL domain Level of independence, whereas gender, age, and time since diagnosis were, in various combinations, related to patients' scores on QOL domains [10]. Sarcoidosis has a considerable impact on patients' QOL, especially in those patients with current symptoms, such as fatigue. This was also shown in three other studies [11–13]. Sarcoidosis patients and rheumatoid arthritis patients had an impaired QOL compared with healthy controls. Fatigue, sleep, activities of daily living, and working capacity were major problems in both patient groups. In addition, rheumatoid arthritis patients had a worse QOL in the domains Physical health and Level of independence compared with the sarcoidosis patients [13]. Another study found that female patients have a lower QOL, except for positive feelings [12]. Finally, recent studies showed that a substantial number of sarcoidosis patients suffer from small fiber neuropathy [14]. In a case report of a patient with

severe small fiber neuropathy, high scores in fatigue, and a low QOL, infliximab, an anti–tumor necrosis factor-α therapy, resulted in such improvement in fatigue and QOL that scores returned to normal values [15].

Sarcoidosis health status

In three studies patients had a worse HS compared with a control group [3,16,17]. In two of these studies patients scored higher on cognitive behavior, home management tasks, recreation and hobbies, sleep, social interaction, and work [3,16]. In the study by Drent and colleagues [3], sarcoidosis patient suffering from symptoms seemed to be responsible for the differences between the sarcoidosis patients and the control group. In a study among Greek sarcoidosis patients with active sarcoidosis, patients reported more dyspnea, more anxiety and depressive symptoms, and a worse HS compared with controls that visited a smoking cessation clinic [17]. In the study by Drent and colleagues [3], the patients with current symptoms reported more depressive symptoms compared with patients without current symptoms. Moreover, whereas the latter subgroup experienced more positive effect, no differences between the two sarcoidosis subgroups were found with regard to negative affect. From the HS aspects, sleep seemed to be associated with depressive symptoms in general and depressive cognitions in particular [3]. Cox and colleagues [18] found that higher scores on depressive symptoms and perceived stress were related to lower HS scores. In another study the relationship between HS and lung function, and respiratory and peripheral muscle function, was examined [16]. Patients with symptoms showed a lower maximum inspiratory pressure, maximum expiratory pressure, and respiratory muscle endurance time compared with those without symptoms. Moreover, correlations were found between respiratory muscle endurance time and the HS aspects mobility and body care and movement. The radiographic stage was related to cognitive and emotional behavior, home management, and social interaction [16]. With regard to the relationship between pulmonary function tests and dyspnea, and HS, most studies find some relationships. Yeager and colleagues [19] found that lower scores on the spirometric tests and more self-reported dyspnea was related to a diminished HS. Furthermore, a study examining the relationship between the 6-minute walk test and HS showed that self-reported dyspnea scores were associated with fatigue scores, the walking distance, and patients' HS. Performance on the 6-minute walk test was predicted by patients' score on the activity scale of the St. George Respiratory Questionnaire, forced vital capacity, and oxygen saturation [20]. In another study self-reported dyspnea and HS was associated with forced expiratory volume in 1 second and forced vital capacity, although it depended on the questionnaires used [17]. In a smaller study [18], spirometric tests and self-reported dyspnea were unrelated to a diminished HS. Finally, Baughman and colleagues [21] examined the usefulness of fluticasone in patients with acute symptomatic pulmonary sarcoidosis. No difference was found between the fluticasone (N = 10) and the placebo group (N = 11) with regard to HS. Oral corticosteroids seemed to be associated with significant complaints, however, whereas inhaled corticosteroids were well tolerated [21].

In a study that aimed to assess the relationship between HS and physiologic impairment [22], patients with various interstitial lung diseases (ILDs) seemed to have a moderately reduced HS. As might be expected, the scores on the applied questionnaires were related to the dyspnea scores of patients and results on their pulmonary function tests.

Discussion

This article focuses on current knowledge of the QOL, HS, and fatigue of sarcoidosis patients. QOL in sarcoidosis is impaired with respect to mobility, working capacity, and activities of daily living, especially in sarcoidosis patients suffering from fatigue and other symptoms, such as breathlessness and arthralgia. HS of sarcoidosis patients is also lower compared with healthy controls, especially in the cognitive aspects, mobility, home management, leisure activities, sleep, social interaction, and work. Patients also displayed more depressive symptoms and, related to this, a lower HS.

Quality of life and health status

The authors distinguished between studies examining QOL and HS, although research often uses the term "QOL" to cover both concepts. HS concerns the impact of disease on functioning, whereas health-related QOL also reflects patients' evaluation of their functioning. It is important to make this distinction when planning and performing intervention studies because QOL and HS measures may provide different results and different conclusions [23].

There are several differences between the types of questions and the meaning of the scores from QOL and HS measures. First, HS may indicate whether there are limitations or not, whereas QOL also reflects to what extent patients experience these limitations as a problem in daily life. Individual expectations regarding health, the ability to cope with limitations, and the threshold for the tolerance of discomfort modulate objective HS facts into subjective values, which represents one's QOL [24]. Consequently, two persons with identical restrictions in functioning (HS) may evaluate these restrictions (QOL) differently. Similarly, a low HS score can coincide with a high score on the corresponding domain of a QOL measure within the same person. Using a HS measure to assess QOL can provide misleading conclusions [25]. This can be illustrated using the social domain. HS measures focus on how often and to what extent physical health and emotional problems have interfered with unspecified social activities. Consequently, patients with few social contacts have a low score and are expected to have an unsatisfactory social life. A QOL measure inquires about patients' satisfaction with their social contacts. Because this is not related to the size of someone's social network, few social contacts may reflect a patient's preference.

Second, HS and QOL measures differ in the level of differentiation. In general, QOL questionnaires assess more aspects of life than HS measures in such a way that it provides more detailed information on patients' life. For example, the psychologic domain of HS measures incorporate a wide spectrum of questions, such as the frequency of feeling nervous, down, calm and quiet, depressed, and happy. Because these questions are aggregated into one score, however, this does not allow the identification of the feelings that are affected. In contrast, a QOL questionnaire assesses a broader range of separate aspects of the domain (eg, negative feelings, positive feelings, and self-esteem).

Third, HS measures only aspects that are directly related to health, whereas QOL instruments measure a broader range of aspects of patients' lives. Measuring a wider scope of aspects is important because patients may feel that aspects that are not directly health-related are very relevant to them and determine their QOL [26]. An example is financial resources, which is often influenced by disease (eg, because patients have to reduce the number of working hours).

Fourth, HS measures are characterized by the tendency to assess infirmity or disability, rather than health [27]. Questions focus on the negative consequences of disease and disregard the positive aspects of life, which are part of QOL measures. The choice for a QOL or HS measure depends on one's aim. In general, if information is wanted about what patients can and cannot do (functioning), a HS measure must be used. If one's interest is in how patients feel about several aspect of their life, however, a QOL measure in indicated. Using the right type of questionnaire to reach one's aim is of the utmost importance, because QOL and HS measures may provide conflicting results. Using a combination of HS and QOL measures has been suggested by several researchers.

Quality of life and health status measures used in sarcoidosis

Until now, only one QOL measure has been used in sarcoidosis: the World Health Organization Quality of Life Assessment Instrument-100 [28,29]. With regard to HS, five different measures have been used in sarcoidosis studies (Table 1). The Chronic Respiratory Questionnaire [30] is a respiratory-specific health-status measure that was originally developed for chronic obstructive pulmonary disease (COPD) patients. It measures four aspects of HS: (1) dyspnea, (2) fatigue, (3) emotional function, and (4) mastery. The questionnaire allows patients to rate the severity of dyspnea associated with individually identified activities. Contrary to the other questionnaires used in sarcoidosis, the Chronic Respiratory Questionnaire is an interviewer-assisted

questionnaire. It seems to be a reliable and valid instrument for COPD and asthma patients [22,30,31]. Chang and coworkers [32] have used the Chronic Respiratory Questionnaire in a validation study among patients with ILD, which included 10 sarcoidosis patients (20% of the total ILD group). They concluded that the Chronic Respiratory Questionnaire was not a good measure for use in ILD.

The Medical Outcome Study Short Form-36 [33] is a 36-item generic health-status measure that assesses health in eight dimensions: (1) physical functioning; (2) social functioning; (3) limitations in usual role activities caused by physical problems (role physical); (4) limitations in usual role activities caused by emotional problems (role emotional); (5) mental health; (6) vitality; (7) bodily pain; and (8) general health perception. In addition, health changes over the last year may be assessed. The Short Form-36 has been widely used and has good psychometric properties [34]. The reliability and validity have been shown to be good in a sample of patients with ILD, which included some sarcoidosis patients [32].

The Sarcoidosis Health Questionnaire [35] is a sarcoidosis-specific HS measure that consists of 29 questions covering three domains: (1) daily functioning, (2) physical functioning, and (3) emotional functioning. The reliability and validity of this questionnaire seems good [3], but further testing is needed. Unfortunately, fatigue, a major symptom of sarcoidosis, is only represented by one question that is part of a domain. Specific information on this symptom cannot be derived from the Sarcoidosis Health Questionnaire. To assess fatigue, another specific fatigue measure needs to be used.

Table 1
Quality of life and health status questionnaires used or examined in sarcoidosis

Questionnaires	QOL/HS measure	Number of items	Required time (min)	Quality in sarcoidosis
CRQ	HS	20	20–30	Not good[a]
SF-36	HS	36	10	Good[a]
SGRQ	HS	76	15–20	Good[a]
SHQ	HS	29	10	Good
SIP	HS	136	20–30	Unknown
WHOQOL-100	QOL	100	15–20	Good

Abbreviations: CRQ, Chronic Respiratory Questionnaire; HS, health status; QOL, quality of life; SF-36, Medical Outcome Study Short Form-36; SGRQ, St. George Respiratory Questionnaire; SHQ, Sarcoidosis Health Questionnaire; SIP, Sickness Impact Profile; WHOQOL-100, World Health Organization Quality of Life Assessment Instrument-100.

[a] Validated in an interstitial lung diseases sample including 10 sarcoidosis patients.

The Sickness Impact Profile [36] is designed to assess sickness-related behavioral dysfunction in 12 categories:

1. Alertness behavior
2. Ambulation
3. Body care and movement
4. Communication
5. Eating
6. Emotional behavior
7. Home management
8. Mobility
9. Recreation and pastimes
10. Sleep and rest
11. Social interaction
12. Employment

It also provides summary scores for physical, psychosocial, and overall behavioral dysfunction. This questionnaire has not been validated for use in sarcoidosis.

The last questionnaire that has been used in sarcoidosis is the St. George Respiratory Questionnaire [37], a measure developed for COPD patients. It contains 76 items with weighted responses covering three components: (1) symptoms, (2) activity, and (3) impacts. The latter two states relate to the patient's current state of health. The St. George Respiratory Questionnaire seems to have good reliability and validity for COPD and asthma patients [37–39]. Moreover, this latter questionnaire was considered a good respiratory-specific measure useful in ILD patients, including 10 sarcoidosis patients [32].

Assessment of fatigue: fatigue assessment scale

Because fatigue has a major impact on QOL in sarcoidosis, establishing the extent of fatigue provides valuable insight regarding patients' QOL [6,10]. There is no objective parameter, however, for assessing fatigue in sarcoidosis [40]. A common way of assessing perceived fatigue is by means of questionnaires. The Fatigue Assessment Scale (FAS) is a promising measure for assessing fatigue in sarcoidosis patients [41]. The FAS is a 10-item questionnaire to assess fatigue (Appendix 1). The response scale is a 5-point scale (1 "never" to 5 "always"); scores on the FAS can range from 10 to 50. The FAS is based on four existing measures, among which is the facet Energy and fatigue from the World Health Organization Quality of Life Assessment Instrument-100, a measure previously used in the authors' fatigue studies among sarcoidosis patients. A group of 134 Dutch sarcoidosis patients

had a significantly higher FAS score compared with a representative sample of the Dutch population (N = 1893). Furthermore, most (80%) of the general population sample scored below the cutoff score of the FAS, whereas 80% of the sarcoidosis patients scored above that score. Moreover, FAS scores seemed not to be related to lung function test results [41]. The reliability and validity of the FAS seemed to be good in persons working at least 20 hours per week and in sarcoidosis patients [41,42].

Current shortcomings

There is a lack of prospective follow-up studies focusing on QOL. Except for the intervention studies, current studies are cross-sectional in nature. Impact on life assessed with QOL measures is an important factor in predicting medical consumption. Appropriate management of sarcoidosis is mandatory because it predominantly affects young adults. Accordingly, the complicated nature of sarcoidosis underlines the need of multidisciplinary evaluation, management, and patient care that pays attention to somatic and psychosocial aspects of the disease.

Clinical implications

Beside physical problems, sarcoidosis has a substantial impact on QOL. There exists no effective treatment for fatigue in sarcoidosis. In a study examining fatigue in two groups of sarcoidosis patients, it seemed that in the group of patient members of the Dutch Sarcoidosis Society, patients using prednisone exhibited higher fatigue scores than patients not using prednisone. In the outpatient group, fatigue was unrelated to prednisone use [40,41]. Several case reports of sarcoidosis patients treated with anti–tumor necrosis factor-α showed a dramatic reduction in fatigue [15]. The positive effect of anti–tumor necrosis factor-α on fatigue has also been demonstrated in other diseases, such as Crohn's disease and rheumatoid arthritis [43,44]. These kinds of drugs, however, cannot be given to patients who are suffering exclusively from fatigue without other evidence of disease activity. Moreover, management of the patient with fatigue requires more than prescribing drugs. It is important for the physician to listen to the patient; it is wise to take seriously what the patient says. Furthermore, patients should be instructed to lead as active and involved a life as possible. Sleeping problems should be treated appropriately [45,46].

When fatigue has a partly psychologic cause, various treatments are available. Patients with clinical depression can be prescribed antidepressants. Some patients may require help to improve coping and self-management of their disease to increase their QOL. Cognitive therapy may be indicated to treat coping problems or stress perception. Furthermore, physical training programs guided by physiotherapists might also improve patients' exercise tolerance and physical fitness [47]. Because what patients can handle is clearly decreased, however, the activities should be adapted accordingly and rehabilitation programs should be developed carefully.

Furthermore, it is very important to guide persons involved in the follow-up of patients with sarcoidosis. It is important to educate employers and physicians who decide about such issues as sick leave that the absence of objective parameters does not always guarantee that persons are healthy.

Summary

The QOL and HS are impaired in patients suffering from sarcoidosis, especially in those with clinical symptoms. Fatigue is an integral part of the clinical picture of sarcoidosis. Although fatigue is a well-known symptom of sarcoidosis, it remains an underestimated problem in clinical practice. Objective test results, such as chest radiographs and laboratory parameters, do not always correlate with the well-being of the patient. Present studies are generally cross-sectional. There is a need for prospective follow-up studies assessing the natural course of patients' disease in relation to symptoms and QOL.

Appendix 1

Fatigue Assessment Scale

The following ten statements refer to how you usually feel. Per statement you can choose one out of five answer categories, varying from never to always. 1 = never, 2 = sometimes; 3 = regularly; 4 = often and 5 = always

		Never	Sometimes	Regularly	Often	Always
1.	I am bothered by fatigue	1	2	3	4	5
2.	I get tired very quickly	1	2	3	4	5
3.	I don't do much during the day	1	2	3	4	5
4.	I have enough energy for everyday life[a]	1	2	3	4	5
5.	Physically, I feel exhausted	1	2	3	4	5
6.	I have problems to start things	1	2	3	4	5
7.	I have problems to think clearly	1	2	3	4	5
8.	I feel no desire to do anything	1	2	3	4	5
9.	Mentally, I feel exhausted	1	2	3	4	5
10.	When I am doing something, I can concentrate quite well[a]	1	2	3	4	5

Based on large representative samples of the Dutch population, the cut-off score of the FAS is 21, ie, scores of ≥ 22 are considered to represent substantial fatigue.

[a] Scores on questions 4 and 10 should be recoded (1 = 5; 2 = 4; 3 = 3; 4 = 2; 5 = 1). Subsequently, the total FAS score can be calculated by summing the scores on all questions (the recoded scores for questions 4 and 10). For a digital version see http://www.ildcare.eu/pages/artsen_informatie_fasen.html.

References

[1] Iannuzzi MC, Rybicki BA, Teirstein AS. Sarcoidosis. N Engl J Med 2007;357:2153–65.

[2] Wirnsberger RM, De Vries J, Wouters EF, et al. Clinical presentation of sarcoidosis in The Netherlands: an epidemiological study. Neth J Med 1998;53:53–60.

[3] Drent M, Wirnsberger RM, Breteler MH, et al. Quality of life and depressive symptoms in patients suffering from sarcoidosis. Sarcoidosis Vasc Diffuse Lung Dis 1998;15:59–66.

[4] Wirnsberger RM, De Vries J, Breteler MH, et al. Evaluation of quality of life in sarcoidosis patients. Respir Med 1998;92:750–6.

[5] De Vries J, Wirnsberger RM. Fatigue, quality of life, and health status in sarcoidosis. Eur Respir Mon 2005;10:92–104.

[6] Michielsen HJ, Peros-Golubicic T, Drent M, et al. Relationship between symptoms and quality of life in a sarcoidosis population. Respiration 2007;74:401–5.

[7] De Vries J. Quality of life assessment. In: Vingerhoets AJJM, editor. Assessment in behavioural medicine. Hove (England): Brunner-Routledge; 2001. p. 353–70.

[8] Curtis JR, Patrick DL. The assessment of health status among patients with COPD. Eur Respir J 2003; 41:36s–45s.

[9] De Vries J, Seebregts A, Drent M. Assessing health status and quality of life in idiopathic pulmonary fibrosis: which measure should be used? Respir Med 2000;94:273–8.

[10] Michielsen HJ, Drent M, Peros-Golubicic T, et al. Fatigue is associated with quality of life in sarcoidosis patients. Chest 2006;130:989–94.

[11] De Vries J, Drent M, Van Heck GL, et al. Quality of life in sarcoidosis: a comparison between members of a patient organization and a random sample. Sarcoidosis Vasc Diffuse Lung Dis 1998;15:183–8.

[12] De Vries J, Van Heck GL, Drent M. Gender differences in sarcoidosis: symptoms, quality of life and medical consumption. Women Health 1999;30:99–114.

[13] Wirnsberger RM, De Vries J, Jansen TL, et al. Impairment of quality of life: rheumatoid arthritis versus sarcoidosis. Neth J Med 1999;54:86–95.

[14] Hoitsma E, Faber CG, Drent M, et al. Neurosarcoidosis: a clinical dilemma. Lancet Neurol 2004;3:397–407.

[15] Hoitsma E, Faber CG, van Santen-Hoeufft M, et al. Improvement of small fiber neuropathy in a sarcoidosis patient after treatment with infliximab. Sarcoidosis Vasc Diffuse Lung Dis 2006;23:73–7.

[16] Wirnsberger RM, Drent M, Hekelaar N, et al. Relationship between respiratory muscle function and quality of life in sarcoidosis. Eur Respir J 1997;10:1450–5.

[17] Antoniou KM, Tzanakis N, Tzouvelekis A, et al. Quality of life in patients with active sarcoidosis in Greece. Eur J Intern Med 2006;17:421–6.

[18] Cox CE, Donohue JF, Brown CD, et al. Health-related quality of life of persons with sarcoidosis. Chest 2004;125:997–1004.

[19] Yeager H, Rossman MD, Baughman RP, et al. Pulmonary and psychosocial findings at enrollment in the ACCESS study. Sarcoidosis Vasc Diffuse Lung Dis 2005;22:147–53.

[20] Baughman RP, Sparkman BK, Lower EE. Six-minute walk test and health status assessment in sarcoidosis. Chest 2007;132:207–13.

[21] Baughman RP, Iannuzzi MC, Lower EE, et al. Use of fluticasone in acute symptomatic pulmonary sarcoidosis. Sarcoidosis Vasc Diffuse Lung Dis 2002;19: 198–204.

[22] Chang JA, Curtis JR, Patrick DL, et al. Assessment of health-related quality of life in patients with interstitial lung disease. Chest 1999;116:1175–82.

[23] Breek JC, De Vries J, Van Heck GL, et al. Assessment of disease impact in patients with intermittent claudication: discrepancy between health status and quality of life. J Vasc Surg 2005;41:443–50.

[24] Testa MA. Methods and applications of quality-of-life measurement during antihypertensive therapy. Curr Hypertens Rep 2000;2:530–7.

[25] Bradley C. Importance of differentiating health status from quality of life. Lancet 2001;357:7–8.

[26] Montazeri A, Milroy R, Gillis CR, et al. Quality of life: perception of lung cancer patients. Eur J Cancer 1996;32A:2284–9.

[27] WHOQOL group. Field trial WHOQOL-100 February 1995; facet definitions and questions. Geneva (IL): WHO(MNH/PSF/95.1.B); 1995.

[28] WHOQOL group. The World Health Organization quality of life assessment (WHOQOL): position paper from the World Health Organization. Soc Sci Med 1995;41:1403–9.

[29] Guyatt GH, Berman LB, Townsend M, et al. A measure of quality of life for clinical trials in chronic lung disease. Thorax 1987;42:773–8.

[30] Guyatt GH, Townsend M, Keller J, et al. Measuring functional status in chronic lung disease: conclusions from a randomised control trial. Respir Med 1989; 83:293–7.

[31] Wijkstra PJ, Ten Vergert EM, Van Altena R, et al. Reliability and validity of the chronic respiratory questionnaire (CRQ). Thorax 1994;49:465–7.

[32] Ware JE Jr, Snow KK, Gandek B. SF-36 health survey. Manual and interpretation guide. Boston: The Health Institute, New England Medical Center; 1993.

[33] Bowling A. Measuring disease: a review of disease-specific quality of life measurement scales. Buckingham (London): Open University Press; 1995.

[34] Cox CE, Donohue JF, Brown CD, et al. The Sarcoidosis Health Questionnaire: a new measure of health-related quality of life. Am J Respir Crit Care Med 2003;168:323–9.

[35] Bergner M, Bobbitt RA, Carter WB, et al. The sickness impact profile: development and final revision of a health-status measure. Med Care 1981;19: 787–805.

[36] Jones PW, Quirk FH, Baveystock CM. The St. George's respiratory questionnaire. Respir Med 1991;85:25–31.

[37] Jones PW, Bosh TK. Quality of life changes in COPD patients treated with salmeterol. Am J Respir Crit Care Med 1997;155:1283–9.

[38] Jones PW, Nedocromil Sodium Quality of Life Study Group. Quality of life, symptoms and pulmonary function in asthma: long-term treatment with

nedocromil sodium examined in a controlled multi-centre trial. Eur Respir J 1994;7:55–62.

[39] Jones PW, Quirk FH, Baveystock CM, et al. A self-complete measure of health status for chronic airflow limitation: the St George's respiratory questionnaire. Am Rev Respir Dis 1992;145:1321–7.

[40] De Vries J, Rothkrantz-Kos S, van Dieijen-Visser MP, et al. The relationship between fatigue and clinical parameters in pulmonary sarcoidosis. Sarcoidosis Vasc Diffuse Lung Dis 2004;21:127–36.

[41] De Vries J, Michielsen HJ, Van Heck L, et al. Measuring fatigue in sarcoidosis: the fatigue assessment scale (FAS). Br J Health Psychol 2004; 9:279–91.

[42] Michielsen HJ, De Vries J, Drent M, et al. Psychometric qualities of the fatigue assessment scale in Croatian sarcoidosis patients. Sarcoidosis Vasc Diffuse Lung Dis 2005;22:133–8.

[43] Lichtenstein GR, Bala M, Han C, et al. Infliximab improves quality of life in patients with Crohn's disease. Inflamm Bowel Dis 2002;8:237–43.

[44] Mittendorf T, Dietz B, Sterz R, et al. Improvement and longterm maintenance of quality of life during treatment with adalimumab in severe rheumatoid arthritis. J Rheumatol 2007;34:2343–50.

[45] Turner GA, Lower EE, Corser BC, et al. Sleep apnea in sarcoidosis. Sarcoidosis Vasc Diffuse Lung Dis 1997;14:61–4.

[46] Verbraecken J, Hoitsma E, van der Grinten CP, et al. Sleep disturbances associated with periodic leg movements in chronic sarcoidosis. Sarcoidosis Vasc Diffuse Lung Dis 2004;21:137–46.

[47] Spruit MA, Thomeer MJ, Gosselink R, et al. Skeletal muscle weakness in patients with sarcoidosis and its relationship with exercise intolerance and reduced health status. Thorax 2005;60:32–8.

ELSEVIER
SAUNDERS

Clin Chest Med 29 (2008) 533–548

CLINICS
IN CHEST
MEDICINE

Treatment of Sarcoidosis

Robert P. Baughman, MD[a],*, Ulrich Costabel, MD[b],
Ronald M. du Bois, MD[c]

[a]Department of Medicine, University of Cincinnati Medical Center, 1001 Holmes, Eden Avenue,
Cincinnati, OH 45267-0565, USA
[b]Department of Pneumology/Allergy, Ruhrlandklinik Essen, Tüschener route 40, D-45239 Essen, Germany
[c]National Jewish Medical Center, 1400 Jackson Street, Denver, CO 80206, USA

The clinical presentation and outcome of sarcoidosis vary considerably. As a result, treatment also varies. The options range from no treatment to a range of agents, including cytotoxic and biological agents [1,2]. Elsewhere in this issue, authors have discussed treatment of various manifestations of sarcoidosis. This reviews specific agents that have been reported as useful in treating sarcoidosis. It also discusses the indications for various agents. For many of the agents, the decision to treat is based on the duration of symptomatic disease and the severity of disease.

Classification of sarcoidosis outcome

The outcome of sarcoidosis can be considered conceptually in three broad and at least partially overlapping groupings:

Acute disease—resolves within 2 to 5 years of time of diagnosis residual defects are fibrosis, not ongoing inflammation
Chronic disease—persists beyond 5 years after diagnosis
Refractory disease—chronic disease that worsens despite adequate systemic therapy

The authors have defined acute disease as disease that resolves within 5 years. Any residual abnormality is not caused by active inflammation but previous inflammation leaving scar tissue. An example of this prolonged effect is the sicca

syndrome, which is a common manifestation of previous lachrymal gland involvement. Chronic disease is considered here to be disease that persists with active inflammation beyond 5 years. Many of these patients will be receiving continuing therapy, but some patients who have chronic disease may not require any systemic therapy. The third group is refractory disease, which is defined as disease that worsens despite adequate systemic therapy. One example of refractory disease is the patient with spinal cord sarcoidosis who develops worsening neurologic deficit despite adequate doses of prednisone with or without immunosuppression [3].

The time at which the disease changes from acute to chronic is debated. Some authors have chosen to use 2 years [4,5]. Others have noted that the rate of resolution of bilateral hilar adenopathy may take up to 5 years [6]. One study proposed an intermediate group, defined as those with resolution between 2 and five 5 after presentation [7]. The decision to use 5 years to separate acute from chronic disease is based on a review of the literature and the results of a task force of the World Association of Sarcoidosis and Other Granulomatous diseases (WASOG). That task force noted that the clinical outcome of patients changed in 40% of cases between years 2 and 5.

One of the early studies systematically examining clinical outcome involved follow-up of a group of 818 sarcoidosis patients and found that some features were associated with resolution within 2 to 5 years, while others were not [4]. Table 1 lists some of the features that characteristically resolve within a few years after diagnosis and those features that are usually more persistent [4,8].

* Corresponding author.
E-mail address: baughmrp@ucmail.uc.edu
(R.P. Baughman).

Table 1
Features associated with acute compared
with chronic disease

Feature	Acute	Chronic
Pulmonary	Hilar adenopathy alone	Pulmonary fibrosis
Cutaneous	Erythema nodosum	Lupus pernio
Ocular	Anterior uveitis	Panuveitis
Neurologic	Isolate seventh nerve paralysis	Mass in head or spine
Cardiac		Congestive heart failure
Calcium metabolism		Nephrolithiasis
Musculoskeletal	Peri articular swelling	Bone cysts
Symptoms	Asymptomatic	Dyspnea

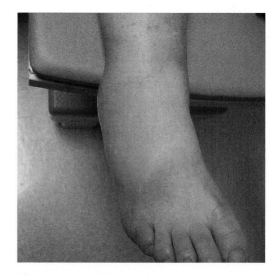

Fig. 1. 51-year-old Caucasian woman with abrupt onset of peri-articular arthritis and red, painful nodules (erythema nodosum). Her chest roentgenogram revealed symmetric hilar adenopathy. Shown are marked swelling of her right ankle and erythema nodosum.

For pulmonary disease, the presence of hilar adenopathy alone usually is associated with a good prognosis [4]. By contrast, the presence of pulmonary fibrosis is associated with chronic disease [4]. Pulmonary fibrosis is also associated with a worse clinical outcome, including pulmonary hypertension [9] and increased mortality [10]. Moderate-to-severe dyspnea at presentation was an independent predictor of the need for systemic therapy for more than 2 years after diagnosis [5].

Erythema nodosum in the Caucasian population is associated with a high rate if resolution [11]. This may be because Caucasian patients who have erythema nodosum often have associated hilar adenopathy and peri-articular arthritis of the lower extremities (Fig. 1). This triad is known as Lofgren's syndrome, in honor of the clinician who described it originally [12]; a good prognosis is associated with this manifestation of the disease. However, up to 20% of patients who have Lofgren's syndrome will develop chronic disease [13]. Recent studies of HLA alleles in the DQ and DR loci have shown that carriage of the DR3/DQB1*0201 haplotype predicts those patients with Lofgren's syndrome who will have a good prognosis, and this carriage may be useful as a clinical screening index [14,15]. Erythema nodosum in the African American and West Indian population is not associated with a high rate of resolution [11], and lupus pernio almost always is associated with a chronic course [16,17]. Although this manifestation is usually in African Americans or West Indians, it can be seen in Caucasians [16]. Lupus pernio also can be refractory to conventional therapy [18].

Anterior uveitis is often a self-limited form of ocular disease [19,20]. Ocular disease is found in more than 60% of Japanese sarcoidosis patients and is associated with a good prognosis in most cases [21]. Posterior and pan uveitis are associated with chronic disease [19,21], and some cases can be refractory to corticosteroids alone [22].

Neurologic and cardiac diseases usually are associated with chronic disease [4]. Patients who have seventh nerve paralysis, however, often have a rapid resolution and usually no significant residual clinical deficit [23]. Patients who have spinal or central nervous system involvement often require years of therapy, and are sometimes refractory to conventional therapy with corticosteroids alone [3,23,24]. Similarly, cardiac disease, especially congestive heart failure, often will require lifetime therapy [25].

Hypercalcemia may resolve without long-term problems. It has been shown, however, that hypercalciuria and associated nephrolithiasis are associated with chronic disease [8,26]. Although this may not lead to refractory disease, steroid alternatives such as chloroquine or hydroxychloroquine often are used because of their low toxicity [27].

Musculoskeletal complaints are common among patients with sarcoidosis. The particular complaint of peri-articular swelling of the ankles (see Fig. 1), however, is associated with Lofgren's syndrome [13]. In men, the swelling may occur without evidence of erythema nodosum [15]. This is associated with a high rate of resolution within a few months [15]. By contrast, bone cysts are associated with a chronic form of the disease [4,28].

The presenting symptoms of the patient are also useful in determining the clinical outcome. The asymptomatic patient usually requires no long-term treatment [29,30]. By contrast, the patient who has moderate-to-severe dyspnea has an increased risk for requiring treatment for 2 years, independent of his or her chest roentgenogram or pulmonary function studies [5].

Treatment strategies

Acute disease

During the first 2 to 5 years after diagnosis, an individual patient can be considered to have acute disease. There are some clinical features that predict chronic disease, but specificity is not total (see Table 1). It is appropriate, therefore, to not assume that chronicity is inevitable because of their presence but to await the passage of time. Fig. 2 demonstrates this approach to the patient who has disease of known duration less than 5 years. A significant percentage of these patients do not have sufficiently severe symptoms to require therapy [5,29–32]. In a recent trial of newly diagnosed patients with sarcoidosis in the United States, it was noted that only half of the patients were receiving systemic therapy within the first 6

months of diagnosis [5]. At 2- year follow-up, only half of the patients on therapy at the initial visit still were receiving treatment. Of the patients not receiving therapy in the first 6 months, only 10% were on therapy at 2 years. Thus a patient presenting with no symptoms has a good chance of never requiring therapy.

For patients who have symptoms from a single organ, topical therapy often can control the disease. This usually means a high-potency topical corticosteroid that has minimal absorption. For the eye, local therapy includes not only eye drops, but also peri-ocular steroid injections [20]. For the skin, topical therapy with fluorinated corticosteroids are often successful [33]. Other reported treatments include topical tacrolimus [34] and laser treatment [35].

Pulmonary disease is the most common manifestation of sarcoidosis [36], and pulmonary symptoms are the most common reason for treatment [5]. The role of topical therapy for pulmonary disease remains unclear, but on balance it is thought to be ineffective when used in isolation. Budesonide has been the most extensively studied inhaled corticosteroid. In a placebo-controlled, randomized trial, budesonide was superior to placebo in improving lung function after 18 months of therapy [37]. Even though therapy was withdrawn after 18 months, the difference remained significant at 5-year follow-up [38]. The study design consisted of 3 months of systemic therapy followed by 15 months of inhaled treatment, so

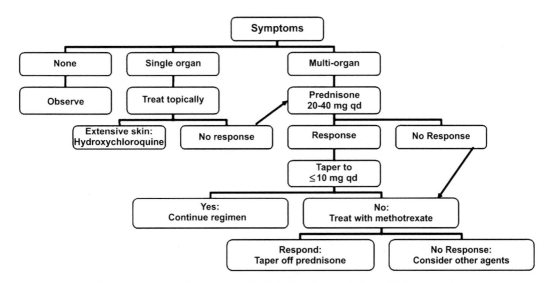

Fig. 2. A suggested treatment strategy for acute sarcoidosis (within 5 years of diagnosis). Severe single organ sarcoidosis, including neuro or cardiac, should be treated the same as multiorgan sarcoidosis.

this study was assessing more than just the efficacy of inhaled therapy. It also was limited to those patients without symptoms requiring systemic therapy. Furthermore, the difference was noted only for those with parenchymal lung disease on chest roentgenogram (Scadding stages 2 and 3). Although others have reported on the benefit of using budesonide for pulmonary sarcoidosis [39–41], others have not seen improvement for symptomatic patients [42]. Two studies of inhaled fluticasone failed to demonstrate any steroid-sparing effect or significant improvement in pulmonary function studies [43,44]. One study suggested inhaled fluticasone might help modify cough in acute sarcoidosis [43].

For extensive cutaneous disease, the antimalarial agents have been useful [45,46]. Chloroquine and hydroxychloroquine have been found to be effective in over half of the reported cases [45]. Other agents used for extensive cutaneous disease, such as thalidomide and infliximab, usually have been given for disease designated as chronic or refractory.

For the patient who has severe single organ (eg, cardiac, neurologic) disease, multiorgan disease, or failing topical therapy, glucocorticoids are considered the first choice of treatment [1,47]. The initial dose of prednisone that is employed is quite variable from center to center, but most clinicians choose between 20 to 40 mg/d of prednisone or the equivalent [47,48]. A key issue with corticosteroid therapy is tapering the dose within an acceptable time period. During this phase of treatment, the clinician is trying to establish the minimal dose associated with control of disease after

achieving maximum improvement [48]. Although no specific guidelines or studies exist that define the recommended rate or method of tapering, one multicenter study found that patient reassessment every 6 weeks with dose halving if improvement was sustained was an acceptable tapering regimen. In 85% of instances, this schedule could be followed at each of the visits [43].

If the patient relapses while reducing the dose of glucocorticoid, or if the symptoms simply cannot be controlled with glucocorticoids alone, a steroid-sparing alternative often is introduced. Methotrexate has been shown to be steroid sparing in acute pulmonary sarcoidosis [49]. Other agents such as chloroquine and azathioprine also may be useful here, although they have not been studied for this indication. For the patient who fails this second line of therapy, the strategies adapted for chronic therapy are appropriate.

Chronic therapy

In a study of unselected cases in the United States, a third of patients required treatment more than 2 years after diagnosis [5], similar to the rate reported by Rizzato and colleagues [32] at a single center. Others have reported a range of chronic disease from 10% [31] to over 60% [30]. This group of patients represents a significant clinical problem, because they will require long-term monitoring not only for response to therapy, but also for toxicity from treatment.

Fig. 3 shows one possible approach to the patient who has chronic disease. The assumption that underpins this strategy is that the patient

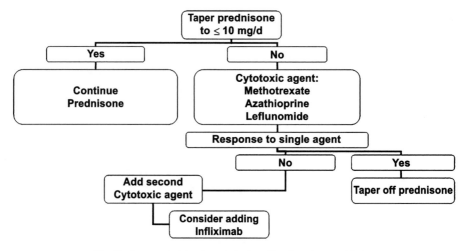

Fig. 3. A suggested treatment strategy for chronic sarcoidosis.

requires systemic therapy for disease control. For those patients who have limited disease, topical therapy may be sufficient. For the patient who requires systemic treatment for symptomatic or severe disease, however, prednisone remains the drug of choice as first line. Again, the physician will try to taper the dose. If the daily dose is less than or equal to 10 mg/d, then it is a reasonable approach to continue this dosage provided that adverse side effect profile is acceptable. If the dose cannot be decreased without worsening disease, however, then steroid-sparing alternatives such as cytotoxic agents should be considered.

The cytotoxic agents commonly considered in chronic sarcoidosis include methotrexate [50,51], azathioprine [52,53], mycophenolate [54], cyclophosphamide, and leflunomide [55]. Chlorambucil has been used with good effect in some cases [56], but is used infrequently because of its higher toxicity; it no longer should be considered. These cytotoxic agents all appear to be about equally effective, although there have been no large formal studies of comparison. The only cytotoxic agent that appears to be more effective than others is cyclophosphamide, for which one study showed that it provided benefit to 9 of 10 cases in which methotrexate did not improve neurosarcoidosis [23].

Although all of these agents have been reported to be useful in treating sarcoidosis, the largest experience has been with methotrexate [50,51,57]. Fig. 4 summarizes the reported response rate for methotrexate in treating pulmonary, cutaneous, ocular, and neurologic disease [23,50,58]. This overall response rate for methotrexate is similar to that reported by other centers [51,59].

Combinations of cytotoxic agents have been used in rheumatologic diseases [60,61]. One report of combination therapy in patients who have sarcoidosis has shown the benefit of adding leflunomide to methotrexate [55]. Combinations of these and other cytotoxic agents require monitoring for cumulative toxicity, including gastrointestinal (GI), hematologic, and hepatic adverse effects.

The antimalarial agents have been reported as useful for chronic cutaneous disease [45,62,63]. The drugs also have proved useful in treating problems with calcium metabolism [27,64]. Given the low toxicity of these agents, they are appealing for treating chronic problems such as nephrolithiasis and chronic skin lesions. One randomized study demonstrated chronic chloroquine therapy reduced the rate of loss of lung function in chronic pulmonary sarcoidosis [65]. Others have reported on the usefulness of antimalarial agents in treating neurosarcoidosis [66].

Refractory disease

The sarcoidosis patient who is failing therapy may be refractory for several reasons:

Noncompliance
Fibrotic disease with no further inflammation

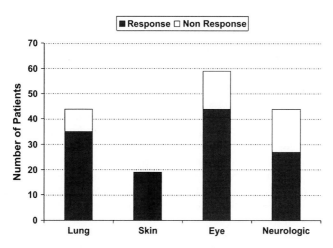

Fig. 4. Results of treatment of various manifestations of sarcoidosis at one institution. Lung response required at least 15% improvement of vital capacity [50]. Other organs were considered improved if there was a greater than 50% resolution of the target lesion and/or reduction of prednisone dose to less than 10 mg/d without worsening of disease [23,50,58].

Secondary complication on disease, including
   pulmonary hypertension, hydrocephalus, or
   cataracts
Complication of therapy
Steroid resistance

Noncompliance to therapy always should be
considered a reason the patient is not doing well,
and noncompliance is often because of the fear of
or development of an adverse effect. The public
knows the toxicity of corticosteroids, and the
profile includes diabetes mellitus, hypertension,
weight gain, osteoporosis, dyspepsia, insomnia,
and mood swings. In one study, one or more of
these effects was noted in more than half the
patients treated with 10 mg or more of prednisone
[49]. The negative impact of corticosteroids
greatly affects the quality of life of the patient
who has sarcoidosis [67].

Patients who have fibrosis without further
inflammation may be considered refractory. In
this situation, the clinician no longer can demonstrate improvement with any anti-inflammatory
regimen. However, they may respond to other
agents. Complications of the disease also may
lead to clinical worsening. Examples include
hydrocephalus, secondary to previous choroid
plexus damage from meningitis [23] that may
require ventriculostomy [68]; pulmonary hypertension (the subject of another article in this issue)
can cause refractory dyspnea [69,70], and complications of therapy can include infection [71].

Steroid resistance also can cause refractory
disease. This phenomenon has been documented
in asthma. In that situation, steroid resistant
asthma is associated with an impairment of
glucocorticoid signaling that normally blocks
cytokine gene transcription [72–74]. In sarcoidosis, one group found that some sarcoidosis
patients showed worsening disease despite corticosteroid therapy [75]. Alveolar macrophages from
these patients were found to be spontaneously
releasing tumor necrosis factor (TNF) at high
levels, implying failure of corticosteroid suppression [75]. This observation has led to the hypothesis that TNF could be a target for treatment in
refractory sarcoidosis patients, although the link
between TNF production and worsening disease
has not been elucidated fully [76].

Thalidomide is a drug with a range of activity,
including anti-TNF effect. It has been shown to be
effective for chronic cutaneous sarcoidosis in
observational studies [16,77]. However, it has
not proved a reliable steroid-sparing agent for

pulmonary disease [16,78]. One of the limitations
of the drug is toxicity, including hypersomnolence
and peripheral neuropathy. Both toxicities are
dose-dependant [16]. Because pulmonary disease
appears to require a higher dose of thalidomide
to have an effect, the role of the agent in pulmonary
disease is unclear [78]. Given the variability of patient response, the agent still may be useful as an
adjunct to therapy in selected refractory cases.

Infliximab is a chimeric monoclonal antibody
against TNF-α, which has been shown to be
effective for refractory sarcoidosis. The initial
positive case reports [18,79] led to a series of clinical series showing benefit for refractory disease,
including extrapulmonary manifestations such as
eye and skin [80–83]. These positive observations
led to two double-blind randomized, placebo-
controlled trials showing benefit for infliximab in
treating chronic pulmonary disease [84,85]. Both
of these studies demonstrated an improvement in
the forced vital capacity (FVC) (Fig. 5). The
larger study demonstrated a significant improvement compared with placebo [84]. A secondary
analysis of the study by Baughman and colleagues
[84] demonstrated a larger improvement for those
patients who had a lower FVC percent predicted
at baseline. The mean improvement in FVC percent predicted was even larger in the study by
Rossman and colleagues [85], who treated patients
with a more severe reduction in FVC.

Other biologic agents with specific anti-TNF
activity include etanerecept and adalimumab. Etanercept is a soluble TNF receptor that binds TNF
in the circulation. It was shown to be effective as
a single agent in pulmonary sarcoidosis in less
than 40% of cases in an open-label trial [86].
That study was discontinued early, because the
authors felt the response rate was too low to
justify the potential adverse effects of the drug.
Patients with refractory sarcoidosis-associated
uveitis who had active disease despite at least
6 months of methotrexate therapy were enrolled
in a double-blind, randomized, placebo-controlled
trial of etanercept [22]. There was no difference in
the response rate.

Adalimumab is a humanized monoclonal antibody against TNF. It is given subcutaneously,
rather than by the intravenous route for infliximab. To date, only a few case reports and one
case series have reported its value in sarcoidosis
[87–89]. The drug seems to have some efficacy, but
the response rate was not as high as that seen with
infliximab [87]. A higher response rate may
be seen with the use of a more intensive dose

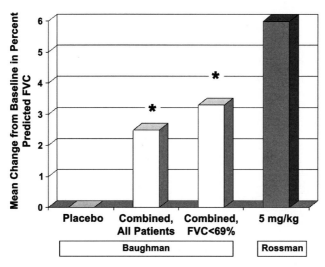

Fig. 5. The mean change from baseline in the percent predicted forced vital capacity (FVC) 6 months after starting therapy, derived from two randomized trials of infliximab. The report by Baughman and colleagues included 138 patients, comprising three treatment groups (placebo, 3 mg/kg, and 5 mg/kg). There was a significant improvement in percent predicted FVC for patients treated with 3 or 5 mg/kg compared with placebo (* = $P < .05$). This difference was larger for those who had a pretreatment FVC less than 69% (the median of all patients in the study) (* = $P < .05$) [84]. The report by Rossman and colleagues comprised 19 patients with chronic pulmonary sarcoidosis who received 5 mg/kg infliximab either initially (13 patients) or delayed (6 patients). For the 13 patients treated with infliximab initially, the mean FVC percent predicted before therapy was 59.6%. The improvement in FVC percent predicted 22 weeks after two treatments with infliximab is shown [85].

regimen, as recently reported for Crohn's disease [90]. Because the drug can be used in patients who are intolerant to infliximab [90], it may have a role for selected patients who are considered for treatment with anti-TNF agents.

Individual agents

Several of the drugs used to treat sarcoidosis have been employed for all three categories of disease (acute, chronic, and refractory). Table 2 summarizes the individual drugs, their indications, their usual doses, common adverse effects, and monitoring recommendations. Most of these recommendations are not evidence-based, because there remains a paucity of randomized clinical trials to support the use of these drugs, and even less information regarding one dose versus another [47,91,92].

Of the glucocorticoids, prednisone is used commonly in the United States, while prednisolone is used commonly in Europe. Prednisone and prednisolone have been studied in widely for treating pulmonary and extrapulmonary sarcoidosis [47,91]. Several randomized trials have compared glucocorticoids with placebo in the

treatment of acute disease [29,93–95]. Although the results of these trials have shown conflicting results, meta-analysis has demonstrated that corticosteroids are associated with significant improvement in chest roentgenogram and diffusion capacity (transfer factor) [91]. This meta-analysis failed to demonstrate a significant improvement in vital capacity with glucocorticoid therapy.

Toxicity is a major concern with chronic glucocorticoid use. For many years, the toxicity of this class of drugs was minimized by physicians. This was in part because there were felt to be few good alternatives. As steroid-sparing agents have become available, physicians have become more careful about toxicity. Weight gain is a problem with prolonged treatment for chronic disease [43,96]. In one trial, the median weight gain after 6 months of prednisone was 25 pounds, with the maximum being 45 pounds [49]. Worsening diabetes and hypertension also were seen in this study [49]. The higher the dose of prednisone, the more weight was gained [43]. Infections are also a complication of chronic corticosteroid use. In a prospective study of 753 sarcoidosis patients followed for 18 months at one sarcoidosis clinic, deep-seated fungal infections were identified in

Table 2
Drugs commonly used to treat sarcoidosis

Drug	Indication	Dosage	Common/important adverse effects	Specific monitoring
Prednisone/ prednisolone	Acute, chronic, refractory	40 mg daily initially; 5–40 mg chronically	Weight gain, diabetes, hypertension, osteoporosis, infection	Bone density, blood glucose/hemoglobin A1c, weight, blood pressure
Hydroxychloroquine	Acute, chronic	200–400 mg daily	Ocular, rash	Eye examination every 6–12 months
Chloroquine	Acute, chronic	250–500 mg daily	Ocular. rash	Eye examination every 6–12 months
Methotrexate	Chronic, refractory	10–15 mg once a week	Nausea, leukopenia, hepatic, pulmonary	CBC, renal, hepatic every 1–3 months; consider liver biopsy every 2–3 years
Azathioprine	Chronic, refractory	50–200 mg daily	Nausea, leukopenia, hepatic infections	CBC, hepatic every 1–3 months
Mycophenolate	Chronic, refractory	500–3000 mg daily	Nausea, diarrhea, leukopenia, infections	CBC, hepatic every 1–3 months
Cyclophosphamide	Refractory	500–2000 mg intravenously every 2–4 weeks	Nausea, leukopenia, infections, hemorrhagic cystitis, cancer	CBC, renal before each dose, Urine analysis once a month Cystoscopy for unexplained hematuria
Thalidomide	Chronic Refractory	50–200 mg orally at night	Teratogenic somnolence, constipation, peripheral neuropathy	Pregnancy testing monthly
Minocycline	Acute, chronic	100–200 mg daily	Nausea, anemia, rash	
Infliximab	Chronic, refractory	3–5 mg/kg initially, 2 weeks later, then every 1–2 months	Infection, allergic reaction, teratogenic	PPD before first dose, careful monitoring during each infusion

Abbreviations: CBC, complete blood counts; liver, liver function tests; PPD, purified protein derivative skin test; renal, renal function including serum creatinine.

seven cases [71]. All seven patients were receiving prednisone, with four patients also receiving methotrexate.

Osteopenia and osteoporosis are recognized complications of chronic glucocorticoid use, even for patients receiving no more than 10 mg/d of prednisone or its equivalent [97,98]. Osteoporosis has been found commonly in sarcoidosis patients treated with corticosteroids [99,100]. Recommendations for screening for osteoporosis include routine use of bone density studies [101,102]. These same groups recommend the use of supplemental calcium and vitamin D for patients at risk for osteoporosis, which includes patients on chronic glucocorticoids [101,102]. For sarcoidosis patients, high levels of endogenous vitamin D3-1,25 question the rationale for calcium and vitamin D supplementation. Their use could lead to hypercalcemia or hypercalciuria [103,104]. As a minimum, serum calcium levels should be monitored regularly, and symptoms suggestive of nephrolithiasis should be elicited by directed questioning in all patients receiving calcium and vitamin D supplements. Less controversial is the use of bisphosphonates for sarcoidosis patients on high doses of glucocorticoids. Studies have demonstrated the safety and efficacy of these drugs for these patients, and it could be argued that they should receive them as first-line protection rather than calcium/vitamin D [105–107].

Antimalarial agents

Only two antimalarial agents have been used widely in sarcoidosis: chloroquine and hydroxychloroquine [46,66,92]. Although both of these drugs have proved useful for sarcoidosis, chloroquine has a higher reported response rate than hydroxychloroquine [45]. Chloroquine also has been demonstrated to slow the progression of chronic pulmonary disease compared with placebo [65]. Chloroquine, however, is associated with more toxicity, especially the potential of direct retinal damage [108,109], with one report of greater than a third of patients on prolonged treatment with chloroquine developing ocular toxicity [110]. Renal dysfunction is a risk factor for ocular toxicity [110]. Hydroxychloroquine is associated with a much lower rate of retinal toxicity, as recently reviewed by Yam and Kwok [111]. Most cases occurred in patients being treated with more than 400 mg/d. For patients treated with anti-malarial agents, screening for ocular toxicity by an ophthalmologist is recommended every 6–12 months [108,112,113].

Methotrexate

This drug is the most widely reported cytotoxic agent used to treat sarcoidosis [47,51]. The drug has been demonstrated to be effective for lung, skin, eye, and neurologic disease [23,45,50,51]. Approximately two thirds of patients will respond to treatment, although higher rates of response have been reported in one large series [51]. The drug is well-tolerated, with nausea and leucopenia the most common adverse effects. These usually respond to dose reduction [114]. Less common but serious complications include pulmonary toxicity [115] and increased risk for opportunistic infections [71]. Hepatotoxicity has been reported with methotrexate, and guidelines have been developed to monitor for hepatoxicity. Although rheumatologists no longer perform routine liver biopsies to monitor for toxicity [116], dermatologists still consider this standard in monitoring methotrexate-treated patients with psoriasis [117]. In sarcoidosis, one group reported on the use of surveillance liver biopsies after every 1 to 1.5 g of cumulative treatment with methotrexate. The rate of methotrexate-related damage was determined to be greater than 10% in this group

[118]. However, none of these patients developed irreversible liver damage. Routine liver function testing every 2 to 3 months should be performed on patients receiving chronic therapy. Persistent elevation of transaminases should be evaluated. Although elevation of alkaline phosphatase is more common with liver involvement from sarcoidosis, transaminase elevation also can be seen as a direct result of sarcoidosis in the liver [118]. If no alternative explanation emerges for chronic elevation of transaminases, than either a liver biopsy should be performed or methotrexate discontinued.

Azathioprine

This agent has been widely used in numerous interstitial lung diseases, including idiopathic pulmonary fibrosis [119,120]. Its use in sarcoidosis appears to be fairly widespread, but there are a limited number of published articles in support of this approach [52,53,121,122]. Although some authors have noted a high response rate [52], others have reported than a less than 20% response [53,122]. This may be a reflection of the circumstances in which it is used. In those studies with a low response rate [53,122], the patients seem to have refractory disease and therefore unlikely to respond. Fig. 6 shows the results of a sequential study of cytotoxic agents for ocular sarcoidosis [58]. For these patients, a nonresponse to methotrexate usually predicted a nonresponse to azathioprine as a single agent. These drugs, however, were effective in more than 70% of cases when used in combination.

The toxicity profile of azathioprine is somewhat similar to methotrexate. It causes nausea and leucopenia, and routine monitoring of the complete blood count is required. Azathioprine is metabolized by thiopurine-methyl-transferase. The enzyme activity is determined genetically, with homozygously deficient patients at risk for severe neutropenia from the drug [123]. Levels of thiopurine-methyl-transferase can be measured and have been used to help direct therapy [124]. An alternative approach, however, is to monitor white counts weeks for 4 weeks, because enzyme-deficient patients will have severe neutropenia soon after commencing treatment. The major advantage of azathioprine is the lower hepatotoxicity reported with the drug than with methotrexate. In patients who have significant hepatic sarcoidosis, azathioprine has been shown to be a very useful steroid-sparing agent, and thus hepatic sarcoidosis is not a contraindication to its use [125].

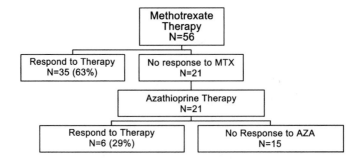

Fig. 6. Outcome of serial treatment of chronic ocular sarcoidosis. Patients initially were treated with methotrexate. After 6 months, patients who had not responded to methotrexate were treated with azathioprine as the only cytotoxic agent. Only six patients who did not respond to methotrexate had a response to azathioprine as a single agent [58].

Leflunomide

This agent was developed as an alternative to methotrexate for rheumatoid arthritis [126]. It has less GI toxicity, but is hepatotoxic. In rheumatoid arthritis, it may be less effective than methotrexate [127]. It has been shown to be effective in treating chronic sarcoidosis [128], with a response rate similar to that reported with methotrexate [55]. Like azathioprine, leflunomide has some differences in toxicity from methotrexate, which can, therefore, make it a reasonable alternative. For example, it has a lower rate of pulmonary toxicity [127], and some patients who have methotrexate-associated pulmonary symptoms have been treated safely with leflunomide [55]. Leflunomide, however, has been associated with pulmonary toxicity in some patients, so patients should be monitored for this potential adverse effect [129]. GI toxicity and hepatotoxicity may occur [127,130]. Although surveillance liver biopsies are not recommended, liver function testing should be done at least every 2 to 3 months. Leflunomide has been shown to be synergistic with methotrexate in treating rheumatoid arthritis [60]. A similar synergism has been observed in sarcoidosis [55].

Mycophenolate

This drug recently has been reported as useful in treating interstitial lung disease associated with collagen vascular disease [131,132]. The drug also has been reported to be effective in treating some patients who have cutaneous [54] or renal [133] sarcoidosis. It is associated with less neutropenia than the traditional cytotoxic agents, but neutropenia can occur. Nausea and diarrhea can be dose-limiting adverse effects of the drug [134].

Cyclophosphamide

This potent cytotoxic agent has been reported to be effective in treating refractory neurosarcoidosis

[23,135]. Both of these reports used intermittent, intravenous treatments. Treatments given every 2 weeks can mimic the effect of daily oral treatment. Toxicity is much lower, however [136]. Major complications include neutropenia, nausea, hemorrhagic cystitis, and increased risk for malignancy. For patients who have Wegener's granulomatosis treated with daily oral cyclophosphamide for more than a year, considerable risk for hemorrhagic cystitis and subsequent bladder cancer has been reported [137]. The drug's toxicity profile limits its use to refractory disease.

Thalidomide

The first reports of the effective treatment of sarcoidosis by thalidomide [138,139] suggested a novel approach [140]. The drug has been shown to suppress TNF release from alveolar macrophages [141,142]. Its effectiveness in sarcoidosis appears to be due to more factors than simply suppression of TNF. In evaluating the treatment of patients who had chronic, cutaneous sarcoidosis, skin biopsies were performed before and after therapy. Oliver and colleagues [143] could not demonstrate a change in TNF levels despite improvement of the skin lesions. The drug appears to affect multiple cytokines involved in the inflammatory response that results in sarcoidosis [142,143]. Thalidomide has been effective in treating chronic disease, such as lupus pernio [16,77,138,139,143,144]. For noncutaneous sarcoidosis, both benefits [77,138] and a limited response [16] have been reported. In this regard, in a study of chronic pulmonary disease, Judson and colleagues found thalidomide was only mildly steroid-sparing [78]. Many of the toxicities of thalidomide, including hypersomnolence, constipation, and peripheral neuropathy, appear to be dose-dependant [16]. Thus, the higher doses needed for some systemic manifestations may not be tolerated. The teratogenicity of thalidomide is not dose-dependant, and patients who receive this drug must not conceive.

Infliximab

The chimeric monoclonal antibody infliximab has been shown to be effective in the treatment of chronic pulmonary sarcoidosis [84,85]. Others have reported its effectiveness for refractory skin [18,81], eye [80], and neurologic [81,145] disease. The drug is given intravenously twice weekly for the first two doses then every 4 to 8 weeks. Efficacy is generally apparent within 6 weeks of commencement of therapy [84,85]. Infusion reactions have been reported in over 20% of patients who have arthritis [146]. An increased risk for infusion reaction was seen in those patients not taking concomitant methotrexate [146]. For patients who had sarcoidosis, the rate of infusion reactions was no different from placebo in one study [84]. These patients, however, were treated for only 6 months. Another concern with infliximab is increased risk for infection [147], especially tuberculosis [148]. The increased risk appears to be for reactivation of latent tuberculosis [148,149]. The anti-TNF biologic agents, including infliximab, have been associated with increased mortality in patients who have advanced congestive heart failure [150]. An unknown factor is the risk for cancer in patients receiving infliximab. For patients treated with infliximab, an increase in lymphoma was found in those with Crohn's disease [151] but not rheumatoid arthritis [152]. Interestingly, there have been cases of sarcoidosis occurring during treatment with infliximab and etanerecept [153,154]. These cases emphasize that symptomatic sarcoidosis is caused by the interactive effects of multiple cytokines and that single therapy is not effective in all patients [155].

The role of other anti-TNF biologic agents for treating sarcoidosis is less clear. The toxicity of these agents is similar to that reported with infliximab, except that there seems to be a lower risk for tuberculosis and other opportunistic infections [148]. There remains a risk of infection, however, but this risk may only be manifest after longer treatment courses [149].

Summary

The use of systemic therapy in sarcoidosis requires a global approach to determine the total effect of drugs on disease symptomatology and time course. Steroid-sparing treatments have become standard for chronic disease. In some cases, refractory disease may require drugs other than corticosteroids. Knowledge of the relative risk and benefits of these agents has to be considered in the care of patients who have sarcoidosis.

References

[1] Hunninghake GW, Costabel U, Ando M, et al. ATS/ERS/WASOG statement on sarcoidosis. American Thoracic Society/European Respiratory Society/World Association of Sarcoidosis and other Granulomatous Disorders. Sarcoidosis Vasc Diffuse Lung Dis 1999;16:149–73.

[2] Baughman RP, du Bois RM, Lower EE. Sarcoidosis. Lancet 2003;361:1111–8.

[3] Bradley DA, Lower EE, Baughman RP. Diagnosis and management of spinal cord sarcoidosis. Sarcoidosis Vasc Diffuse Lung Dis 2006;23(1):58–65.

[4] Neville E, Walker AN, James DG. Prognostic factors predicting the outcome of sarcoidosis: an analysis of 818 patients. Q J Med 1983;208: 525–33.

[5] Baughman RP, Judson MA, Teirstein A, et al. Presenting characteristics as predictors of duration of treatment in sarcoidosis. QJM 2006;99(5):307–15.

[6] Nagai S, Shigematsu M, Hamada K, et al. Clinical courses and prognoses of pulmonary sarcoidosis. Curr Opin Pulm Med 1999;5(5):293–8.

[7] Pietinalho A, Furuya K, Yamaguchi E, et al. The angiotensin-converting enzyme DD gene is associated with poor prognosis in Finnish sarcoidosis patients. Eur Respir J 1999;13:723–6.

[8] Rizzato G, Fraioli P, Montemurro L. Nephrolithiasis as a presenting feature of chronic sarcoidosis. Thorax 1995;50(5):555–9.

[9] Sulica R, Teirstein AS, Kakarla S, et al. Distinctive clinical, radiographic, and functional characteristics of patients with sarcoidosis-related pulmonary hypertension. Chest 2005;128(3):1483–9.

[10] Baughman RP, Winget DB, Bowen EH, et al. Predicting respiratory failure in sarcoidosis patients. Sarcoidosis 1997;14:154–8.

[11] Mana J, Marcoval J. Erythema nodosum. Clin Dermatol 2007;25(3):288–94.

[12] Sharma OP. Sarcoidosis: a historical perspective. Clin Dermatol 2007;25(3):232–41.

[13] Mana J, Gomez VC, Montero A, et al. Lofgren's syndrome revisited: a study of 186 patients. Am J Med 1999;107(3):240–5.

[14] Sato H, Grutters JC, Pantelidis P, et al. HLA-DQB1*0201: a marker for good prognosis in British and Dutch patients with sarcoidosis. Am J Respir Cell Mol Biol 2002;27(4):406–12.

[15] Grunewald J, Eklund A. Sex-specific manifestations of Lofgren's syndrome. Am J Respir Crit Care Med 2007;175(1):40–4.

[16] Baughman RP, Judson MA, Teirstein AS, et al. Thalidomide for chronic sarcoidosis. Chest 2002; 122:227–32.

[17] Spiteri MA, Matthey F, Gordon T, et al. Lupus pernio: a clinico–radiological study of thirty-five cases. Br J Dermatol 1985;112(3):315–22.

[18] Baughman RP, Lower EE. Infliximab for refractory sarcoidosis. Sarcoidosis Vasc Diffuse Lung Dis 2001;18:70–4.

[19] Chan SM, Hudson M, Weis E. Anterior and intermediate uveitis cases referred to a tertiary centre in Alberta. Can J Ophthalmol 2007;42(6):860–4.

[20] Bradley DA, Baughman RP, Raymond L, et al. Ocular manifestations of sarcoidosis. Semin Respir Crit Care Med 2002;23:543–8.

[21] Ohara K, Judson MA, Baughman RP. Clinical aspects of ocular sarcoidosis. In: Drent M, Costabel U, editors. Sarcoidosis. Wakefield (UK): The Charlesworth Group; 2005. p. 188–209.

[22] Baughman RP, Lower EE, Bradley DA, et al. Etanercept for refractory ocular sarcoidosis: results of a double-blind randomized trial. Chest 2005; 128(2):1062–7.

[23] Lower EE, Broderick JP, Brott TG, et al. Diagnosis and management of neurologic sarcoidosis. Arch Intern Med 1997;157:1864–8.

[24] Agbogu BN, Stern BJ, Sewell C, et al. Therapeutic considerations in patients with refractory neurosarcoidosis. Arch Neurol 1995;52:875–9.

[25] Deng JC, Baughman RP, Lynch JP. Cardiac involvement in sarcoidosis. Semin Respir Crit Care Med 2002;23:513–28.

[26] Rizzato G, Colombo P. Nephrolithiasis as a presenting feature of chronic sarcoidosis: a prospective study. Sarcoidosis 1996;13:167–72.

[27] Adams JS, Diz MM, Sharma OP. Effective reduction in the serum 1,25-dihydroxyvitamin D and calcium concentration in sarcoidosis-associated hypercalcemia with short-course chloroquine therapy. Ann Intern Med 1989;111(5):437–8.

[28] Rohatgi PK. Osseous sarcoidosis. Semin Respir Med 1992;13:468–88.

[29] Gibson GJ, Prescott RJ, Muers MF, et al. British Thoracic Society Sarcoidosis study: effects of long-term corticosteroid treatment. Thorax 1996; 51(3):238–47.

[30] Gottlieb JE, Israel HL, Steiner RM, et al. Outcome in sarcoidosis. The relationship of relapse to corticosteroid therapy. Chest 1997;111(3): 623–31.

[31] Hunninghake GW, Gilbert S, Pueringer R, et al. Outcome of the treatment for sarcoidosis. Am J Respir Crit Care Med 1994;149(4 Pt 1):893–8.

[32] Rizzato G, Montemurro L, Colombo P. The late follow-up of chronic sarcoid patients previously treated with corticosteroids. Sarcoidosis 1998;15: 52–8.

[33] Volden G. Successful treatment of chronic skin diseases with clobetasol propionate and a hydrocolloid occlusive dressing. Acta Derm Venereol 1992;72(1):69–71.

[34] Katoh N, Mihara H, Yasuno H. Cutaneous sarcoidosis successfully treated with topical tacrolimus. Br J Dermatol 2002;147(1):154–6.

[35] Cliff S, Felix RH, Singh L, et al. The successful treatment of lupus pernio with the flashlamp pulsed dye laser. J Cutan Laser Ther 1999;1(1):49–52.

[36] Baughman RP, Teirstein AS, Judson MA, et al. Clinical characteristics of patients in a case–control study of sarcoidosis. Am J Respir Crit Care Med 2001;164:1885–9.

[37] Pietinalho A, Tukiainen P, Haahtela T, et al. Oral prednisolone followed by inhaled budesonide in newly diagnosed pulmonary sarcoidosis: a double-blind, placebo-controlled, multicenter study. Chest 1999;116:424–31.

[38] Pietinalho A, Tukiainen P, Haahtela T, et al. Early treatment of stage II sarcoidosis improves 5-year pulmonary function. Chest 2002;121:24–31.

[39] Alberts C, van der Mark TW, Jansen HM. Inhaled budesonide in pulmonary sarcoidosis: a double-blind, placebo-controlled study. Dutch Study Group on Pulmonary Sarcoidosis. Eur Respir J 1995;8(5):682–8.

[40] Spiteri MA, Newman SP, Clarke SW, et al. Inhaled corticosteroids can modulate the immunopathogenesis of pulmonary sarcoidosis. Eur Respir J 1989;2(3):218–24.

[41] Zych D, Pawlicka L, Zielinski J. Inhaled budesonide vs prednisone in the maintenance treatment of pulmonary sarcoidosis. Sarcoidosis 1993;10: 56–61.

[42] Milman N, Graudal N, Grode G, et al. No effect of high-dose inhaled steroids in pulmonary sarcoidosis: a double-blind, placebo-controlled study. J Intern Med 1994;236(3):285–90.

[43] Baughman RP, Iannuzzi MC, Lower EE, et al. Use of fluticasone in acute symptomatic pulmonary sarcoidosis. Sarcoidosis Vasc Diffuse Lung Dis 2002;19(3):198–204.

[44] du Bois RM, Greenhalgh PM, Southcott AM, et al. Randomized trial of inhaled fluticasone propionate in chronic stable pulmonary sarcoidosis: a pilot study. Eur Respir J 1999;13(6):1345–50.

[45] Baughman RP, Lower EE. Evidence-based therapy for cutaneous sarcoidosis. Clin Dermatol 2007; 25(3):334–40.

[46] Siltzbach LE, Teirstein AS. Chloroquine therapy in 43 patients with intrathoracic and cutaneous sarcoidosis. Acta Med Scand 1964;425:302S–8S.

[47] Baughman RP, Selroos O. Evidence-based approach to the treatment of sarcoidosis. In: Gibson PG, Abramson M, Wood-Baker R, editors. Evidence-based respiratory medicine. Malden (MA): Blackwell Publishing Ltd.; 2005. p. 491–508.

[48] Judson MA. An approach to the treatment of pulmonary sarcoidosis with corticosteroids: the six phases of treatment. Chest 1999;115(4):1158–65.

[49] Baughman RP, Winget DB, Lower EE. Methotrexate is steroid sparing in acute sarcoidosis: results of a double blind, randomized trial. Sarcoidosis Vasc Diffuse Lung Dis 2000;17:60–6.

[50] Lower EE, Baughman RP. Prolonged use of methotrexate for sarcoidosis. Arch Intern Med 1995; 155:846–51.

[51] Vucinic VM. What is the future of methotrexate in sarcoidosis? A study and review. Curr Opin Pulm Med 2002;8(5):470–6.

[52] Muller-Quernheim J, Kienast K, Held M, et al. Treatment of chronic sarcoidosis with an azathioprine/prednisolone regimen. Eur Respir J 1999; 14(5):1117–22.

[53] Lewis SJ, Ainslie GM, Bateman ED. Efficacy of azathioprine as second-line treatment in pulmonary sarcoidosis. Sarcoidosis Vasc Diffuse Lung Dis 1999;16:87–92.

[54] Kouba DJ, Mimouni D, Rencic A, et al. Mycophenolate mofetil may serve as a steroid-sparing agent for sarcoidosis. Br J Dermatol 2003;148(1):147–8.

[55] Baughman RP, Lower EE. Leflunomide for chronic sarcoidosis. Sarcoidosis Vasc Diffuse Lung Dis 2004;21:43–8.

[56] Kataria YP. Chlorambucil in sarcoidosis. Chest 1980;78:36–42.

[57] Baughman RP, Lower EE. Alternatives to corticosteroids in the treatment of sarcoidosis. Sarcoidosis 1997;14:121–30.

[58] Baughman RP, Lower EE, Bradley DA, et al. Use of cytotoxic therapy for chronic opthalmic sarcoidosis. Sarcoidosis Vasc Diffuse Lung Dis 1999;16: S17.

[59] Gedalia A, Molina JF, Ellis GS, et al. Low-dose methotrexate therapy for childhood sarcoidosis. J Pediatr 1997;130:25–9.

[60] Kremer JM, Genovese MC, Cannon GW, et al. Concomitant leflunomide therapy in patients with active rheumatoid arthritis despite stable doses of methotrexate. A randomized, double-blind, placebo-controlled trial. Ann Intern Med 2002; 137(9):726–33.

[61] Weinblatt ME, Kremer JM, Coblyn JS, et al. Pharmokinetics, safety, and efficacy of combination treatment with methotrexate and leflunomide in patients with active rheumatoid arthritis. Arthritis Rheum 1999;42:1322–8.

[62] Chloroquine in the treatment of sarcoidosis. A report from the Research Committee of the British Tuberculosis Association. Tubercle 1967;48(4): 257–72.

[63] Jones E, Callen JP. Hydroxychloroquine is effective therapy for control of cutaneous sarcoidal granulomas. J Am Acad Dermatol 1990;23(3 Pt 1): 487–9.

[64] O'Leary TJ, Jones G, Yip A, et al. The effects of chloroquine on serum 1,25-dihydroxyvitamin D and calcium metabolism in sarcoidosis. N Engl J Med 1986;315(12):727–30.

[65] Baltzan M, Mehta S, Kirkham TH, et al. Randomized trial of prolonged chloroquine therapy in advanced pulmonary sarcoidosis. Am J Respir Crit Care Med 1999;160(1):192–7.

[66] Sharma OP. Effectiveness of chloroquine and hydroxychloroquine in treating selected patients with sarcoidosis with neurologic involvement. Arch Neurol 1998;55:1248–54.

[67] Cox CE, Donohue JF, Brown CD, et al. The sarcoidosis health questionnaire. A new measure of health-related quality of life. Am J Respir Crit Care Med 2003;168:323–9.

[68] Benzagmout M, Boujraf S, Gongora-Rivera F, et al. Neurosarcoidosis which manifested as acute hydrocephalus: diagnosis and treatment. Intern Med 2007;46(18):1601–4.

[69] Baughman RP, Engel PJ, Meyer CA, et al. Pulmonary hypertension in sarcoidosis. Sarcoidosis Vasc Diffuse Lung Dis 2006;23:108–16.

[70] Shorr AF, Helman DL, Davies DB, et al. Pulmonary hypertension in advanced sarcoidosis: epidemiology and clinical characteristics. Eur Respir J 2005;25(5):783–8.

[71] Baughman RP, Lower EE. Fungal infections as a complication of therapy for sarcoidosis. Q J Med 2005;98:451–6.

[72] Barnes PJ. Corticosteroid resistance in airway disease. Proc Am Thorac Soc 2004;1(3):264–8.

[73] Hew M, Bhavsar P, Torrego A, et al. Relative corticosteroid insensitivity of peripheral blood mononuclear cells in severe asthma. Am J Respir Crit Care Med 2006;174(2):134–41.

[74] Goleva E, Hauk PJ, Boguniewicz J, et al. Airway remodeling and lack of bronchodilator response in steroid-resistant asthma. J Allergy Clin Immunol 2007;120(5):1065–72.

[75] Ziegenhagen MW, Rothe ME, Zissel G, et al. Exaggerated TNF-alpha release of alveolar macrophages in corticosteroid resistant sarcoidosis. Sarcoidosis Vasc Diffuse Lung Dis 2002:185–90.

[76] Baughman RP, Iannuzzi M. Tumour necrosis factor in sarcoidosis and its potential for targeted therapy. BioDrugs 2003;17(6):425–31.

[77] Nguyen YT, Dupuy A, Cordoliani F, et al. Treatment of cutaneous sarcoidosis with thalidomide. J Am Acad Dermatol 2004;50(2):235–41.

[78] Judson MA, Silvestri J, Hartung C, et al. The effect of thalidomide on corticosteroid-dependent pulmonary sarcoidosis. Sarcoidosis Vasc Diffuse Lung Dis 2006;23(1):51–7.

[79] Yee AM, Pochapin MB. Treatment of complicated sarcoidosis with infliximab antitumor necrosis-alpha therapy. Ann Intern Med 2001;135:27–31.

[80] Baughman RP, Bradley DA, Lower EE. Infliximab for chronic ocular inflammation. Int J Clin Pharmacol Ther 2005;43:7–11.

[81] Doty JD, Mazur JE, Judson MA. Treatment of sarcoidosis with infliximab. Chest 2005;127(3): 1064–71.

[82] Saleh S, Ghodsian S, Yakimova V, et al. Effectiveness of infliximab in treating selected patients with sarcoidosis. Respir Med 2006;100(11):2053–9.

[83] Sweiss NJ, Welsch MJ, Curran JJ, et al. Tumor necrosis factor inhibition as a novel treatment for refractory sarcoidosis. Arthritis Rheum 2005;53(5):788–91.

[84] Baughman RP, Drent M, Kavuru M, et al. Infliximab therapy in patients with chronic sarcoidosis and pulmonary involvement. Am J Respir Crit Care Med 2006;174(7):795–802.

[85] Rossman MD, Newman LS, Baughman RP, et al. A double-blind, randomized, placebo-controlled trial of infliximab in patients with active pulmonary sarcoidosis. Sarcoidosis Vasc Diffuse Lung Dis 2006;23:201–8.

[86] Utz JP, Limper AH, Kalra S, et al. Etanercept for the treatment of stage II and III progressive pulmonary sarcoidosis. Chest 2003;124(1):177–85.

[87] Baughman RP. Tumor necrosis factor inhibition in treating sarcoidosis: the American experience. Reyista Portuguesa de Pneumonologia 2007;13(2): 547–50.

[88] Callejas-Rubio JL, Ortego-Centeno N, Lopez-Perez L, et al. Treatment of therapy-resistant sarcoidosis with adalimumab. Clin Rheumatol 2006;25:596–7.

[89] Heffernan MP, Smith DI. Adalimumab for treatment of cutaneous sarcoidosis. Arch Dermatol 2006;142(1):17–9.

[90] Sandborn WJ, Rutgeerts P, Enns R, et al. Adalimumab induction therapy for Crohn's disease previously treated with infliximab: a randomized trial. Ann Intern Med 2007;146(12):829–38.

[91] Paramothayan S, Jones PW. Corticosteroid therapy in pulmonary sarcoidosis: a systematic review. JAMA 2002;287:1301–7.

[92] Paramothayan S, Lasserson T, Walters EH. Immunosuppressive and cytotoxic therapy for pulmonary sarcoidosis. Cochrane Database Syst Rev 2003;(3):CD003536.

[93] Israel HL, Fouts DW, Beggs RA. A controlled trial of prednisone treatment of sarcoidosis. Am Rev Respir Dis 1973;107:609–14.

[94] Pietinalho A, Lindholm A, Haahtela T, et al. Inhaled budesonide for treatment of pulmonary sarcoidosis. Results of a double-blind, placebo-controlled, multicentre study. Eur Respir J 1996; 9:406s.

[95] Selroos O, Sellergren TL. Corticosteroid therapy of pulmonary sarcoidosis. Scand J Respir Dis 1979; 60:215–21.

[96] Everhart JE, Lombardero M, Lake JR, et al. Weight change and obesity after liver transplantation: incidence and risk factors. Liver Transpl Surg 1998;4(4):285–96.

[97] Habib GS, Haj S. Bone mineral density in patients with early rheumatoid arthritis treated with corticosteroids. Clin Rheumatol 2005;24(2):129–33.

[98] Ton FN, Gunawardene SC, Lee H, et al. Effects of low-dose prednisone on bone metabolism. J Bone Miner Res 2005;20(3):464–70.

[99] Adler RA, Funkhouser HL, Petkov VI, et al. Glucocorticoid-induced osteoporosis in patients with sarcoidosis. Am J Med Sci 2003;325(1):1–6.

[100] Rizzato G, Tosi G, Mella C, et al. Prednisone-induced bone loss in sarcoidosis: a risk especially frequent in postmenopausal women. Sarcoidosis 1988;5(2):93–8.

[101] American College of Rheumatology Ad Hoc Committee on Glucocorticoid-Induced Osteoporosis. Recommendations for the prevention and treatment of glucocorticoid-induced osteoporosis: 2001 update. Arthritis Rheum 2001;44(7): 1496–503.

[102] Adler RA, Hochberg MC. Suggested guidelines for evaluation and treatment of glucocorticoid-induced osteoporosis for the Department of Veterans Affairs. Arch Intern Med 2003;163(21): 2619–24.

[103] Rizzato G. Clinical impact of bone and calcium metabolism changes in sarcoidosis. Thorax 1998; 53(5):425–9.

[104] Sharma OP. Vitamin D, calcium, and sarcoidosis. Chest 1996;109(2):535–9.

[105] Gallacher SJ, Fenner JA, Anderson K, et al. Intravenous pamidronate in the treatment of osteoporosis associated with corticosteroid-dependent lung disease: an open pilot study. Thorax 1992;47(11): 932–6.

[106] Rizzato G, Montemurro L. Reversibility of exogenous corticosteroid-induced bone loss. Eur Respir J 1993;6(1):116–9.

[107] Gonnelli S, Rottoli P, Cepollaro C, et al. Prevention of corticosteroid-induced osteoporosis with alendronate in sarcoid patients. Calcif Tissue Int 1997;61(5):382–5.

[108] Bartel PR, Roux P, Robinson E, et al. Visual function and long-term chloroquine treatment. S Afr Med J 1994;84:32–4.

[109] Raiza-Casillas R, Cardenas F, Morales Y, et al. Factors associated with chloroquine-induced retinopathy in rheumatic diseases. Lupus 2004; 13(2):119–24.

[110] Leecharoen S, Wangkaew S, Louthrenoo W. Ocular side effects of chloroquine in patients with rheumatoid arthritis, systemic lupus erythematosus, and scleroderma. J Med Assoc Thai 2007; 90(1):52–8.

[111] Yam JC, Kwok AK. Ocular toxicity of hydroxychloroquine. Hong Kong Med J 2006;12(4): 294–304.

[112] Marmor MF, Carr RE, Easterbrook M, et al. Recommendations on screening for chloroquine and hydroxychloroquine retinopathy: a report by the American Academy of Ophthalmology. Ophthalmology 2002;109(7):1377–82.

[113] Silman A, Shipley M. Ophthalmological monitoring for hydroxychloroquine toxicity: a scientific review of available data. Br J Rheumatol 1997; 36(5):599–601.

[114] Baughman RP, Lower EE. A clinical approach to the use of methotrexate for sarcoidosis. Thorax 1999;54:742–6.

[115] Zisman DA, McCune WJ, Tino G, et al. Drug-induced pneumonitis: the role of methotrexate-Sarcoidosis Vasc Diffuse Lung Dis 2001;18(3): 243–52.

[116] Kremer JM, Alarcon GS, Lightfoot RW Jr, et al. Methotrexate for rheumatoid arthritis. Suggested guidelines for monitoring liver toxicity. American College of Rheumatology. Arthritis Rheum 1994; 37(3):316–28.

[117] Roenigk HH, Auerbach R, Maibach HI, et al. Methotrexate guidelines revised. J Am Acad Dermatol 1982;6:145–55.

[118] Baughman RP, Weber FL, Bejarano PB, et al. Methotrexate for chronic sarcoidosis: hepatotoxicity assessed by liver biopsy. Am J Respir Crit Care Med 1999;159:A342.

[119] Demedts M, Behr J, Buhl R, et al. High-dose acetylcysteine in idiopathic pulmonary fibrosis. N Engl J Med 2005;353(21):2229–42.

[120] Raghu G, Depaso WJ, Cain K, et al. Azathioprine combined with prednisone in the treatment of idiopathic pulmonary fibrosis: a prospective double-blind, randomized, placebo-controlled clinical trial. Am Rev Respir Dis 1991;144(2): 291–6.

[121] Baughman RP, Lower EE. Steroid-sparing alternative treatments for sarcoidosis. Clin Chest Med 1997;18:853–64.

[122] Mosam A, Morar N. Recalcitrant cutaneous sarcoidosis: an evidence-based sequential approach. J Dermatolog Treat 2004;15(6):353–9.

[123] Escousse A, Mousson C, Santona L, et al. Azathioprine-induced pancytopenia in homogenous thiopurine methyltransferase-deficient renal transplant recipients: a family study. Transplant Proc 1995;27: 1739–42.

[124] Soria-Royer C, Legendre C, Mircheva J, et al. Thiopurine-methyl-transferase activity to assess azathioprine myelotoxicity in renal transplant recipients. Lancet 1993;341(8860):1593–4.

[125] Kennedy PT, Zakaria N, Modawi SB, et al. Natural history of hepatic sarcoidosis and its response to treatment. Eur J Gastroenterol Hepatol 2006;18(7): 721–6.

[126] Osiri M, Shea B, Robinson V, et al. Leflunomide for the treatment of rheumatoid arthritis: a systematic review and meta analysis. J Rheumatol 2003; 30(6):1182–90.

[127] Emery P, Breedveld FC, Lemmel EM, et al. A comparison of the efficacy and safety of leflunomide and methotrexate for the treatment of rheumatoid arthritis. Rheumatology (Oxford) 2000;39(6): 655–65.

[128] Majithia V, Sanders S, Harisdangkul V, et al. Successful treatment of sarcoidosis with leflunomide. Rheumatology (Oxford) 2003;42(5):700–2.

[129] Savage RL, Highton J, Boyd IW, et al. Pneumonitis associated with leflunomide: a profile of New Zealand and Australian reports. Intern Med J 2006; 36(3):162–9.

[130] Chan V, Tett SE. How is leflunomide prescribed and used in Australia? Analysis of prescribing and adverse effect reporting. Pharmacoepidemiol Drug Saf 2006;15(7):485–93.

[131] Swigris JJ, Olson AL, Fischer A, et al. Mycophenolate mofetil is safe, well-tolerated, and preserves lung function in patients with connective tissue disease-related interstitial lung disease. Chest 2006;130(1):30–6.

[132] Zamora AC, Wolters PJ, Collard HR, et al. Use of mycophenolate mofetil to treat scleroderma-associated interstitial lung disease. Respir Med 2008102(1):150–5.

[133] Moudgil A, Przygodzki RM, Kher KK. Successful steroid-sparing treatment of renal limited sarcoidosis with mycophenolate mofetil. Pediatr Nephrol 2006;21(2):281–5.

[134] Baughman RP, Peddi R, Lower EE. Therapy: general issues. In: Baughman RP, du Bois RM, Lynch JP III, editors. Diffuse lung disease: a practical approach. London: Arnold; 2004. p. 78–90.

[135] Doty JD, Mazur JE, Judson MA. Treatment of corticosteroid-resistant neurosarcoidosis with a short-course cyclophosphamide regimen. Chest 2003;124(5):2023–6.

[136] Baughman RP, Lower EE. Use of intermittent, intravenous cyclophosphamide for idiopathic pulmonary fibrosis. Chest 1992;102(4):1090–4.

[137] Talar-Williams C, Hijazi YM, Walther MM, et al. Cyclophosphamide-induced cystitis and bladder cancer in patients with Wegener granulomatosis. Ann Intern Med 1996;124:477–84.

[138] Carlesimo M, Giustini S, Rossi A, et al. Treatment of cutaneous and pulmonary sarcoidosis with thalidomide. J Am Acad Dermatol 1995; 32(5 Pt 2):866–9.

[139] Lee JB, Koblenzer PS. Disfiguring cutaneous manifestation of sarcoidosis treated with thalidomide: a case report. J Am Acad Dermatol 1998; 39(5 Pt 2):835–8.

[140] Baughman RP, Lower EE. Newer therapies for cutaneous sarcoidosis: the role of thalidomide and other agents. Am J Clin Dermatol 2004;5(6):385–94.

[141] Tavares JL, Wangoo A, Dilworth P, et al. Thalidomide reduces tumour necrosis factor-alpha production by human alveolar macrophages. Respir Med 1997;91(1):31–9.

[142] Ye Q, Chen B, Tong Z, et al. Thalidomide reduces IL-18, IL-8, and TNF-alpha release from alveolar

macrophages in interstitial lung disease. Eur Respir J 2006;28(4):824–31.

[143] Oliver SJ, Kikuchi T, Krueger JG, et al. Thalidomide induces granuloma differentiation in sarcoid skin lesions associated with disease improvement. Clin Immunol 2002;102(3):225–36.

[144] Haley H, Cantrell W, Smith K. Infliximab therapy for sarcoidosis (lupus pernio). Br J Dermatol 2004; 150(1):146–9.

[145] Sollberger M, Fluri F, Baumann T, et al. Successful treatment of steroid-refractory neurosarcoidosis with infliximab. J Neurol 2004;251(6):760–1.

[146] Kapetanovic MC, Larsson L, Truedsson L, et al. Predictors of infusion reactions during infliximab treatment in patients with arthritis. Arthritis Res Ther 2006;8(4):R131.

[147] Kroesen S, Widmer AF, Tyndall A, et al. Serious bacterial infections in patients with rheumatoid arthritis under anti-TNF-alpha therapy. Rheumatology (Oxford) 2003;42(5):617–21.

[148] Keane J, Gershon S, Wise RP, et al. Tuberculosis associated with infliximab, a tumor necrosis factor-alpha neutralizing agent. N Engl J Med 2001; 345:1098–104.

[149] Gomez-Reino JJ, Carmona L, Angel DM. Risk of tuberculosis in patients treated with tumor necrosis factor antagonists due to incomplete prevention of reactivation of latent infection. Arthritis Rheum 2007;57(5):756–61.

[150] Chung ES, Packer M, Lo KH, et al. Randomized, double-blind, placebo-controlled, pilot trial of infliximab, a chimeric monoclonal antibody to tumor necrosis factor-alpha, in patients with moderate-to-severe heart failure: results of the Anti-TNF Therapy Against Congestive Heart Failure (ATTACH) trial. Circulation 2003;107(25): 3133–40.

[151] Hansen RA, Gartlehner G, Powell GE, et al. Serious adverse events with infliximab: analysis of spontaneously reported adverse events. Clin Gastroenterol Hepatol 2007;5(6):729–35.

[152] Wolfe F, Michaud K. The effect of methotrexate and antitumor necrosis factor therapy on the risk of lymphoma in rheumatoid arthritis in 19,562 patients during 89,710 person–years of observation. Arthritis Rheum 2007;56(5):1433–9.

[153] Almodovar R, Izquierdo M, Zarco P, et al. Pulmonary sarcoidosis in a patient with ankylosing spondylitis treated with infliximab. Clin Exp Rheumatol 2007;25(1):99–101.

[154] Gonzalez-Lopez MA, Blanco R, Gonzalez-Vela MC, et al. Development of sarcoidosis during etanercept therapy. Arthritis Rheum 2006;55(5): 817–20.

[155] Sweiss NJ, Baughman RP. Tumor necrosis factor inhibition in the treatment of refractory sarcoidosis: slaying the dragon? J Rheumatol 2007;34: 2129–31.

ELSEVIER
SAUNDERS

CLINICS
IN CHEST
MEDICINE

Clin Chest Med 29 (2008) 549–563

Pulmonary Hypertension Caused by Sarcoidosis

Enrique Diaz-Guzman, MD[a], Carol Farver, MD[b],
Joseph Parambil, MD[a], Daniel A. Culver, DO[a],*

[a]Department of Pulmonary and Critical Care Medicine, Respiratory Institute, Cleveland Clinic,
9500 Euclid Avenue, Cleveland, OH 44195, USA
[b]Department of Anatomic Pathology, Division of Pathology and Laboratory Medicine, Cleveland Clinic,
9500 Euclid Avenue, Cleveland, OH 44195, USA

...the lungs, heart, and circulation should be thought of as a single apparatus for the transfer of oxygen and carbon dioxide between the atmosphere and the working tissues [1].

Pulmonary hypertension (PH) is defined as a mean pulmonary artery pressure (mPAP) higher than 25 mm Hg at rest or 30 mm Hg with exercise [2,3]. The disease can be idiopathic (familial or sporadic) or associated with several disorders that ultimately induce remodeling of the pulmonary circulation and result in a permanent elevation of the pulmonary vascular resistance. Idiopathic pulmonary arterial hypertension is a rare disease affecting 6 to 15 individuals per million [4,5]; nonidiopathic forms are considered to be much more common, particularly in patients with chronic respiratory disorders.

Sarcoidosis is a multisystem granulomatous disorder that affects the lungs in 90% to 95% of patients [6]. The disease has an estimated incidence of 10 to 35 cases per 100,000 people in the United States, with an overall mortality of 1% to 5% [7,8]. Initially considered a rare manifestation of long-standing sarcoidosis, sarcoidosis-associated pulmonary hypertension (SAPH) is now being recognized as an important complication that can result in significant morbidity and

mortality. Although SAPH occurs more frequently in patients with evidence of advanced parenchymal fibrosis, it can also be present despite no apparently significant interstitial lung disease. Severe untreated pulmonary arterial hypertension carries an extremely poor prognosis and is associated with higher mortality in patients with interstitial lung diseases and sarcoidosis [9,10]. Early diagnosis and consideration of treatment options may be keys to improve patient outcomes.

History

The modern history of sarcoidosis probably began in 1898, when Hutchinson [11], a London dermatologist, described a case of a patient with "Mortimer's malady," allegedly a patient with evidence of cutaneous disease. In the initial description, the disease was thought to be a form of cutaneous lupus. Sarcoidosis was recognized as a distinct pathologic entity a year later, when Boeck [12] described the histology of the "sarkoid" granulomas. By 1929, Bernstein [13] had described cardiopulmonary system involvement by sarcoidosis, the same year that Forssman [14] revolutionized the study of cardiac and pulmonary hemodynamics by demonstrating that cardiac catheterization was possible in human beings.

Between 1930 and 1950, several clinical, radiologic, and pathologic studies established that the involvement of the lung was common in patients with sarcoidosis [15–17]. Furthermore, right ventricular failure was recognized as an explanation for dyspnea, cyanosis, and death in patients with advanced lung disease. In 1948, for example,

D.A. Culver's work is supported by NIH grant HL081538, from the National Heart Lung and Blood Institute.

D.A. Culver and J. Parambil are site investigators on an investigator-sponsored trial (Actelion).

* Corresponding author.
E-mail address: culverd@ccf.org (D.A. Culver).

Mallory [18] described six patients with granulo-matous pneumonitis consistent with sarcoidosis and parenchymal fibrosis. In this article, the investigator presented evidence of invasion and thrombosis of the pulmonary vasculature. Two years later, the clinical relevance of these findings was suggested by Austrian [19], who noted elevated pulmonary artery pressures in two patients with sarcoidosis. In the following decades, several small cohorts of patients with SAPH began to elucidate the frequency, pathophysiology, and prognosis of pulmonary hypertension in sarcoidosis patients. In the past decade, with the advent of specific medications for treatment of pulmonary arterial hypertension (PAH), interest in SAPH has burgeoned dramatically.

Epidemiology

The actual prevalence of SAPH has not been established. In patients with significant parenchymal lung disease, the disease was historically thought to be rare, with involvement of the pulmonary vasculature in less than 5% of the cases. Unfortunately, most of the early cohorts were identified retrospectively based on autopsies or case series of patients with clinically diagnosed right heart failure. For example, Mayock and colleagues [20] performed a review of 145 patients with sarcoidosis from nine published series, and found only six (4.1%) patients with evidence of pulmonary hypertension and cor pulmonale. Similarly, a series of 320 autopsies in Japanese patients with sarcoidosis revealed 18 cases of cor pulmonale (5.6%) [21]. No hemodynamic measurements were made in any of these reports.

It is clear that the measurement technique and the entry criteria for performing screening influence the ascertained prevalence of SAPH. It is also probable that ethnicity affects development of the disease. Thus, estimates of prevalence have been widely variable (Table 1). Separate reviews of right heart catheterization (RHC) results among 104 subjects in Italy and Poland suggested that the prevalence of resting PH is 6% to 23% [22–24]. Higher chest radiograph (CXR) stage was associated with increased risk in all three series, with approximately one-half of those with stage III CXR demonstrating at least mild elevations of mPAP. When the screening is limited to patients with more advanced parenchymal disease, the prevalence is substantially higher. Emirgil and colleagues [25] reported 15 patients with

sarcoid-related pulmonary fibrosis who had RHC, of whom 10 (67%) had evidence of PH at rest. In a retrospective evaluation of 106 subjects with sarcoidosis, Sulica and colleagues [26] found that 51% of the subjects with a pre-existing clinical indication for performing echocardiography had evidence of PH by transthoracic echocardiography (TTE). In this study, the majority of subjects also had radiographic evidence of advanced disease. Finally, in a cohort of 363 sarcoidosis patients listed for lung transplantation between 1995 and 2002, 74% of the group who had RHC had some form of PH; approximately one third of the patients had severe PH (mPAP ≥ 40 mm Hg) [27].

In a prospective observational study using TTE, 246 Japanese patients with predominantly chronic sarcoidosis but good overall lung function were evaluated at a referral center [28]. Of the 212 patients with adequate echocardiograms, only 12 (5.7%) had PH (defined as systolic PAP ≥ 40 mm Hg). Restrictive pulmonary physiology was the only independent risk factor for SAPH. In contrast, when only patients with unexplained dyspnea are studied, the prevalence appears to be higher. For example a recent single-center retrospective review of 53 subjects with sarcoidosis found that 25 out of 53 (47%) of the subjects with persistent dyspnea had a mean PAP greater than or equal to 25 mm Hg [29]. Importantly, only 69% of the subjects in this study had evidence of CXR stage III or IV sarcoidosis. A recent review of Danish patients prospectively characterized with right heart catheterization at the time of referral for lung transplantation reported that 79% (19 out of 24 subjects) had a mPAP greater than 25 mm Hg [30]. These subjects had severe pulmonary sarcoidosis, as evidenced by chronicity (median duration 11 years), CXR stage (75% with stage IV) and forced vital capacity (FVC) (median 41% predicted).

A subgroup of patients with sarcoidosis appears to have excessive elevations of pulmonary arterial pressures during exercise. In an Italian cohort of 62 sarcoidosis subjects published more than two decades ago, 10 subjects with normal resting hemodynamics exhibited exercise-induced PH [22]. Two subsequent studies from the same group in Poland demonstrated similar findings. In the first study, 3 of 10 subjects with stage II CXR developed PA pressure elevation of 20 mm Hg above baseline, and all 10 subjects with stage III CXR had increases greater than 10 mm Hg [23]. Some of the subjects demonstrated very

Table 1
Ascertained prevalence of sarcoidosis-associated pulmonary hypertension in several populations

Author	Location	Population	Number	Method	Prevalence (%)
Handa [28]	Single center, Japan	Prospective study of unselected clinic patients	212[a]	TTE	5.7
Rizzato [22]	Single center, Italy	Unspecified patients who had RHC	50	RHC	6[b]
Gluskowski [24]	Single center, Poland	Prospective study of CXR stage II and III	24	RHC	12.5[b]
Gluskowski [23]	Single center, Poland	Unspecified patients who had RHC	30	RHC	23
Baughman [29]	Single center, United States	Subjects with dyspnea disproportionate to PFTs	53	RHC	47
Sulica [26]	Single center, United States	Retrospective review of patients who had TTE for clinical indications	106	TTE	51
Emirgil [25]	Single center, United States	Series of severe sarcoidosis patients	15	RHC	67
Shorr [27]	UNOS database, United States	All lung transplant candidates who also had RHC	363	RHC	74[c]
Milman [30]	Single center, Denmark	All lung transplant candidates who also had RHC	24	RHC	79

Abbreviations: PFT, pulmonary function test; RHC, right heart catheterization; TTE, transthoracic echocardiography; UNOS, United Network for Organ Sharing.

[a] 34 out of 246 subjects had no evaluable tricuspid regurgitation jet.

[b] Additional 20% to 33% of subjects had exercise-induced PH (mPAP $\geq$ 30 mm Hg).

[c] 36% had severe PH (mPAP > 40 mm Hg).

dramatic (50 mm Hg–100 mm Hg) elevations of mPAP with exercise, despite normal resting PA pressures. A prospective follow-up study of unselected patients with stage II or III CXR, persistence of disease for at least 6 months, and mild average restriction (mean FVC 82 ± 17% predicted) revealed an even higher prevalence [24]. Based on a threshold of 10-mm Hg increase in mPAP with exercise, 18 of 24 subjects demonstrated exercise-induced SAPH. Finally, using multiple-uptake gated acquisition scans in subjects with unremarkable echocardiograms, Baughman and colleagues [31] noted 12 of 14 had a significant drop in the right ventricular ejection fraction associated with exercise and attributed to the development of PH.

Most of the available studies have shown an average age at the time of diagnosis of 40 to 60 years. In the United States, SAPH appears to be more common in females and African Americans, but this finding reflects only the overall demographic trends for sarcoidosis, and neither gender nor race has been independently associated with the disease. In the Japanese experience, male gender was associated with SAPH in univariate analysis, although the total number was small [28]. Finally, although some reports have suggested that the incidence of SAPH may be even higher when including hemodynamic evaluations with exercise, the prevalence of exercise-induced SAPH in larger cohorts of unselected sarcoidosis patients is currently unknown.

In conclusion, currently, ascertainment bias has confounded efforts to accurately assess the true prevalence of PH in patients with sarcoidosis. Almost all the published data are derived from referral centers, and most of the data are from selected patient populations within these institutions. Translating the findings in the Japanese and European centers to the United States experience is also problematic, because ethnicity substantially influences sarcoidosis phenotype. For example, in

Japan cardiac involvement is extremely common and could contribute to SAPH. In general, the lack of prospective surveys, reliance on echocardiography, and selection bias have led to poorly generalizable estimation of the overall prevalence.

Pathophysiology

The World Health Organization (WHO) currently classifies pulmonary hypertension into five groups, with sarcoidosis included as Class V (miscellaneous) [32]. Compared with idiopathic pulmonary fibrosis, where pulmonary hypertension is probably caused by fibrotic destruction of the distal capillary bed, several mechanisms may be relevant in SAPH. Thus, it is not incorrect to state that the mechanisms for SAPH could be grouped into all five WHO categories [33].

The granulomatous inflammation in sarcoidosis involves the lung in a lymphatic distribution. This distribution places the granulomas adjacent to the pulmonary artery in the bronchovascular area and to the veins that run within the interlobular septae (Fig. 1). Because of this proximity, the pulmonary arteries are commonly involved by granulomas (Fig. 2A) or giant cells (see Fig. 2B) in pulmonary sarcoidosis. This vascular involvement may involve the adventitia, media, or intima of the pulmonary arteries. Pathologic studies have shown that 69% to 100% of subjects have invasion of the vessel walls by granulomas that result in occlusive changes, perivascular fibrosis, or granulomatous pulmonary angiitis [34,35]. Similarly, scarring and occlusion by granulomas and giant cells may occur in the pulmonary veins (Fig. 3), mimicking pulmonary veno-occlusive disease from a hemodynamic

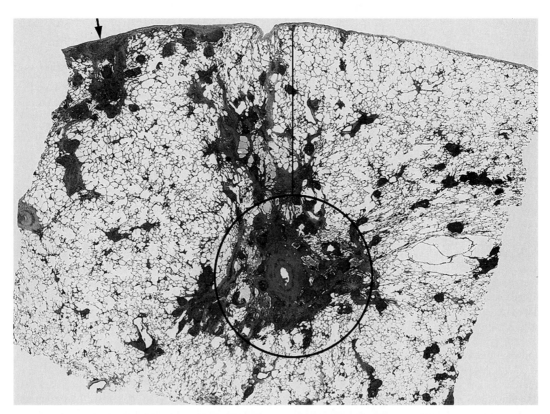

Fig. 1. Distribution of granulomas in pulmonary sarcoidosis. Sarcoidosis granulomas are found in a lymphatic distribution, including surrounding the bronchovascular bundle (*circled area*), the interlobular septae which also contain the pulmonary veins (adjacent to the line), and the subpleural area (*arrow*). Because of this anatomic orientation, granulomatous inflammation frequently encroaches on the vascular structures, even in the absence of overt fibrosis or vascular wall inflammation (Hematoxylin and eosin stain). (*From* Farver CF. Sarcoidosis. In: Tomashefski JF, Cagle PT, Farver CF, et al, editors. Dail and Hammar's pulmonary pathology. New York: Springer-Verlag; 2008; with permission.)

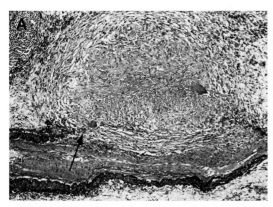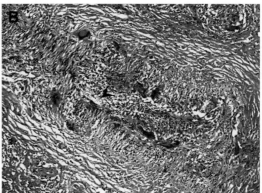

Fig. 2. Granulomatous arteritis in sarcoidosis. (*A*) Movat pentachrome stain showing granulomas obliterating the internal and external elastic laminae and smooth muscle (*arrow*) of medium size artery. There is secondary intimal fibroplasia seen in the center of the artery. (Movat pentachrome stain) (*B*) In some cases, only giant cells and mononuclear cell infiltrates may be seen in sarcoidosis-associated arteritis. Arrowhead indicates the vascular lumen. Numerous giant cells may be seen in the vessel wall (Hematoxylin and eosin).

standpoint [34–37]. Obliteration of these vessels by either active granulomatous inflammation and by fibrosis affords one mechanism for development of pulmonary hypertension in patients with advanced radiographic stages. Furthermore, this preferential location of the granulomas adjacent to these vessels may explain the presence of SAPH, even in patients with little apparent radiologic involvement of the lung parenchyma.

Although the hypothesis that SAPH results from fibrotic or granulomatous obliteration of the pulmonary microvasculature in advanced disease fits most patients, this may not fully explain why

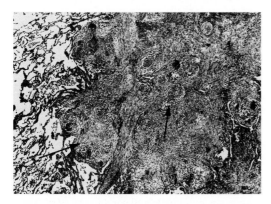

Fig. 3. Obliteration of pulmonary venous drainage by exuberant granuloma formation. Movat pentachrome stain of an interlobular septum showing extensive fibrosis and obliteration of the venous structures by granulomas. Perivenular distribution of granulomas is typical in sarcoidosis. Arrows indicate compressive granulomas (Movat pentachrome stain).

some individuals with no radiographic evidence of interstitial lung disease develop PH [38,39]. In a recent retrospective review of 22 patients with SAPH, 32% of the patients developed pulmonary hypertension in the absence of overt parenchymal fibrosis [40]. Fifty percent of the patients had an elevation in the mPAP that was considered out of proportion to the changes in lung mechanics [40]. An isolated case study described the presence of plexiform lesions in patients with SAPH, but the significance of this observation is unclear because these lesions have not been observed in larger series of SAPH [40,41]. Several reports suggest other possible mechanisms, including extrinsic compression of pulmonary arteries by enlarged hilar lymph nodes (Fig. 4) [40,42,43], diastolic or systolic dysfunction from myocardial sarcoidosis [44,45], and hypoxic vasoconstriction. Obstructive sleep apnea, which is common in sarcoidosis patients [46], may also contribute to the development of elevated pulmonary resistance. Finally, although the possibility of isolated vasoreactivity has been deemed to be a sufficient explanation for some cases of SAPH [47], this concept continues to be mainly hypothetical in the absence of corresponding pathologic data demonstrating that there is not granulomatous inflammation in these subjects.

Endothelin has been implicated in the development of idiopathic pulmonary hypertension. Endothelin-1 (ET-1) is found in abundance in the lung, where it is produced by smooth muscle, endothelial, and airway epithelial cells [48]. Binding of ET-1 with its receptor, ET_A, induces

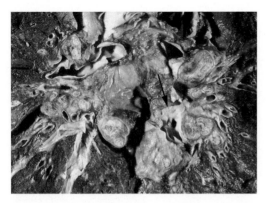

Fig. 4. Compression of central pulmonary vascular structures by bulky lymph nodes. Coronal section of thorax of post-mortem specimen from a patient who died from end-stage SAPH. There is extensive hilar compression of the main pulmonary arteries. Arrow denotes the left lower lobe pulmonary artery, which is subtotally occluded by extrinsic compression of calcified lymph nodes that are present throughout the mediastinum. (*From* Farver CF. Sarcoidosis. In: Tomashefski JF, Cagle PT, Farver CF, et al, editors. Dail and Hammar's pulmonary pathology. New York: Springer-Verlag; 2008; with permission.)

significant pulmonary vasoconstriction; in addition, ET-1 promotes proliferation of smooth muscle cells and fibroblasts, and in animal models has been linked to development of pulmonary fibrosis [49,50]. Urinary and plasma levels of ET-1 are elevated in patients with sarcoidosis, and in some instances treatment with corticosteroids is associated with a normalization of the plasma ET-1 levels [51]. Similarly, ET-1 levels appear to be elevated in bronchoalveolar lavage (BAL) fluid from patients with sarcoidosis, systemic sclerosis, and idiopathic pulmonary fibrosis [52]. A study that limited BAL analysis to 22 subjects with sarcoidosis found approximately 25% had elevated levels of ET-1 [53]. Immunostaining in these patients suggested that alveolar macrophages may be an important source for ET-1. However, it is currently unknown whether ET-1 is only a biomarker for the severity of inflammation or an important mediator of vascular remodeling in sarcoidosis.

Clinical presentation

Pulmonary hypertension should be suspected in any sarcoidosis patient with dyspnea, hypoxemia, or clinical evidence suggesting right heart failure, particularly if symptoms appear to be out of proportion to the degree of parenchymal lung disease. Unfortunately, these symptoms are often present in patients without PH. Other considerations when patients present with unexplained dyspnea or exercise limitation include myopathy (skeletal or respiratory muscle), large airway obstruction, occult cardiac disease, depression, and anemia [54–56].

The most common symptom in patients with SAPH is progressive dyspnea on exertion. Other common complaints include cough, chest pain, palpitations, and symptoms suggesting right heart failure, such as lower extremity edema and syncope. Only the signs of right heart failure are independent predictors of elevated right-sided pressures, but their sensitivity is low. In a retrospective analysis of 106 patients who had echocardiography for clinical reasons, only 21% of the patients with SAPH had pretest evidence of right heart failure (elevated jugular venous pressure, lower extremity edema or right ventricular heave) compared with none of the patients without pulmonary hypertension [26].

Other rare reported presentations of SAPH include sudden death because of compression of large pulmonary arteries [57], main pulmonary vein occlusion caused by intravascular sarcoidosis [58], and combined SAPH and portal hypertension [59]. Although there are case reports of SAPH simulating pulmonary veno-occlusive disease (PVOD) [36,37,40,60], the authors believe that this simply represents the usual distribution of granulomatous inflammation, as the pulmonary venous drainage is closely approximated with the lymphatics. The histopathology of the reported sarcoid-induced PVOD more closely resembles burned-out sarcoidosis than actual PVOD (see Fig. 3). The term PVOD associated with sarcoidosis therefore represents a misnomer and should be avoided.

Imaging studies

Pulmonary hypertension may be present despite the absence of overt fibrotic changes on chest imaging, but the great majority of patients with SAPH appear to have stage III or IV chest radiographs. In an initial study of subjects with chronic cor pulmonale and sarcoidosis, 30% were found to have only perihilar infiltrates [61]. Subsequent studies have confirmed that fibrosis is present in approximately two thirds of subjects, and the CXR may be normal in 9% to 10% [26,40]. High resolution computed tomography of the chest may suggest additional mechanisms. For example, 3 of 14 (21%) of a series of SAPH sub-jects with pulmonary fibrosis also had extrinsic compression of large pulmonary arteries [40]. Overall, however, specific high-resolution chest CT findings are not generally helpful for predict-ing the presence versus absence of SAPH [28].

A common clinical strategy is to measure the main pulmonary artery diameter, the ratio of the pulmonary artery to ascending aorta, or the ratio of segmental artery to bronchus to detect the presence of PH in patients with parenchymal lung disease. Unfortunately, this strategy appears to be unreliable in pulmonary fibrosis [62] and sarcoid-osis [29].

Pulmonary function tests and oxygenation

Depending on the degree of parenchymal involvement, patients with SAPH typically exhibit hypoxemia, decreased carbon monoxide diffusing capacity (DLCO), and restrictive physiology. Most patients with SAPH require at least some supplemental oxygen; among lung transplant candidates, a requirement for 3 L or more of supplemental oxygen more than doubled the risk of PH [27]. In the same cohort, 93.4% of the sub-jects with mPAP greater than 40 mm Hg required at least some supplemental oxygen. In the experi-ence at Mt. Sinai hospital in New York, all pa-tients identified with SAPH by TTE exhibited exercise-induced desaturation [26]. Based on these reports, it can be concluded that the absence of desaturation below 90% with exercise suggests a low likelihood of significant SAPH.

In radiographic stages 0 to 3, SAPH patients classically exhibit a mild restrictive defect with a disproportionate decrease in DLCO. In the Mt. Sinai series, of the 46 subjects without pulmonary fibrosis, the ratio of percent predicted FVC to percent predicted DLCO was 1.9 plus or minus 1.1 in SAPH versus 1.3 plus or minus 0.6 in subjects without PH [26]. The scleroderma experi-ence suggests that serial decline in DLCO despite FVC greater than 70% predicted portends the de-velopment of pulmonary hypertension [63]; the utility of serial PFT data has not been reported in SAPH. In patients with pulmonary fibrosis, there is characteristically a marked reduction in FVC, forced expiratory volume in the first second of expiration, DLCO, and PaO_2. However, these abnormalities may be more pronounced in SAPH, compared with patients without pulmo-nary hypertension [26,40]. It is important to rec-ognize that pulmonary function tests, while more

severely impaired in patients with SAPH [28], may not correlate well with measured pulmonary artery pressures [29,40].

Finally, the 6-minute walk test is useful only when it is normal, as there are multiple reasons for abnormal tests in sarcoidosis patients. It is prob-ably most helpful for serial measurements of cardiopulmonary function. A prospective study of 142 consecutive patients seen a tertiary center evaluated the utility of the 6-minute walk [64]. The 14 patients with proven SAPH had a shorter 6-min-ute walk distance (median, 280 m; range, 61 to 404) than those without proven SAPH (median, 411 m; range, 46 to 747; $P < .0001$). Although the lowest oxygen saturation was correlated with 6-minute walk distance, the presence of PH was not an inde-pendent risk factor in this series.

Hemodynamics

The gold standard for the diagnosis of SAPH is direct measurement of the pulmonary artery pressures with RHC. Pulmonary hypertension is present when the mPAP exceeds 25 mm Hg at rest or 30 mm Hg with exercise. Measurement of the transpulmonary gradient (the difference between the mPAP and the pulmonary capillary wedge pressure or PCWP) is useful to exclude left ventricular disease associated with cardiac sar-coidosis or other causes. However, because left ventricular end-diastolic volume may be impaired by septal flattening in severe pulmonary hyper-tension, it is mandatory to correlate PCWP measurements with echocardiographic assessment of interventricular dependence.

The importance of RHC was emphasized by a recent series of 53 subjects who had both echocardiography and RHC [29]. In these sub-jects, TTE was unable to establish the diagnosis of elevated right ventricular systolic pressure (RVSP) in 16 out 53 (30%) of the subjects with in-creased pulmonary artery pressures. In addition, 24% of the subjects with elevated pulmonary pres-sures had a PCWP greater than 20 mm Hg. These findings suggest that intrinsic cardiac disease (eg, diastolic left ventricular dysfunction) should be excluded before diagnosing SAPH. Despite the presence of increased PAP with exercise in a subset of sarcoidosis patients, the role of routine exercise testing during RHC is unknown.

Echocardiography

Doppler echocardiography is frequently used to evaluate patients with pulmonary hypertension.

Although studies have reported that Doppler analysis of the tricuspid regurgitant velocity by echocardiography may be used to estimate pulmonary pressures [65], many patients with PH have no evidence of tricuspid regurgitation. When useful data are obtained, the sensitivity and specificity of TTE for diagnosing any degree of pulmonary hypertension has varied from 0.69 to 1.0 and 0.68 to 0.98, respectively, in idiopathic PH; correlation coefficients between echocardiography and RHC are generally robust for PAP between 50 mm Hg and 100 mm Hg [66–69]. These data have generated enthusiasm among clinicians for use of TTE as a screening tool when PH is suspected.

However, patients with parenchymal lung disease pose a challenge, because the presence of lung disease may obscure echocardiographic windows and render accurate estimation of PAP difficult [70]. In these patients, the correlation between RVSP and PAP is highly variable, and TTE may underestimate peak right ventricular pressures, particularly in patients with severe PH [71,72]. In a large study that included 374 transplant candidates, estimation of the RVSP was possible in only 44% [73]. Moreover, although the overall correlation between echocardiogram-estimated systolic PAP and RHC was moderately good (r = 0.69), approximately half of the pressure estimations were inaccurate by more than 10 mm Hg. Echocardiographic estimation of PAP thus appears to have inadequate positive and negative predictive value in patients with advanced lung disease. A more recent single-center review of patients with sarcoidosis who had RHC when persistent dyspnea was deemed disproportionate to PFT abnormalities showed a similar correlation between TTE and RHC (r = 0.79) [29]. Nevertheless, the investigators reported that seven out of nine patients for whom RVSP could not be assessed by TTE had SAPH confirmed by pulmonary artery catheterization.

In patients with SAPH, echocardiography can establish the presence of other cardiac causes of dyspnea, such as left ventricular systolic or diastolic dysfunction, valvular abnormalities, pericardial effusion, or the presence of right to left shunts. In the absence of tricuspid regurgitation, the diagnosis of SAPH should be suspected when there are echocardiographic findings of right ventricular pressure overload, including right ventricular hypertrophy, systolic dysfunction, flattening of the interventricular septum, or an abnormal ratio of the interventricular septum to posterior left ventricular wall thickness [74]. The absence of these findings, nevertheless, does not exclude the possibility of SAPH [22], and therefore RHC is currently still considered necessary for definitive diagnosis.

Management

The optimal management strategy for pulmonary hypertension associated with sarcoidosis is unknown. Treatment has typically involved use of systemic anti-inflammatory medications, anticoagulants, pulmonary vasodilators, endothelin receptor antagonists, and supplemental oxygen. The available literature regarding these therapeutic strategies is limited to small cohort studies, retrospective analyses, and case reports.

Immunomodulating medications

Theoretically, anti-inflammatory medications could have a major impact on some patients with SAPH [75,76]. The results of the available trials, however, have not demonstrated consistent benefits from use of immunosuppressants in SAPH. In a small study of 24 subjects, the effects of corticosteroid treatment on pulmonary hemodynamics were evaluated by RHC [24]. The subjects were treated with an initial dose of 60 mg per day of prednisolone, tapered to 25 mg at 6 months, and continued for 1 year. Only two of four subjects with PH at rest had significant improvement of pulmonary pressures after 1 year of therapy. Interestingly, although almost all patients had improvement in pulmonary function, elevated exercise-induced pulmonary pressures decreased in only half of the group. Other investigators have noted similar results, with hemodynamic improvements noted in 0% to 30% after corticosteroid treatment [29,40].

Although these results suggest that corticosteroids may be helpful in a subset of patients with SAPH, it appears that the benefits are difficult to predict. Based on the available data, corticosteroids or other immunomodulators may be most useful for patients with evidence of active inflammation or compression of central vascular structures by bulky lymph nodes. The role of steroids in patients with established parenchymal fibrosis is less clear. To the authors' knowledge, there are no available studies that have systematically addressed the use of other immune modulating agents in SAPH.

Pulmonary vasodilators

Currently available vasodilators include prostacyclin analogs, calcium channel blockers, and phosphodiesterase inhibitors. Use of these agents in patients with pulmonary fibrosis has been controversial, given concerns for severe hypoxemia or pulmonary edema caused by intrapulmonary shunting [77–79]. Because SAPH is often caused by fibrosis with end-stage pulmonary microcirculatory "fixed" abnormalities, it has also been unclear whether these agents have any beneficial impact on the pulmonary vascular resistance.

To address this issue, Preston and colleagues [44] treated eight subjects with SAPH using intravenous epoprostenol (EPO), inhaled nitric oxide (iNO), or calcium channel blockers (Table 2). All subjects had advanced sarcoidosis (CXR stages III and IV) and severe pulmonary hypertension (average mPAP, 55 mm Hg). The acute response in mPAP was greater for those receiving iNO (decrease of 18 ± 4%) compared with patients that received EPO at doses of 2 ng/kg to 8 ng/kg per minute (6 ± 2% decrease). No subjects had an acute response with nifedipine. Five subjects continued treatment with iNO at 100 ppm to 200 ppm and one received iNO plus EPO; follow-up showed that patients were able to maintain stable functional class, although both mPAP and pulmonary vascular resistance (PVR) tended to increase. Other reports that included patients with sarcoidosis and parenchymal fibrosis who received low dose epoprostenol therapy reported favorable hemodynamic responses without worsening hypoxemia [80]. A more recent study that included two subjects with severe SAPH reported an excellent initial hemodynamic response (40% decrease in mPAP) in one subject [29].

Fatal pulmonary edema has been reported after initiation of intravenous prostacyclin agents in patients with pulmonary hypertension associated with PVOD or other fibrotic lung diseases, such as scleroderma [81,82]. Fisher and colleagues [83] reported one patient out of seven who developed non-cardiogenic pulmonary edema after treatment with epoprostenol. Given that patients with SAPH may have significant impairment of the pulmonary venous system, therapy with pulmonary vasodilators should be started with caution. However, the available literature does not indicate that patients with SAPH have an excessively elevated risk of developing this complication.

Little is known about the use of other inhaled agents in SAPH. In the article by Nunes and colleagues [40], one patient with SAPH and pulmonary fibrosis was treated with inhaled iloprost without any clinical benefit.

In the authors' center, eight patients received treatment with prostanoid agents alone or in combination with endothelin antagonists, in addition to standard therapy with immunosuppressants [84]. Despite a high proportion of patients with evidence of severe parenchymal scarring (63%), none experienced episodes of vasodilator-induced shunting. Significant short-term benefits of vasoactive therapy were observed among most of the patients, especially those with preserved vital capacity (FVC ≥ 70% of predicted). However, progression to lung transplant or death over 12 to 18 months was extremely common.

The largest published long-term experience with prostanoids, however, suggests that circumspection is warranted before use of these agents [83]. In this study, which included mainly patients with severe restrictive physiology, six of seven subjects demonstrated an acute vasodilator response to low doses of EPO (75% had ≥25% drop in PVR). Six subjects were subsequently treated with EPO and one subject received treatment with subcutaneous treprostinil. However, one subject developed pulmonary edema and another subject died hours after administration of EPO. After a mean follow-up of 29 months, only four subjects enjoyed transplant-free survival, with continued EPO dose titration (mean dose 55 ng/kg per minute).

In summary, most of the available literature regarding the use of pulmonary vasodilators includes patients with advanced stage sarcoidosis. The experience is greatest with the use of epoprostenol. In many cases, it has been used as a palliative measure or a "bridge" to transplantation. The limited evidence suggests that some patients with SAPH may respond well to prostanoid therapy, but that a few individuals do develop pulmonary edema. For the remainder, the therapy appears to be well tolerated, despite use of high doses, and long-term outcomes may be improved. It is still unknown if the potential benefits from prostanoids differ between patients with or without advanced parenchymal disease.

Endothelin antagonists

There is some evidence that endothelin may play a role in the pathogenesis of SAPH.

Table 2
Reports of vasodilator therapy in sarcoidosis

	Number treated	FVC%[a]	mPAP[a] (mm Hg)	Treatment (number)	Follow up (mo)	Outcome	Observations
Preston [44]	8	48	55	iNO (5) CCB (2)	6–24	5 out of 8 subjects died in 0–18 months	Acute vasodilator response in 7 out of 8 subjects
Culver [84]	11	57	76[b]	EPO (4) EPO + Bos (4) Bos (3)	2–30	8 out of 11 subjects died or required lung transplant Short-term hemodynamic or functional benefit observed in all subjects	Hemodynamic response most evident in patients with FVC ≥70%
Foley [85]	1	64	55	Bosentan	24	mPAP decreased to 23 mm Hg at 6 months	Improved functional class (NYHA IV to II)
Sharma [86]	1	40	78[c]	Bosentan	12	Improved 6-minute walk distance	Improved functional class (NYHA IV to II)
Nunes [40]	1	N/A	N/A	Iloprost (1)	4	Died awaiting lung transplant	—
Baughman [29]	7	64	83	EPO (1) EPO + Bos (1) Bos (4) CCB (1)	6	Significant decrease in mPAP after 6 months in 5 out of 7 patients	Immunosupressive therapy was increased
Fisher [83]	7	59	57	EPO (7)	0–49	The majority of subjects responded to EPO therapy; 4 out of 7 subjects alive and without transplant	One episode of pulmonary edema; One sudden death 4 hours after EPO initiation
Milman [30]	12	41	36	Sildenafil	1–12	mPAP decreased >20% in 50% of subjects; cardiac output improved in 86%	No benefit on 6- minute walk test

Abbreviations: Bos, bosentan; CCB, calcium channel blocker; NYHA, New York Heart Association.
[a] Mean or median value for the entire reported population, including those treated with vasodilators.
[b] Right ventricular systolic pressure estimate by echocardiogram.
[c] Systolic pulmonary artery pressure.

Bosentan, a specific endothelin-1 antagonist, has been approved by the Food and Drug Administration for the treatment idiopathic PAH and scleroderma-related PAH. The experience with bosentan in SAPH is limited to scattered case reports, often in combination with other agents [29,85,86].

At the authors' institution, seven patients with SAPH who were treated with bosentan were identified [84]. Three subjects received bosentan and four received bosentan in addition to prostanoid therapy. Four of the subjects demonstrated objective improvement after short-term (6–18 months) follow-up, but the other three died from their disease. A similar report that included four subjects treated with bosentan alone showed a significant drop in the pulmonary pressures after 6 months follow-up [29]. These reports are too few to provide guidance for clinicians, but they generally demonstrate the possibility of efficacy for some SAPH patients. The role of endothelin antagonists in combination with other pulmonary vasodilators, such as epoprostenol or sildenafil, remains unclear. As for other causes of PH, it seems reasonable to limit the first-line use of endothelin antagonists to patients with mild to moderate (New York Heart Association functional class II and III) dyspnea.

Phosphodiesterase inhibitors

Sildenafil, a potent phosphodiesterase type 5 inhibitor, has theoretic benefits in pulmonary hypertension caused by parenchymal lung disease, as it may preserve ventilation-perfusion matching better than prostanoids [79]. Small case series have suggested benefits in idiopathic pulmonary fibrosis [79], scleroderma [87], and cystic fibrosis [88]. Moreover, in patients with end-stage chronic obstructive pulmonary disease and idiopathic pulmonary fibrosis-associated pulmonary hypertension, the beneficial hemodynamic effects of sildenafil may also impact exercise tolerance and 6-minute walk distance [89,90]. A recent series described the use of sildenafil in Danish patients listed for lung transplant because of end-stage sarcoidosis [30]. The subjects had severe restrictive lung disease (mean FVC 41% predicted). Twelve subjects with mPAP greater than 25 mm Hg were treated with oral sildenafil (median dose 150 mg daily) for 1 to 12 months. Although the 6-minute walk time did not improve, there were substantial reductions in mPAP (48 ± 15 mm Hg versus 39 ± 13 mm Hg), PVR (10.7 ± 4.8 versus

5.6 ± 4.0 Wood units), and improved cardiac index (2.3 ± 0.5 L/m^2 versus 2.9 ± 1.0 L/m^2 per minute). Although these findings are encouraging, the role of sildenafil compared with prostanoids or endothelin antagonists for SAPH is currently unknown.

Prognosis

Sarcoidosis is generally considered a disease with a favorable long-term prognosis. Although the disease remits spontaneously in nearly two-thirds of patients, about 1% to 5% of patients die from progressive respiratory failure, central nervous system disease, or myocardial involvement [8,91,92]. Right ventricular failure has been described in up to 30% of sarcoidosis-related deaths [20,93]. Patients with substantial pulmonary fibrosis have a particularly elevated risk. A single-center retrospective cohort study of 41 subjects with stage III and IV disease listed for orthotopic lung transplantation suggested that right atrial pressure greater than 15 mm Hg was the strongest independent predictor of mortality in this population [94]. Kaplan-Meier analysis estimated survival of 51% at 1 year and 25% at 2 years when mPAP was greater than or equal to 35 mm Hg. Right arterial pressure greater than or equal to 15 mm Hg increased the risk of death by 5.2-fold. A follow-up analysis of the United Network Organ System database confirmed that higher pulmonary artery pressures portend lower survival among patients awaiting lung transplant [10,95]. These reports have led the International Society for Heart and Lung Transplantation to recommend early assessment for lung transplantation in patients with SAPH [96]. However, these recommendations are limited by the ascertainment bias of the reports from which they are derived.

Compared to patients with radiographic evidence of advanced stage, little is known about the natural history and prognosis of SAPH in the absence of significant pulmonary fibrosis. A recent report proposed that the subset of patients with SAPH and no evidence of pulmonary fibrosis may have a shorter time between diagnosis of sarcoidosis and diagnosis of PH, as well as higher pulmonary vascular resistance compared with patients with parenchymal fibrosis [40]. However, ascertainment bias again is likely influencing this observation. It is currently not known if these patients represent a subgroup in early stages of the disease or if they have a different natural history compared with patients with severe interstitial lung disease. The profound heterogeneity in this group of patients suggests that clinical caution and close follow-up for evidence of progression are warranted. Whether patients with SAPH without pulmonary fibrosis who are treated with pulmonary vasodilators or endothelin antagonists have better outcomes compared with patients with parenchymal fibrosis is also currently not known.

In conclusion, the presence of pulmonary hypertension appears to confer poor prognosis in patients with sarcoidosis. Particularly at risk are patients with evidence of severe parenchymal disease. Clinicians must be vigilant for the development of SAPH, as this complication appears to be associated with worse outcomes. Prompt recognition and referral to an experienced center for consideration of initiation of specific therapy or transplant evaluation are important considerations.

Summary

The authors conclude that SAPH may be present irrespective of the degree of parenchymal involvement. It may account for a substantial proportion of dyspnea among all sarcoidosis patients, and appears to be common in those with severe parenchymal disease. A major gap in current clinical practice is identification of a cost-effective, reliable, noninvasive method to screen for the presence of SAPH. Further studies are needed to characterize the natural history more closely, to establish whether there is a role for routine trials of augmented immunosuppression and to define the effects of the therapeutic options. Early identification of patients at risk for developing this complication might facilitate preventive efforts.

Variable response rates to different agents or combinations of drugs reflect the fact that this particular complication of sarcoidosis may be the consequence of quite complex underlying mechanisms, including granulomatous fibrosis, sarcoid-induced occlusive venopathy, and granulomatous inflammation of pulmonary arteries. Although the presence of pulmonary fibrosis may indicate the possibility of irreversible derangement and portend a worse outcome, its presence should not preclude a cautious therapeutic trial. If the patient is a candidate, concomitant evaluation for lung transplantation should be considered as well.

References

[1] Henderson LJ. Blood: a study in general physiology. London: Oxford University Press; 1928.

[2] Simonneau G, Galie N, Rubin LJ, et al. Clinical classification of pulmonary hypertension. J Am Coll Cardiol 2004;43:5S–12S.

[3] Rubin LJ. Diagnosis and management of pulmonary arterial hypertension: ACCP evidence-based clinical practice guidelines. Chest 2004;126:7S–10S.

[4] Jing ZC, Xu XQ, Han ZY, et al. Registry and survival study in Chinese patients with idiopathic and familial pulmonary arterial hypertension. Chest 2007;132:373–9.

[5] Humbert M, Sitbon O, Chaouat A, et al. Pulmonary arterial hypertension in France: results from a national registry. Am J Respir Crit Care Med 2006;173:1023–30.

[6] Baughman RP, Teirstein AS, Judson MA, et al. Clinical characteristics of patients in a case control study of sarcoidosis. Am J Respir Crit Care Med 2001;164:1885–9.

[7] Rybicki BA, Major M, Popovich J Jr, et al. Racial differences in sarcoidosis incidence: a 5-year study in a health maintenance organization. Am J Epidemiol 1997;145:234–41.

[8] Hunninghake GW, Costabel U, Ando M, et al. ATS/ERS/WASOG statement on sarcoidosis. American Thoracic Society/European Respiratory Society/World Association of Sarcoidosis and Other Granulomatous Disorders. Sarcoidosis Vasc Diffuse Lung Dis 1999;16:149–73.

[9] Ryu JH, Krowka MJ, Pellikka PA, et al. Pulmonary hypertension in patients with interstitial lung diseases. Mayo Clin Proc 2007;82:342–50.

[10] Shorr AF, Davies DB, Nathan SD. Outcomes for patients with sarcoidosis awaiting lung transplantation. Chest 2002;122:233–8.

[11] Hutchinson J. Cases of Mortimer's malady (lupus vulgaris multiplex non ulcerans et non serpiginosis). Arch Surg 1898;9:307–14.

[12] Boeck C. Multiple benign sarkoid of the skin. Journal of Cutaneous and Genito-urinary Diseases 1899; 17:543–50.

[13] Bernstein M, Konzlemann FW, Sidlick DM. Boeck's sarcoid: report of a case with visceral involvement. Arch Intern Med 1929;44:721–34.

[14] Forssmann W. Die soniderung des rechten herzens. Klinische Wochenschrift 1929;8:2085.

[15] Ricker W, Clark M. Sarcoidosis: a clinicopathologic review of three hundered cases, including twenty-two autopsies. Am J Clin Pathol 1949;19:725–49.

[16] Reisner D. Boeck's sarcoid and systemic sarcoidosis: a study of thirty-five cases. Am Rev Tuberc 1944;49: 289–307.

[17] Freiman DG. Medical progress: sarcoidosis. N Engl J Med 1948;239:664–71, 709–16, 743–9.

[18] Mallory TB. Pathology of pulmonary fibrosis, including chronic pulmonary sarcoidosis. Radiology 1948;51:468.

[19] Austrian R, McClement JH, Renzetti AD Jr, et al. Clinical and physiologic features of some types of pulmonary diseases with impairment of alveolar-capillary diffusion: the syndrome of "alveolar-capillary block". Am J Med 1951;11:667–85.

[20] Mayock RL, Bertrand P, Morrison CE, et al. Manifestations of sarcoidosis. Analysis of 145 patients, with a review of nine series selected from the literature. Am J Med 1963;35:67–89.

[21] Iwai K, Tachibana T, Takemura T, et al. Pathological studies on sarcoidosis autopsy. I. Epidemiological features of 320 cases in Japan. Acta Pathol Jpn 1993;43(7-8):372–6.

[22] Rizzato G, Pezzano A, Sala G, et al. Right heart impairment in sarcoidosis: haemodynamic and echocardiographic study. Eur J Respir Dis 1983;64(2):121–8.

[23] Gluskowski J, Hawrylkiewicz I, Zych D, et al. Pulmonary haemodynamics at rest and during exercise in patients with sarcoidosis. Respiration 1984; 46(1):26–32.

[24] Gluskowski J, Hawrylkiewicz I, Zych D, et al. Effects of corticosteroid treatment on pulmonary haemodynamics in patients with sarcoidosis. Eur Respir J 1990;3:403–7.

[25] Emirgil C, Sobol BJ, Herbert WH, et al. The lesser circulation in pulmonary fibrosis secondary to sarcoidosis and its relationship to respiratory function. Chest 1971;60:371–8.

[26] Sulica R, Teirstein AS, Kakarla S, et al. Distinctive clinical, radiographic, and functional characteristics of patients with sarcoidosis-related pulmonary hypertension. Chest 2005;128:1483–9.

[27] Shorr AF, Helman DL, Davies DB, et al. Pulmonary hypertension in advanced sarcoidosis: epidemiology and clinical characteristics. Eur Respir J 2005;25: 783–8.

[28] Handa T, Nagai S, Miki S, et al. Incidence of pulmonary hypertension and its clinical relevance in patients with sarcoidosis. Chest 2006;129:1246–52.

[29] Baughman RP, Engel PJ, Meyer CA, et al. Pulmonary hypertension in sarcoidosis. Sarcoidosis Vasc Diffuse Lung Dis 2006;23:108–16.

[30] Milman N, Burton CM, Iversen M, et al. Pulmonary hypertension in end-stage pulmonary sarcoidosis: therapeutic effect of sildenafil? J Heart Lung Transplant 2008;27:329–34.

[31] Baughman RP, Gerson M, Bosken CH. Right and left ventricular function at rest and with exercise in patients with sarcoidosis. Chest 1984;85:301–6.

[32] Farber HW, Loscalzo J. Pulmonary arterial hypertension. N Engl J Med 2004;351:1655–65.

[33] Baughman RP. Pulmonary hypertension associated with sarcoidosis. Arthritis Res Ther 2007; 9(Suppl 2):S8.

[34] Rosen Y, Moon S, Huang CT, et al. Granulomatous pulmonary angiitis in sarcoidosis. Arch Pathol Lab Med 1977;101:170–4.

[35] Takemura T, Matsui Y, Oritsu M, et al. Pulmonary vascular involvement in sarcoidosis: granulomatous angiitis and microangiopathy in transbronchial lung biopsies. Virchows Arch A Pathol Anat Histopathol 1991;418:361–8.

[36] Hoffstein V, Ranganathan N, Mullen JB. Sarcoidosis simulating pulmonary veno-occlusive disease. Am Rev Respir Dis 1986;134:809–11.

[37] Schachter EN, Smith GJ, Cohen GS, et al. Pulmonary granulomas in a patient with pulmonary veno-occlusive disease. Chest 1975;67:487–9.

[38] Levine BW, Saldana M, Hutter AM. Pulmonary hypertension in sarcoidosis. A case report of a rare but potentially treatable cause. Am Rev Respir Dis 1971; 103:413–7.

[39] Smith LJ, Lawrence JB, Katzenstein AA. Vascular sarcoidosis: a rare cause of pulmonary hypertension. Am J Med Sci 1983;285:38–44.

[40] Nunes H, Humbert M, Capron F, et al. Pulmonary hypertension associated with sarcoidosis: mechanisms, haemodynamics and prognosis. Thorax 2006;61:68–74.

[41] Tayal S, Voelkel NF, Rai PR, et al. Sarcoidois and pulmonary hypertension—a case report. Eur J Med Res 2006;11:194–7.

[42] Westcott JL, DeGraff AC Jr. Sarcoidosis, hilar adenopathy, and pulmonary artery narrowing. Radiology 1973;108:585–6.

[43] Damuth TE, Bower JS, Cho K, et al. Major pulmonary artery stenosis causing pulmonary hypertension in sarcoidosis. Chest 1980;78:888–91.

[44] Preston IR, Klinger JR, Landzberg MJ, et al. Vasoresponsiveness of sarcoidosis-associated pulmonary hypertension. Chest 2001;120:866–72.

[45] Bargout R, Kelly RF. Sarcoid heart disease: clinical course and treatment. Int J Cardiol 2004;97:173–82.

[46] Turner GA, Lower EE, Corser BC, et al. Sleep apnea in sarcoidosis. Sarcoidosis Vasc Diffuse Lung Dis 1997;14:61–4.

[47] Barst RJ, Ratner SJ. Sarcoidosis and reactive pulmonary hypertension. Arch Intern Med 1985;145: 2112–4.

[48] Fagan KA, McMurtry IF, Rodman DM. Role of endothelin-1 in lung disease. Respir Res 2001;2: 90–101.

[49] Yang Z, Krasnici N, Luscher TF. Endothelin-1 potentiates human smooth muscle cell growth to PDGF: effects of ETA and ETB receptor blockade. Circulation 1999;100:5–8.

[50] Hocher B, Schwarz A, Fagan KA, et al. Pulmonary fibrosis and chronic lung inflammation in ET-1 transgenic mice. Am J Respir Cell Mol Biol 2000; 23:19–26.

[51] Letizia C, Danese A, Reale MG, et al. Plasma levels of endothelin-1 increase in patients with sarcoidosis and fall after disease remission. Panminerva Med 2001;43:257–61.

[52] Reichenberger F, Schauer J, Kellner K, et al. Different expression of endothelin in the bronchoalveolar lavage in patients with pulmonary diseases. Lung 2001;179:163–74.

[53] Terashita K, Kato S, Sata M, et al. Increased endothelin-1 levels of BAL fluid in patients with pulmonary sarcoidosis. Respirology 2006;11:145–51.

[54] Spruit MA, Thomeer MJ, Gosselink R, et al. Skeletal muscle weakness in patients with sarcoidosis and its relationship with exercise intolerance and reduced health status. Thorax 2005;60:32–8.

[55] Kabitz HJ, Lang F, Walterspacher S, et al. Impact of impaired inspiratory muscle strength on dyspnea and walking capacity in sarcoidosis. Chest 2006; 130:1496–502.

[56] Chambellan A, Turbie P, Nunes H, et al. Endoluminal stenosis of proximal bronchi in sarcoidosis: bronchoscopy, function, and evolution. Chest 2005;127:472–81.

[57] Martin JM, Dowling GP. Sudden death associated with compression of pulmonary arteries in sarcoidosis. CMAJ 1985;133:423–4.

[58] Padia SA, Budev M, Farver CF, et al. Intravascular sarcoidosis presenting as pulmonary vein occlusion: CT and pathologic findings. J Thorac Imaging 2007; 22:268–70.

[59] Salazar A, Mana J, Sala J, et al. Combined portal and pulmonary hypertension in sarcoidosis. Respiration 1994;61:117–9.

[60] Portier F, Lerebours-Pigeonniere G, Thiberville L, et al. [Sarcoidosis simulating a pulmonary veno-occlusive disease]. Rev Mal Respir 1991;8:101–2 [in French].

[61] Battesti JP, Georges R, Basset F, et al. Chronic cor pulmonale in pulmonary sarcoidosis. Thorax 1978; 33:76–84.

[62] Zisman DA, Karlamangla AS, Ross DJ, et al. High-resolution chest CT findings do not predict the presence of pulmonary hypertension in advanced idiopathic pulmonary fibrosis. Chest 2007;132:773–9.

[63] Steen V, Medsger TA Jr. Predictors of isolated pulmonary hypertension in patients with systemic sclerosis and limited cutaneous involvement. Arthritis Rheum 2003;48:516–22.

[64] Baughman RP, Sparkman BK, Lower EE. Six-minute walk test and health status assessment in sarcoidosis. Chest 2007;132:207–13.

[65] Berger M, Haimowitz A, Van Tosh A, et al. Quantitative assessment of pulmonary hypertension in patients with tricuspid regurgitation using continuous wave Doppler ultrasound. J Am Coll Cardiol 1985; 6:359–65.

[66] McGoon M, Gutterman D, Steen V, et al. Screening, early detection, and diagnosis of pulmonary arterial hypertension: ACCP evidence-based clinical practice guidelines. Chest 2004;126:14S–34S.

[67] Chan KL, Currie PJ, Seward JB, et al. Comparison of three Doppler ultrasound methods in the prediction of pulmonary artery pressure. J Am Coll Cardiol 1987;9:549–54.

[68] Yock PG, Popp RL. Noninvasive estimation of right ventricular systolic pressure by Doppler ultrasound in patients with tricuspid regurgitation. Circulation 1984;70:657–62.

[69] Currie PJ, Seward JB, Chan KL, et al. Continuous wave Doppler determination of right ventricular pressure: a simultaneous Doppler-catheterization study in 127 patients. J Am Coll Cardiol 1985;6: 750–6.

[70] Homma A, Anzueto A, Peters JI, et al. Pulmonary artery systolic pressures estimated by echocardiogram vs cardiac catheterization in patients awaiting lung transplantation. J Heart Lung Transplant 2001; 20:833–9.

[71] Bossone E, Duong-Wagner TH, Paciocco G, et al. Echocardiographic features of primary pulmonary hypertension. J Am Soc Echocardiogr 1999;12: 655–62.

[72] Brecker SJ, Gibbs JS, Fox KM, et al. Comparison of Doppler derived haemodynamic variables and simultaneous high fidelity pressure measurements in severe pulmonary hypertension. Br Heart J 1994; 72:384–9.

[73] Arcasoy SM, Christie JD, Ferrari VA, et al. Echocardiographic assessment of pulmonary hypertension in patients with advanced lung disease. Am J Respir Crit Care Med 2003;167:735–40.

[74] Bossone E, Bodini BD, Mazza A, et al. Pulmonary arterial hypertension: the key role of echocardiography. Chest 2005;127:1836–43.

[75] Rodman DM, Lindenfeld J. Successful treatment of sarcoidosis-associated pulmonary hypertension with corticosteroids. Chest 1990;97:500–2.

[76] Davies J, Nellen M, Goodwin JF. Reversible pulmonary hypertension in sarcoidosis. Postgrad Med J 1982;58:282–5.

[77] Castro PF, Bourge RC, McGiffin DC, et al. Intrapulmonary shunting in primary pulmonary hypertension: an observation in two patients treated with epoprostenol sodium. Chest 1998;114:334–6.

[78] Olschewski H, Ghofrani HA, Walmrath D, et al. Inhaled prostacyclin and iloprost in severe pulmonary hypertension secondary to lung fibrosis. Am J Respir Crit Care Med 1999;160:600–7.

[79] Ghofrani HA, Wiedemann R, Rose F, et al. Sildenafil for treatment of lung fibrosis and pulmonary hypertension: a randomised controlled trial. Lancet 2002;360:895–900.

[80] Jones K, Higenbottam T, Wallwork J. Pulmonary vasodilation with prostacyclin in primary and secondary pulmonary hypertension. Chest 1989;96: 784–9.

[81] Palmer SM, Robinson LJ, Wang A, et al. Massive pulmonary edema and death after prostacyclin infusion in a patient with pulmonary veno-occlusive disease. Chest 1998;113:237–40.

[82] Farber HW, Graven KK, Kokolski G, et al. Pulmonary edema during acute infusion of epoprostenol in a patient with pulmonary hypertension and limited scleroderma. J Rheumatol 1999;26:1195–6.

[83] Fisher KA, Serlin DM, Wilson KC, et al. Sarcoidosis-associated pulmonary hypertension: outcome with long-term epoprostenol treatment. Chest 2006;130:1481–8.

[84] Culver DA, Minai OA, Chapman JT, et al. Treatment of pulmonary hypertension in sarcoidosis. Proc Am Thorac Soc 2005;2:A862.

[85] Foley RJ, Metersky ML. Successful treatment of sarcoidosis-associated pulmonary hypertension with bosentan. Respiration 2008;75(2):211–4.

[86] Sharma S, Kashour T, Philipp R. Secondary pulmonary arterial hypertension: treated with endothelin receptor blockade. Tex Heart Inst J 2005; 32:405–10.

[87] Rosenkranz S, Diet F, Karasch T, et al. Sildenafil improved pulmonary hypertension and peripheral blood flow in a patient with scleroderma-associated lung fibrosis and the Raynaud phenomenon. Ann Intern Med 2003;139:871–3.

[88] Montgomery GS, Sagel SD, Taylor AL, et al. Effects of sildenafil on pulmonary hypertension and exercise tolerance in severe cystic fibrosis-related lung disease. Pediatr Pulmonol 2006;41:383–5.

[89] Madden BP, Allenby M, Loke TK, et al. A potential role for sildenafil in the management of pulmonary hypertension in patients with parenchymal lung disease. Vascul Pharmacol 2006;44:372–6.

[90] Collard HR, Anstrom KJ, Schwarz MI, et al. Sildenafil improves walk distance in idiopathic pulmonary fibrosis. Chest 2007;131:897–9.

[91] Gideon NM, Mannino DM. Sarcoidosis mortality in the United States 1979–1991: an analysis of multiple-cause mortality data. Am J Med 1996;100:423–7.

[92] Takada K, Ina Y, Noda M, et al. The clinical course and prognosis of patients with severe, moderate or mild sarcoidosis. J Clin Epidemiol 1993;46:359–66.

[93] Sones M, Israel HL. Course and prognosis of sarcoidosis. Am J Med 1960;29:84–93.

[94] Arcasoy SM, Christie JD, Pochettino A, et al. Characteristics and outcomes of patients with sarcoidosis listed for lung transplantation. Chest 2001;120:873–80.

[95] Shorr AF, Davies DB, Nathan SD. Predicting mortality in patients with sarcoidosis awaiting lung transplantation. Chest 2003;124:922–8.

[96] Orens JB, Estenne M, Arcasoy S, et al. International guidelines for the selection of lung transplant candidates: 2006 update—a consensus report from the Pulmonary Scientific Council of the International Society for Heart and Lung Transplantation. J Heart Lung Transplant 2006;25:745–55.

ELSEVIER
SAUNDERS

Clin Chest Med 29 (2008) 565–574

CLINICS
IN CHEST
MEDICINE

Outcome of Sarcoidosis

Sonoko Nagai, MD, PhD[a],*, Tomohiro Handa, MD, PhD[b],
Yutaka Ito, MD, PhD[b], Kousuke Ohta, MD[a], Manabu Tamaya, MD[c],
Takateru Izumi, MD, PhD[a,d]

[a]Central Clinic/Research Center, Masuyacho 56-58, Sanjou-Takakura, Nakagyoku, Kyoto, 604-8111, Kyoto, Japan
[b]Department of Respiratory Medicine, Graduate School of Medicine, Kyoto University, 54 Kawahara-machi,
Shogoin, Sakyoku, Kyoto, 606-8507, Japan
[c]Division of Respiratory Medicine, First Department of Internal Medicine, Osaka Medical College, Osaka, Japan
[d]Department of Respiratory Medicine, Kyoto University, Kawahara cho 54, Shogoin, Sakyoku, Kyoto, 606-8507, Japan

Sarcoidosis is a chronic granulomatous inflammatory disease of unknown etiology with heterogeneous outcome. Based on the natural history or clinical treatment course, the outcomes of cases can be divided into two wings: spontaneous regression (self-limited disease) or progression of extensive fibrotic lesions as a postgranulomatous fibrosis [1–3]. Löfgren's syndrome (LS) is a typical self-limiting form of sarcoidosis [4]. Sarcoidosis generally is characterized as chronic disease. If treatments with corticosteroids or immunosuppressive drugs are indicated, they must be continued for more than 2 years after the initial diagnosis [5]. In occasional cases, on the other hand, long-term treatment may affect prognosis adversely [2]. Nonepithelioid cell granuloma surrounded by mononuclear cells, one of the hallmarks of sarcoidosis, is thought to be the product of antigen-specific immune responses (Th1 type). It remains unclear whether immunosuppressive therapies delay the processes that resolve this condition. There also have been ongoing debates as to whether the therapies influence the outcome of sarcoidosis positively or negatively, and whether those receiving early treatment can expect a better outcome than those receiving late treatment, or vice versa [6]. Based on Siltzbach's hypothesis proposed in 1965,

a susceptible host can undergo a Th1 immune burst during adolescence, then either spontaneously regress within 2 years or suffer from persistent lesions for 7 years. A subgroup of the chronic cases may deteriorate [1]. Given that some patients who have sarcoidosis spontaneously regress, the authors note that it may be difficult to credit any changes in indexes to the therapies the patients receive.

In spite of various concerns with regard to the sarcoidosis outcome, the authors recognized that postgranulomatous fibrosis results in incurable, deteriorated course in a portion of patients even after intensive treatment [7]. Lung transplantation is the only treatment that will save a patient who has deterioration in the lungs [8]. Although overall mortality is low in patients who have sarcoidosis, it remains a critical challenge to avoid deterioration early in the course of the disease [2].

A statement on sarcoidosis reported in 1999 includes the following description on the course and prognosis [2]:

> "the course and prognosis may correlate with the mode of onset and the extent of the disease. An acute onset with erythema nodosum or asymptomatic bilateral hilar lymphadenopathy usually heralds a self-limiting course, whereas an insidious onset, especially with multiple extrapulmonary lesions, may be followed by relentless, progressive fibrosis of the lungs and other organs."

This article reviews the clinical outcomes in patients who have pulmonary sarcoidosis in

This work was supported by a Grant from the Central Clinic/Research Center Foundation.

* Corresponding author.
E-mail address: nagai@chuo-c.jp (S. Nagai).

relation to the presence of extrathoracic involvements. It does not review specific extrathoracic involvements or their outcomes, respectively.

Spontaneous regression

The clinical expression, natural history, and prognosis of sarcoidosis are highly variable [2]. Spontaneous regression occurs in nearly two thirds of patients, but Siltzbach's scheme and the authors' experience suggest that this takes several years in most cases. Clarification of the natural history of sarcoidosis is confounded by the influence of corticosteroid therapy, which usually is offered to patients who have signs and symptoms. In the classic report from Katz [9], 60% to 80% of patients who had stage 1 sarcoidosis spontaneously regressed within 1 to 2 years after detection.

The authors' group measured the duration of bilateral hilar lymphadenopathy (BHL), from detection to resolution, in a series of patients from Japan. The authors selected two contrasting patient groups: patients less than 26 years old who had BHL but no extrathoracic lesions at the time of detection (n = 112), and patients older than 38 years who had both pulmonary involvement and extrathoracic lesions at the time of detection (n = 9). As shown in Table 1, the rate of remnant shadows at 10 years after detection was only 1% in the BHL group, versus 33% in the patients who had both pulmonary lesions and extrathoracic involvement. The rate of remnant shadows on chest radiograph decreased linearly within the first 5 years after detection, then remained largely unchanged from 5 to 10 years [3]. Based on this evidence, the authors proposed a 5-year interval

Table 1
Corticosteroid, age, and extrathoracic lesions as factors that relate to a persistence of sarcoidosis

	<26 years old, BHL, no extrathoracic lesions: 112	>38 years old, lung, extrathoracic lesions: 9
Male/female	66/4	2/7
Age	21.4 years	50.0 years
Steroid	24%	78%
10 years after		
Cleared	96%	11%
Reduced	2%	33%
Unchanged	1%	22%
Progressed	1%	33%

after onset/detection in association with spontaneous regression.

Persistence and chronicity

In most patients, sarcoidosis evolves into chronic courses. Acute onset with good prognosis can be expected in cases with erythema nodosum (EN), anterior uveitis, and acute arthritis. There has been discussion on how long patients who have sarcoidosis should be followed to identify cases in the chronic stage.

In the authors' study, they selected a special population of patients who were asymptomatic, whose disease had been detected when they were in their 20s, and who had no extrathoracic lesions. The authors then divided them into a steroid treatment group and a nonsteroid treatment group. The results showed no difference between the two groups in the rates of remnant shadows on chest radiographs at detection. There were, however, statistically significant differences between the groups in the rates of remnant shadows at both 3 and 5 years after detection. The rates of remnant shadows were higher in the treated patients than in the nontreated ones, and were unchanged from 5 to 10 years after detection in both groups, as shown in Fig. 1 [3].

In another series, 337 patients who had pulmonary sarcoidosis were followed from the time of detection to more than 10 years after detection. From overall follow-up, the rates of remnant shadows on chest radiograph decreased linearly within 5 years after detection, but thereafter did not change significantly [3]. Based on these studies, the chronic stage can be assumed to begin after a duration of more than 5 years after detection in both treated and untreated patients [3].

In the authors' series of 337 patients, a higher mean age, the presence of symptoms, the presence of extrathoracic involvement, and a history of treatment with corticosteroids before detection were associated with remnant shadows but not with the disappearance of chest opacity (Table 2). These factors that related to chronicity in terms of the persistence of chest opacities, however, did not relate to further deterioration (Table 3).

In a long-term follow-up report on the same group, 61% of patients (both treated and untreated) were stable; 31% had improved, and only 8% had deteriorated from the baseline [10]. The British Thoracic Society performed a prospective follow-up study on patients who had stage 2 or

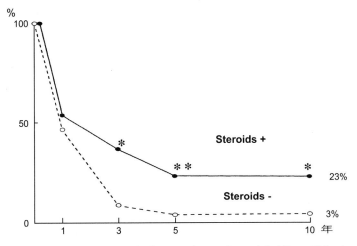

Fig. 1. Serial change in the rates of the remnant shadows on chest radiograph in bilateral hilar lymphadenopathy sarcoidosis patients whose age is in the 20s and who have no extrathoracic lesions. Abscissa: years from the time of detection. Ordinate: the rates of the remnant shadows on chest radiograph (%). Asterisks: * statistically significant ($P < .01$) when compared with untreated patients. ** statistically significant ($P < .05$) when compared with untreated patients.

3 disease. After a 6-month observation, 33 patients needed corticosteroid therapy, and 58 patients showed radiographic improvement over this period. The remaining 58 patients were allocated into a long-term steroid treatment group (group L) and a selected treatment group (group S) [11]. Group L showed greater improvements in symptoms, respiratory function, and radiographic appearance than group S. Thus, this study demonstrated the importance of long-term corticosteroid treatment in cases with stage 2 or 3 pulmonary lesions. There are no data, however, on the further longitudinal outcomes in this report.

Relapse and recurrence

In most the large series published to date, one third to one half of patients who had sarcoidosis were treated with corticosteroids [10]. Patients stabilize or improve with treatment, but 16% to 74% of them relapse when the corticosteroids are tapered or discontinued [7,10,12].

In a large study from the United States, 337 patients who had sarcoidosis were divided into three groups: spontaneous remission, corticosteroid-induced remission, and recalcitrant [13]. The rate of relapse was 74% in the induced remission group, versus only 8% in the spontaneous remission group. The prognosis of sarcoidosis in various patient populations varies with patient characteristics and clinical manifestations such as age, sex, race, chest stage, number of extrathoracic involvements, and so on. The tapering of corticosteroids and presence of extrathoracic involvement may play key roles in association with relapse of sarcoidosis. One report identified 17 patients who suffered recurrences (24 recurrences in total) after having remained stable for at least 3 years without therapy [14]. To evaluate relapse, a long-term follow-up is needed, even in patients who have inactive disease.

Table 2
Comparison of the parameters at the time of initial examination. Between the patients with the persistence of shadows on chest radiograph (remained) and those without shadows during following (disappeared)

	Male/female	Age (years)	Symptoms	Stage 1	Extrathoracic lesions	Therapy[a]
Disappeared	145/110	26.1 ± 9.1	77	209	75	97
Remained	36/47	37.9 ± 13.6	47	58	46	65
p value	ns	$P < .001$	$P < .01$	$P < .01$	$P < .01$	$P < .01$

Symptoms include both pulmonary and extrapulmonary.

Abbreviation: ns, not statistically significant.

[a] Therapy means previous therapy with corticosteroids.

Table 3
The parameters at the time of initial examination, which predicted chronicity, did not predict further deterioration after 10 years observation to the patients who have the remnant shadows

	Male/female	Age (years)	Symptoms	Stage 1	Extrathoracic lesions	Therapy[a]
Reduced	1526	39.0 ± 14.2	24	26	25	33
Unchanged	1211	38.1 ± 14.1	10	21	10	15
Progressed	99	35.6 ± 11.0	12	10	11	17
p value	ns	ns	ns	ns	ns	ns

Among the remained shadow group divided into 3 groups: Reduced: the shadows on chest radiograph reduced after 10 years. Unchanged: the shadows on chest radiograph unchanged after 10 years. Progressed: the shadows on chest radiograph progressed after 10 years.
 [a] Therapy means previous therapy with corticosteroids.

In patients receiving single-lung transplantations for end-stage pulmonary sarcoidosis, sarcoidosis recurred in the transplanted lung in about 50% of the cases within 3 to 6 months after the transplantation [8]. This recurrence, however, had no significant impact on lung function or short-term outcome (including survival or risk of complication). The authors have no data on the longitudinal outcomes of these transplanted hosts in whom sarcoidosis recurred.

Deterioration

Deterioration usually means a progression of pulmonary fibrosis, cardiac failure, prominent decrease in visual acuity, and impaired activity of daily living caused by neuromuscular lesions in patients who have sarcoidosis.

One study reported 17 deaths by sarcoidosis among a population of 254 patients followed for 27 years from the initial diagnosis at admission [15]. In this report, respiratory symptoms at presentation were independently related to overall mortality. A similar result has been reported in a 7-year follow-up of 479 patients; 13 patients who had visible fibrotic changes on chest radiographs and vital capacities of less than 1.5 died of respiratory failure [16]. In the authors' series, 18 of 337 patients deteriorated. Respiratory failure occurred more than 10 years after detection in all of the deteriorated patients whose chest radiographs were stage 3 at the time of detection. In this group, 67% of the patients were symptomatic, and 89% were treated with corticosteroids at the time of detection. The interval from deterioration to death seemed quite long, and during the interval, the patients frequently suffered from complications such as fungal, nontuberculous mycobacterial or *Pseudomonas aeruginosa* infections in segments with bronchiectatic or bronchial distorted areas [7,17]. The risk of pulmonary infection or other adverse events tends to increase in patients who have pulmonary deterioration lesions that require treatment by corticosteroids. Myocardial involvement and extensive bronchiectasis with or without mycetomas are typical clinical features of intolerable sarcoidosis in patients who have end-stage pulmonary lesions.

These reports indicate that deterioration takes place in a small number of patients who have sarcoidosis, and only after a relatively long time has passed from the initial detection. Corticosteroids are apparently ineffective at stopping the further deterioration of fibrotic lesions in patients who have sarcoidosis.

In the report from the Copenhagen National Lung Transplant Group, a population of 362 adult lung disease patients who received lung transplantations between 1992 and 2003 included seven patients who had sarcoidosis (1.9%) [18]. This figure suggests that that patients who have sarcoidosis have relatively low rates of deterioration, when compared with patients who have other pulmonary diseases.

One retrospective cohort study of 405 patients listed for lung transplantation in the United States between 1995 and 2000 sheds some light on prognostic factors in sarcoidosis patients awaiting lung transplantation [19]. In that population, 111 patients died while awaiting the transplantation. Race (African American), pulmonary hypertension, and oxygen use were all positively associated with mortality risk. The timing of transplantation for sarcoidosis patients is challenging, as mortality rates are high (27% to 53%) among sarcoid patients awaiting lung transplantation.

Mortality and morbidity

According to death certificate reports of 26,866,600 people who died from 1979 to 1991 in the United States, 5791 deaths were caused by sarcoidosis or a complication of the disease. This mortality rate seems to be low. The reported mortality caused by sarcoidosis varies by region, sex, and race. The age-adjusted mortality rates increased from 1.3 deaths per 1 million population in 1979 to 1.6 deaths per 1 million population in 1991 among men, and from 1.9% to 2.5%, respectively, among women. Though the age-adjusted mortality was consistently higher among African Americans than among Caucasians it remains to be solved whether this difference is related to race or to the disease itself [20]. Based on the results of a nationwide survey conducted in 1972 and 1984, the age-adjusted mortality in Japan decreased gradually from 0.2 to 0.1 deaths per 1 million population [21]. It remains unclear whether the change in mortality reflects improved treatment or proper management after diagnosis at the early stage.

Regarding the mortality rate, it seems to be difficult to estimate precisely, as a substantial number of patients would be missing from the statistics, partly because of higher frequency of regression, and partly because of cases that are not diagnosed definitely before death. The incidence in autopsy was estimated to be six to nine times higher than the clinically recognized incidence [22].

In the statement on sarcoidosis, overall mortality is described as 1% to 5%.

Differing mortality rates may reflect differences in disease severity, referral bias, and diverse genetic and epidemiologic factors. Studies in the nonreferral settings collectively showed a lower mortality rate of less than 1% in association with few serious morbidities [2]. Reports from referral centers, on the other hand, showed higher rates for both morbidity and mortality. Fatalities generally occur in patients who have respiratory failure, or central nervous system or myocardial involvement [3,12,23,24].

Organ involvement of sarcoidosis and outcomes

A large population of sarcoidosis patients (818) was analyzed retrospectively to study the prognoses for individual manifestations of the disease [24]. EN, acute arthritis, and BHL were confirmed to have good prognoses, while cor pulmonale, nephrocalcinosis, lupus pernio, and upper respiratory mucosal involvement had unfavorable clinical courses. Hepatomegaly carried a worse prognosis than splenomegaly or pulmonary involvement without BHL. These results

reflected the classical understanding about the outcome of sarcoidosis.

In the Case Control Etiologic Study of Sarcoidosis, 736 incident sarcoidoses were accumulated in 10 affiliated institutions in the United States, within 6 months of diagnosis using standardized diagnostic instruments [25]. The study clarified several important points for evaluating outcomes in patients who have sarcoidosis. Based on the standardized diagnostic methods, the study concluded that the initial clinical manifestation relates to age at the time of detection, sex, and race [26]. Women were more likely to have eye and neurologic involvement, and to be age 40 years or over, whereas men were more likely to be hypercalcemic. These clinical characteristics are similar to those observed in the Japanese sarcoidosis patients from the authors' series.

Clinical phenotypes

The WASOG (World Association of Sarcoidosis and Other Granulomatous Disorders) task group tried to define clinical phenotypes in association with clinical outcomes in sarcoidosis patients diagnosed according to the standardized diagnostic instrument proposed by the ACCESS study [25]. The clinical phenotypes were defined at least 5 years after detection or onset. Five years was identified as the start of a chronic phase, based on rates of remnant shadows on chest radiographs (see Fig. 1). At the time of evaluation, disease activities can be divided into three parts: resolved, minimal, and persistent. Minimal activities are defined as less than 25% of the initial activities. Persistent phases are divided into two groups: not currently treated (never treated or no treatment for more than 12 months) and currently treated (asymptomatic, no worsening in the prior 12 months, and worsening in the prior 12 months). The use of systemic therapy was classified as never (included patients treated with intermittent corticosteroids for a disease other than sarcoidosis), current, or none in the past year. Patients who received systemic therapy in the past year were considered on current therapy. Patients who had required an increase in their medication in the past year were considered worsening. Thus, nine clinical phenotypes are proposed to have relevant associations with clinical courses, as shown in Figs. 2 and 3.

Four-hundred patients from eight different geographic areas worldwide were allocated to these clinical phenotypes. Although nearly 40%

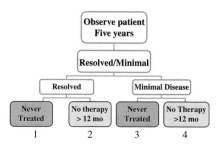

Fig. 2. Clinical phenotypes of patients with sarcoidosis. Clinical phenotypes were defined based on the diagnosis using the standardized diagnostic instrument from the A Case Control Etiologic Study of Sarcoidosis. Clinical phenotypes were applied to patients who have been followed more than 5 years after the detection. Remission was defined as less than 25% of maximal disease.

of the patients were receiving treatment, only 8% of them showed progression under treatment. Spontaneous regression was observed in about 8% of this study population, and minimal lesions remained in 8%. The other cases were grouped into the chronic–persistent subgroup, but most of these patients were not currently treated. This distribution of clinical phenotypes was found to be similar in the authors' series of 130 Japanese patients who had sarcoidosis (Tables 4 and 5) when the authors applied the same clinical phenotypes. In this series, both spontaneous regression and deterioration tended to be found in the younger males (20s or 30s) [27].

Genotypes, clinical phenotypes, and clinical outcomes

An interplay between genetic and environmental factors has been considered in the pathogenesis of sarcoidosis. No single causative environmental factor has been identified from the ACCESS study. Family clustering and differences in the racial incidence of sarcoidosis support an inherited susceptibility. Although several susceptibility genes have been reported, few of them are associated with clinical outcomes. As part of the ACCESS study, one group tested the hypothesis that sibling pairs who share genes and environmental exposures might have similar phenotypic expression of sarcoidosis. This multicenter family study resulted in mostly a minimal concordance between the phenotypic features and clinical outcomes of sarcoidosis in sibling pairs, although significant concordance was observed in ocular and liver involvements [28]. In another study using microarray analysis, the genes coding for affectors of the Th1 immune response were overexpressed in patients who had progressive sarcoidosis [29].

The sarcoidosis genetic analysis (SAGA) study identified eight chromosomal regions with suggestive evidence for linkage to sarcoidosis susceptibility in African American siblings. Using these eight chromosomal regions, a multipoint linkage analysis was performed with covariates based on pulmonary and organ involvement phenotypes. According to the results, the genes influencing clinical presentation of sarcoidosis in African Americans are likely to differ from those that underlie disease susceptibility [30].

Toll-like receptor gene polymorphism also was examined as another potential trigger of immune responses to bacterial components, in Dutch patients and controls. No differences were found, however, in the allelic distributions between patients and controls, or within the different clinical entities of the sarcoidosis group [31].

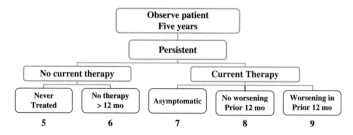

Fig. 3. Clinical phenotypes of patients with sarcoidosis. Clinical phenotypes were defined based on the diagnosis using the standardized diagnostic instrument from the A Case Control Etiologic Study of Sarcoidosis. Clinical phenotypes were applied to patients who have been followed more than 5 years after the detection. The use of systemic therapy was classified as never (included patients treated with intermittent corticosteroids for a disease other than sarcoidosis), current, or none in the past year. Patients who received systemic therapy in the past year were considered on current therapy. Patients who had required an increase in their medication in the past year were considered worsening.

Table 4
Japanese study: 130 patients who have sarcoidosis who have been followed more than 5 years

Phenotypes	Women	Men
1	0	4.5
2	0	2.3
3	12.8	15.9
4	24.4	13.6
5	7.0	4.6
6	15.1	31.8
7	20.9	15.9
8	16.3	2.3
9	3.5	9.1

Phenotypes: Clinical phenotypes proposed by the World Association of Sarcoidosis and Other Granulomatous Disorders task groups.

A group of researchers from Sweden tried to investigate the relationship between the HLA haplotype and clinical courses (nonchronic and chronic, based on the monitoring for up to 10 years) using a polymerase chain reaction (PCR) method [32]. HLA-DR17(3) was found in 65% of nonchronic patients, while DR14(6) and DR15(2) were associated with chronic diseases.

One study demonstrated that HLA DQB*0201 is a strong marker for mild sarcoidosis and has clear associations with LS and a reduced risk of disease progression [33]. Another study demonstrated that one cytokine gene polymorphism, the TNFB*1 allele, is a marker for prolonged clinical course in patients who have sarcoidosis [34].

All of these genetic studies seem to link a persistence of abnormalities with the progression of sarcoidosis. Yet according to the authors' clinical follow-up studies, the factors that relate to the persistence of abnormalities may differ from those that relate to deterioration. If this is correct, the detected genetic evidence may be associated solely with chronicity. The genetic factors that actually contribute to deterioration of sarcoidosis remain to be definitively identified.

Pulmonary hypertension as a prognostic factor

Pulmonary hypertension can be associated with sarcoidosis, although this is generally uncommon. Most cases are detected in patients who have advanced pulmonary fibrotic lesions or prominent hilar lymphadenopathy, and very few are found in association with veno-occlusive disease [35–38]. This clinical manifestation is not constelled adequately in the current clinical phenotypes or in the organ involvement standardized by ACCESS. When pulmonary hypertension is diagnosed in a patient who has sarcoidosis, it is an unfavorable prognostic factor for the patient's outcome.

A large retrospective study found that 73.8% of sarcoidosis patients listed for transplants had pulmonary hypertension [39]. Several other studies found pulmonary hypertension to be associated mainly with advanced sarcoidosis, although the frequency in nonfibrotic disease was not low [35–38,40]. Destruction of vasculature caused by fibrotic lung disease often has been identified as the most likely cause, although other mechanisms have been proposed [37,41]. In one small study, pulmonary venous occlusive disease was observed in the explanted lungs [39]. Several studies have found an association of pulmonary function with the incidence of pulmonary hypertension [36–38]. Right heart failure was seen in 21% to 23% of patients in one population [39]. Corticosteroids were effective in treating some sarcoidosis patients with associated pulmonary hypertension [39]. Inhaled nitric oxide, epoprostenol, and bosentan have been shown to be efficacious in a small number of patients [42–44].

Table 5
Japanese study: 130 patients with sarcoidosis who have been followed more than 5 years

Generation/CPS	1	2	3	4	5	6	7	8	9
10–19	50.0	0	0	0	0	0	4.0	0	0
20–29	50.0	0	11.1	22.2	0	11.1	28.0	6.7	42.9
30–39	0	100	22.2	29.6	12.5	11.1	8.0	6.7	14.3
40–49	0	0	33.3	11.1	25.0	25.9	16.0	26.7	14.3
50–59	0	0	22.2	25.9	50.0	40.7	16.0	33.3	14.3
60–69	0	0	11.1	11.1	12.5	7.4	28.0	20.0	14.3
70–	0%	0%	0%	0%	0%	3.7%	0%	6.7%	0%

Abbreviation: CPS; clinical phenotypes proposed by the World Association of Sarcoidosis and Other Granulomatous Disorders task groups.

Considering the pulmonary hypertension associated with sarcoidosis apparently manifests through heterogeneous pathophysiologic processes, more aggressive screening for pulmonary hypertension is warranted.

Novel drug therapy and the outcome of sarcoidosis

Corticosteroid is a standard therapeutic drug for sarcoidosis patients whose clinical phenotype requires treatment. Some reports demonstrate favorable responses, although there has been debate as to whether corticosteroids should be introduced earlier or later in the clinical course [11,45–47]. The wide distribution of the organ involvement, the presence of extrathoracic lesions, and several other prognostic factors suggest that a portion of patients in the subgroup requiring corticosteroid treatment can expect an unfavorable outcome. Sarcoidosis patients treated with corticosteroids also frequently relapse. Long-term treatment in relapsed cases may induce adverse effects. It remains unconfirmed whether corticosteroids prolong the disease by delaying resolution.

Some patients have been administered immunosuppressants such as methotrexate and azathioprine together with corticosteroids. In the global context, however, additive therapy with immunosuppressants is adopted commonly in the United States. In a nonrandomized interventional study of patients who had chronic sarcoidosis treated with methotrexate for at least 2 years, the therapy was found to confer steroid-sparing effects and good efficacy for chronic cases [48]. Its long-term effects on the clinical outcomes remain to be clarified, however. Large-scale clinical trials may help to ascertain long-term effects with possible influences on clinical courses of patients who are refractory to corticosteroids.

Novel drugs have been introduced for treating patients who have chronic deteriorating sarcoidosis and patients refractory to corticosteroid therapy. The antirheumatic drug (anticytotoxic drug) leflunomide was well-tolerated by 32 patients who had chronic sarcoidosis (ocular and lung), some of whom were unable to tolerate methotrexate [49]. The authors concluded that the patient response was better than that to methotrexate, with less toxicity. There is no evidence, however, that this drug influences the long-term outcome of sarcoidosis. Infliximab (a chimeric monoclonal antibody that specifically inhibits

tumor necrosis factor α) therapy to 138 patients who had chronic pulmonary sarcoidosis brought about a statistically significant improvement in the predicted percent of vital capacity at 24 weeks in a phase 2, multicenter, randomized, double-blind, placebo-controlled study [50]. The clinical significance in terms of the efficacy for long-term outcome remains to be evaluated.

A critical challenge will be warranted to clarify whether there is a subgroup of sarcoidosis cases with unfavorable clinical outcome, based on genetic or clinical backgrounds. On the other hand, several clinical phenotypes associated with favorable outcome are known. After dividing patients into several significant clinical or genetic phenotypes, the long-term outcomes with and without treatment can be clarified in sarcoidosis patients with diverse clinical courses.

Summary

Clinical outcomes of sarcoidosis include spontaneous regression, improvement with treatment, persistence of lesions (chronicity), relapse/recurrence, and deterioration. Based on the proposed clinical phenotypes, most patients are in the chronic stage, and more than 40% of patients are under treatment. Spontaneous regression and deterioration have similar frequencies. Several factors can be detected as prognostic factors associated with chronicity or deterioration. No definite relation can be found between genetic data and long-term clinical outcome. It remains to be determined whether sarcoidosis, as a syndrome, comprises both genetic and clinically diverse phenotypes that relate to outcomes.

Acknowledgments

The article was approved by the ethical committee in Central Clinic/Research Center. The authors thank Mr. Simon Johnson for his linguistic review.

References

[1] Siltzbach LE. Sarcoidosis: clinical features and management. Med Clin North Am 1967;51:483–502.
[2] American Thoracic Society (ATS), The European Respiratory Society (ERS), and the World Association of sarcoidosis and other granulomatous disorders (WASOG). Statement of sarcoidosis. Am J Respir Crit Care Med 1999;160:736–55.

[3] Nagai S, Shigematsu M, Hamada K, et al. Clinical courses and prognoses of pulmonary sarcoidosis. Curr Opin Pulm Med 1999;5:293–8.

[4] Mana J, Gomez-Vaquero C, Montero A, et al. Lofgren's syndrome revisited: a study of 186 patients. Am J Med 1999;107:240–5.

[5] Baughman RP, Judson MA, Teirstein A, et al. Presenting characteristics as predictors of duration of treatment in sarcoidosis. Q J Med 2006;99:307–15.

[6] Turner-Warwick M. Treatment of pulmonary sarcoidosis. State of the art. In: Grassi C, Rizzato G, Pozzi E, editors. Sarcoidosis and other granulomatous disorders. Proceedings of the XI World Congress on Sarcoidosis, and other granulomatous disorders. Milan, 1987. International Congress series. 756. Amsterdam: Excerpta Medica; 1988. p. 621–9.

[7] Lynch JP III, Kazerooni EA, Gay SE. Pulmonary sarcoidosis. Clin Chest Med 1997;18:755–85.

[8] Shah L. Lung transplantation in sarcoidosis. Semin Respir Crit Care Med 2007;28(1):134–40.

[9] Katz S. Clinical presentation and natural history of sarcoidosis. In: Fanburg BL, editor. Sarcoidosis and other granulomatous diseases of the lung. New York: Marcel Dekker; 1983. p. 3–36.

[10] Hunninghake GW, Gilbert S, Pueringer R, et al. Outcome of the treatment for sarcoidosis. Am J Respir Crit Care Med 1994;149:893–8.

[11] Gibson GJ, Prescott RJ, Muers MF, et al. British Thoracic Society Sarcoidosis Study; effects of long-term corticosteroid treatment. Thorax 1996;51: 238–47.

[12] Takada K, Ina Y, Noda M, et al. The clinical course and prognosis of patients with severe, moderate, or mild sarcoidosis. J Clin Epidemiol 1993;46(4): 359–66.

[13] Gottlieb JE, Israel HL, Steiner RM, et al. Outcome in sarcoidosis. The relationship of relapse to corticosteroid therapy. Chest 1997;111:623–31.

[14] Mana J, Montero A, Vidal M, et al. Recurrent sarcoidosis: a study of 17 patients with 24 episodes of recurrence. Sarcoidosis Vasc Diffuse Lung Dis 2003;20:212–21.

[15] Vestbo J, Viskum K. Respiratory symptoms at presentation and long-term vital prognosis in patients with pulmonary sarcoidosis. Sarcoidosis 1994;11: 123–5.

[16] Baughman RP, Winget DB, Bowen EH, et al. Predicting respiratory failure in sarcoidosis patients. Sarcoidosis Vasc Diffuse Lung Dis 1997;14:154–8.

[17] Lewis NM, Mortelliti MP, Yeager H Jr, et al. Clinical bronchiectasis complicating pulmonary sarcoidosis: case series of seven patients. Sarcoidosis Vasc Diffuse Lung Dis 2002;19:154–9.

[18] Burton CM, Milman N, Carlsen J, et al. The Copenhagen National Lung Transplant Group: survival after single-lung, double-lung, and heart–lung transplantation. J Heart Lung Transplant 2005;24: 1834–43.

[19] Shorr AF, Davies DB, Nathan SD. Predicting mortality in patients with sarcoidosis awaiting lung transplantation. Chest 2003;124:922–8.

[20] Gideon NM, Mannino DM. Sarcoidosis mortality in the United States, 1979–1991; an analysis of multiple-cause mortality data. Am J Med 1996;100: 423–7.

[21] Yamaguchi M, Hosoda Y, Sasaki I, et al. Epidemiological study on sarcoidosis in Japan. Recent trends in incidence and prevalence rates and changes in epidemiological features. Sarcoidosis 1989;6:138–46.

[22] Iwai K. Morbid anatomy of sarcoidosis in Japan. Sarcoidosis 1992;9(Suppl 1):9–15.

[23] Perry A, Vuitch F. Causes of death in patients with sarcoidosis. A morphologic study of 38 autopsies with clinicopathologic correlations. Arch Pathol Lab Med 1995;119(2):167–72.

[24] Neville E, Walker AN, James DG. Prognostic factors predicting the outcome of sarcoidosis. An analysis of 818 patients. Q J Med 1983;52(208):525–38.

[25] Judson MA, Baughman RP, Teirstein AS, et al. Defining organ involvement in sarcoidosis: the ACCESS proposed instrument. Sarcoidosis Vasc Diffuse Lung Dis 1999;16:75–86.

[26] Baughman RP, Teirstein AS, Judson MA, et al. Clinical characteristics of patients in a case–control study of sarcoidosis. Am J Respir Crit Care Med 2001;164:1885–9.

[27] Nagai S, Baughman RP, Costabel U, et al, WASOG task group. Clinical phenotypes of sarcoidosis. Japanese Journal of Sarcoidosis and Other Granulomatous Disorders 2005;25:93–8.

[28] Judson MA, Hirst K, Iyengar SK, et al. Comparison of sarcoidosis phenotypes among affected African American siblings. Chest 2006;130:855–62.

[29] Schischmanoff PO, Naccache JM, Carrere A, et al. Progressive pulmonary sarcoidosis is associated with overexpression of TYK2 and p21Wafl/Cip1. Sarcoidosis Vasc Diffuse Lung Dis 2006;23:101–7.

[30] Rybicki BA, Sinha R, Iyengar S, et al. Genetic linkage analysis of sarcoidosis phenotypes: the sarcoidosis genetic analysis (SAGA) study. Genes Immun 2007;8:379–86.

[31] Veltkamp M, Grutters JC, van Moorsel CH, et al. Toll-like receptor (TLR) 4 polymorphism Asp299Gly is not associated with disease course in Dutch sarcoidosis patients. Clin Exp Immunol 2006;145:215–8.

[32] Berlin M, Fogdell-Hahn A, Olerup O, et al. HLA-DR predicts the prognosis in Scandinavian patients with pulmonary sarcoidosis. Am J Respir Crit Care Med 1997;156:1601–5.

[33] Sato H, Grutters JC, Pantelidis P, et al. HLA-DQB *0201: a marker for good prognosis in British and Dutch patients with sarcoidosis. Am J Respir Cell Mol Biol 2002;27:406–12.

[34] Yamaguchi E, Itoh A, Hizawa N, et al. The gene polymorphism of tumor necrosis factor-beta, but not that of tumor necrosis factor-alpha, is associated

with the prognosis of sarcoidosis. Chest 2001;119: 753–61.

[35] Baughman RP, Engel PJ, Meyer CA, et al. Pulmonary hypertension in sarcoidosis. Sarcoidosis Vasc Diffuse Lung Dis 2006;23(2):108–16.

[36] Handa T, Nagai S, Izumi T, et al. Incidence of pulmonary hypertension and its clinical relevance in patients with sarcoidosis. Chest 2006;129(5):1246–52.

[37] Nunes H, Humbert M, Capron F, et al. Pulmonary hypertension associated with sarcoidosis: mechanisms, haemodynamics, and prognosis. Thorax 2006;61(1):68–74.

[38] Sulica R, Teirstein AS, Kakarla S, et al. Distinctive clinical, radiographic, and functional characteristics of patients with sarcoidosis-related pulmonary hypertension. Chest 2005;128(3):1483–9.

[39] Shigemitsu H, Nagai S, Sharma OP. Pulmonary hypertension and granulomatous vasculitis in sarcoidosis. Curr Opin Pulm Med 2007;13(5):434–8.

[40] Shorr AF, Helman DL, Davies DB, et al. Pulmonary hypertension in advanced sarcoidosis: epidemiology and clinical characteristics. Eur Respir J 2005;25(5): 783–8.

[41] Padia SA, Budev M, Farver CF, et al. Intravascular sarcoidosis presenting as pulmonary vein occlusion: CT and pathologic findings. J Thorac Imaging 2007; 22(3):268–70.

[42] Fisher KA, Serlin DM, Wilson KC, et al. Sarcoidosis-associated pulmonary hypertension: outcome with long-term epoprostenol treatment. Chest 2006;130(5):1481–8.

[43] Baughman RP. Pulmonary hypertension associated with sarcoidosis. Arthritis Res Ther 2007; 9(Suppl 2):s8.

[44] Preston IR, Klinger JR, Landzberg MJ, et al. Vasoresponsiveness of sarcoidosis-associated pulmonary hypertension. Chest 2001;120(3):866–72.

[45] Johns CJ, Schonfeld SA, Scott PP, et al. Longitudinal study of chronic sarcoidosis with low-dose maintenance corticosteroid therapy. Outcome and complications. Ann N Y Acad Sci 1986;465:702–12.

[46] Sugisaki K, Yamaguchi T, Nagai S, et al. Clinical characteristics of 195 Japanese sarcoidosis patients treated with oral corticosteroids. Sarcoidosis Vasc Diffuse Lung Dis 2003;20:222–6.

[47] Petinalho A, Tukiainen P, Haahtela T, et al. Early treatment of stage II sarcoidosis improves 5-year pulmonary function. Chest 2002;121:24–31.

[48] Lower EE, Baughman RP. Prolonged use of methotrexate for sarcoidosis. Arch Intern Med 1995;155: 846–51.

[49] Baughman RP, Lower EE. Leflunomide for chronic sarcoidosis. Sarcoidosis Vasc Diffuse Lung Dis 2004; 21:43–8.

[50] Baughman RP, Drent M, Kavuru M, et al. Infliximab therapy in patients with chronic sarcoidosis and pulmonary involvement. Am J Respir Crit Care Med 2006;174(7):795–802.

**ELSEVIER
SAUNDERS**

Clin Chest Med 29 (2008) 575–583

CLINICS IN CHEST MEDICINE

Index

Note: Page numbers of article titles are in **boldface** type.

A

A Case Control Etiologic Study of Sarcoidosis (ACCESS), 360, 365, 369, 392, 493, 509

Ablation, radiofrequency, in cardiac sarcoidosis management, 503–504

ACCESS (A Case Control Etiologic Study of Sarcoidosis), 360, 365, 369, 392, 493, 509

ACE. See *Angiotensin-converting enzyme (ACE)*.

Adalimumab, for refractory sarcoidosis, 538–539

Airway(s), sarcoidosis of, 463

American Thoracic Society, 509

Angiotensin-converting enzyme (ACE), in sarcoidosis, 400–401
  as marker of inflammation, 445–446

Anterior uveitis, 534
  ocular sarcoidosis and, 512–514

Antiarrhythmic agents, for cardiac sarcoidosis, 503

Anti-inflammatory drugs, for SAPH, 556

Antimalarial agents, for sarcoidosis, 541
  chronic, 537

Apoptosis, in sarcoidosis, 383

Arrhythmia(s)
  atrial, in cardiac sarcoidosis, 495
  ventricular, in cardiac sarcoidosis, 495
    risk assessment for, 502–503

Arthritis, sarcoid, early onset, 403–404

Atrial arrhythmias, in cardiac sarcoidosis, 495

Azathioprine
  for sarcoidosis, 540, 541
    chronic, 537
  in neurosarcoidosis management, 487

B

BAL. See *Bronchoalveolar lavage (BAL)*.

B-cell lymphoma, case example, 423–424

Biopsy
  endomyocardial, in cardiac sarcoidosis diagnosis, 501–502
  in hepatic sarcoid diagnosis, 511

Blau syndrome, 403–404, 425–426

Bone(s), sarcoidosis in, 421

Bone marrow, sarcoidosis in, 421

Brain, MRI of, in neurosarcoidosis diagnosis, 479–481

Bronchoalveolar lavage (BAL), in sarcoidosis diagnosis, 418

Bronchoalveolar lavage (BAL) fluid, T cells in, in sarcoidosis, 384

C

Calcium, metabolism of, sarcoidosis effects on, 453

Candidate genes, in sarcoidosis, 395–396

Cardiac sarcoidosis, **493–508**
  atrial arrhythmias in, 495
  clinical manifestations of, 495–496
  conduction abnormalities in, 495
  congestive heart failure in, 495–496
  diagnosis of, 496–502
    ECG in, 496–497
    echocardiography in, 497–499
    endomyocardial biopsy in, 501–502
    gallium-67 scintigraphy in, 498–500
    MRI in, 498, 500–501
    noninvasive imaging in, 497–501
    nuclear imaging in, 498, 499
    PET in, 498, 500